Keratoconus

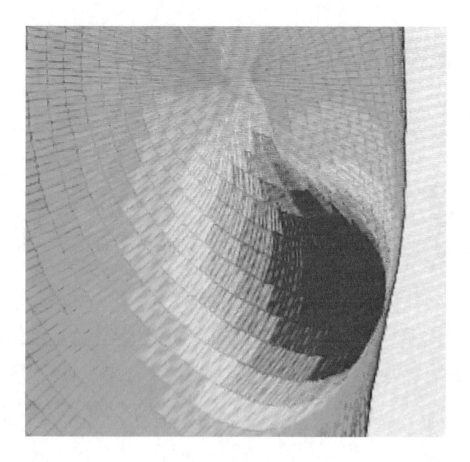

Ashraf Armia · Cosimo Mazzotta
Editors

Keratoconus

Current and Future State-of-the-Art

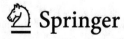 Springer

Editors
Ashraf Armia
Watany Eye Hospital
Cairo, Egypt

Cosimo Mazzotta
Ophthalmology Unit
Department of Medical
Surgical and Experimental Sciences
Italy and Siena Crosslinking Center
Italy, University of Sassari
Siena, Italy

ISBN 978-3-030-84508-7   ISBN 978-3-030-84506-3   (eBook)
https://doi.org/10.1007/978-3-030-84506-3

This Springer imprint is published by the registered company Springer Nature Switzerland AG
The registered company address is: Gewerbestrasse 11, 6330 Cham, Switzerland

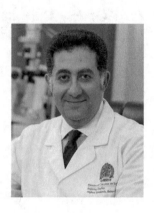

Dedicated to Vivian, Carol, Karim and my great father Armia and All Authors

Ashraf Armia MD, MSc, FRSC, FACS

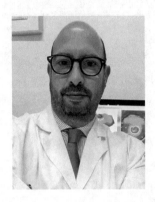

Dedicated to my mother Anna, my Family and to University of Sassari, Italy

Prof. Cosimo Mazzotta MD, Ph.D, Associate Professor of Ophthalmology, Department of Medical, Surgical and Experimental Sciences University of Sassari, Italy Head and Founder of the Siena Crosslinking Center, Siena, Italy

Preface

I was both honoured and delighted to be invited to write the preface for this volume. A book devoted to recent findings in the field of Keratoconus has been long overdue and therefore this volume fills a substantial void. The Editors are World authorities in this field and have used their reputations to secure a huge range of international expertise to cover every aspect of our current understanding of Keratoconus. This work excels in bringing together clinicians with extensive international experience in caring for such a disparate group of patients while at the same time integrating the latest endeavours of scientists who are actively involved in understanding the genetics, aetiology and prognosis of this condition. A cursory study of the chapter headings will convince the reader of the wide-ranging nature of this book and its systematic approach to defining the problems, the current situation in the clinic and the potential future of clinical management in relation to a variety of research approaches. While the old debate of nature versus nurture continues, molecular biology and biophysics have begun to tilt the discussion in favour of genetic predisposition with the discovery of numerous genes concerned with controlling the structural integrity of the cornea. A more detailed understanding of these processes is fundamental to the continued provision of safe refractive surgery. Comprehensive studies of the cellular and structural integrity of the cornea and the underlying mechanisms of cross-linking are also fundamental to extending the use and development of this technique. All these subjects are covered in the various chapters of this volume together with the special problems of addressing refractive errors in patients with significantly deformed corneas. The range of international authorship provides a comprehensive update for individuals moving into this area and a means of rapidly assimilating new information for those established in the field. I congratulate my many friends and colleagues for completing this work during such a strange time in world medicine and commend the volume to all interested in Keratoconus.

London, UK   John Marshall
April 2021

Contents

Current Advances in Keratoconus Imaging

Shady T. Awwad and Lara Asroui

1 Introduction

Keratoconus imaging has evolved dramatically over the past decade. Scheimpflug imaging, a major advent and add-on to placido-based technology that dominated the 80s and 90s, is still the dominant technology, allowing the clinician to evaluate both the anterior and posterior posterior curvature and compare corneal thickness at every point of the cornea. However, with the dawn of this new decade, a new contender has emerged and will seemingly overtake other technologies by the end of this decade: optical coherence tomography (OCT). The latter has been gaining widespread adoption in anterior segment imaging, but it is not until recently that several well-designed devices successfully incorporated this technology into routine and efficient assessment of the cornea and anterior segment. Interestingly, the time-honored videokeratography technology might continue as a mainstay of the anterior curvature imaging, at least for some time, in combination with optical scanning tomography, whether scheimpflug or OCT-based, due to its fast and high-resolution capture ability. Additionally, major strides have been realized in accurate biomechanical assessment of the cornea, through high frequency Scheimpflug sampling of the corneal shape and response to air puffs, and more recently through light assessment technology such as the briouillin microscopy. Along with these technologies, complex algorithms, some based on finite element analysis, logistic regressions, machine learning decision trees, and deep learning, have been developed to better make sense of the findings displayed by various platforms, and significantly improve detection sensitivities and specificities.

S. T. Awwad (✉) · L. Asroui
Department of Ophthalmology, American University of Beirut Medical Center, Beirut, Lebanon

A. Armia and C. Mazzotta (eds.), *Keratoconus*,
https://doi.org/10.1007/978-3-030-84506-3_1

1

2   Videokeratoscopy

Videokeratoscopy relies on reflection-based principle to measure the anterior curvature of the cornea, a concept first introduced in 1854 by Von Helmohtz [1].

The introduction of computerized videokeratography, with the advent of personal computing, jumpstarted the corneal imaging revolution, and had set the stage
for a more accurate screening and diagnosis of keratoconus. Since then, algorithms
and analyses derived from the axial curvature have been tested and validated, like
the Maeda's Keratoconus Index and the Keratoconus Prediction Index (KPI) [2, 3],
Rabinowitz KISA% index among other indices [4–6], and Roberts and Mahmoud's
Cone Location and Magnitude Index (CLMI) [7]. Axial curvature maps, however,
while useful for refractive corneal power calculations, are not ideal in locating the
cone, which is often off-center. Instead, tangential or instantaneous curvature maps
show better corneal apex and cone location and their refractive impact, which is
helpful in planning surgical procedures and monitoring their outcomes via subtraction mapping. Gaussian maps, first proposed for corneal topography by Barsky
et al. [8] represent the product of the steepest and flattest curvature at any given
point, and they were shown to even better locate the corneal apex and cone,
independent of the videokeratographic (VK) normal (i.e. patient's fixation). They
were initially introduced on the Keratron topographer (Optikon, Rome, Italy) and
were recently adopted by modern platforms such as the MS-39 (CSO, Florence,
Italy) (Fig. 1).

3   Scheimpflug Optical Scanning Tomography

Optical scanning tomography using Scheimpflug imaging directly measures the
sagittal height of the front and the back surface fo the cornea by using the principle
of light scattering. The data is displayed as elevation points referenced to a best-fit
surface (BFS), or a best-fit toric asphere (BFTA), and corneal thickness is derived at
every single point of the cornea by subtracting the elevation of the posterior surface
from anterior one. This technology has revolutionized the diagnosis, monitoring,
and treatment of keratoconus, and has dominated the field of corneal imaging for
almost two decades. Limitations, however, include sensitivity to corneal opacities
and scatter, which can lead to inaccurate measurements of corneal pachymetry and
posterior corneal surface [9, 10]. In addition, corneal curvature is derived from
elevation data, but its resolution is lower than the one that can be achieved from
reflection-based videokeratoscopy. Hence, this prompted some manufacturers to
produce a combined placido and Scheimpflug machines, allowing direct measurement of the anterior corneal curvature as well as direct measurement of the
anterior and posterior corneal elevations with pachymetry derivation.

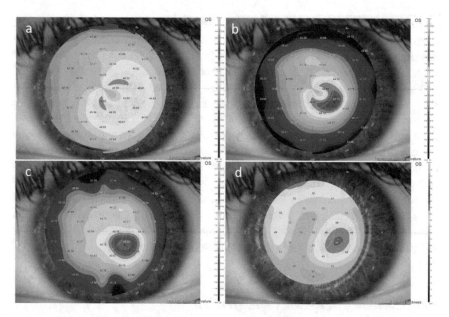

Fig. 1 a Axial curvature map of a keratoconus cornea. The exact location of the cone is hard to determine. **b** Instantaneous or tangential curvature map of the same cornea. The location of the cone is easier to define. **c** Gaussian curvature map of the same cornea, showing a more precise delineation of the corneal apex and cone, ideal for therapeutic laser refractive procedures on keratoconus eyes. **d** Epithelial map, showing thinning over the cone, with great concordance in location with the Gaussian map, and close similarity with the instantaneous one

3.1 The Posterior Corneal Surface

Scheimpflug imaging allowed for evaluation of the corneal posterior surface. For years, elevation-based representation was considered the norm, based on the fact that they are less dependent on patient's fixation than curvature maps [11]. Elevation maps however, as opposed to curvature map, tend to somehow "smoothen out" surface irregularities and reference them to a BFS or BFTA. The advantages of the latter is that the reference sphere more closely resembles the shape of the analyzed cornea, and hence tends to more snugly "hug" the measured corneal surface shape. Hence, small areas of elevation and irregularities, representing early ectatic areas, can be detected easier. An index of BFTA asymmetry has been described on the Galilei platform (Ziemer, Port, Switzerland), the asphericity asymmetry index, (AAI), which subtracts the lowest negative point of a BFTA hemisphere from the highest positive point on the opposite hemisphere [12]. Smadja et al. have used this index, together with corneal volume, to build a decision tree to distinguish normal eyes from keratoconus eyes [13]. One issue with the BFTA is its strong dependence on the angle alpha chord, which can lead to false positive values in any index built on it, when the corneal vertex and the geometric center of the cornea are not closely aligned. Another profile of the posterior surface is posterior curvature. Curvature analysis had long been considered as inferior to elevation under the claim that it was heavily dependent on centration and patient fixation [11]. However, drastic enhancements in topographers and tomographers' auto-centration and tracking have markedly improved centration. On the other hand, we have found that elevation maps were more dependent on patients' fixation vis-à-vis the angle alpha chord than curvature maps [14]. Eyes with large angle alpha chord often display a horizontally deviated corneal vertex with respect to the geometric center of the corneal (typically nasal deviation), with less prominent vertical deviation (typically inferior), hence, boosting the temporal elevation datapoint values and minimizing the nasal ones [14]. The Cone Location and Magnitude Index (CLMI-X) index developed by Cynthia Roberts on the Galilei (Ziemer, Port, Switzerland) makes good use of the anterior and posterior axial and instantaneous curvatures, among other parameters like the posterior BFS elevation and pachymetry, to distinguish keratoconus eyes from normal [15].

3.2 Corneal Pachymetry Progression

Renato Ambrosio introduced the concept of corneal thickness profile on the Pentacam tomographer (Oculus, Wetzlar, Germany), detailing how the cornea gets thicker spatially towards the periphery [16, 17]. The relational thickness indices combine the thinnest value and the fastest, slowest, and the horizontal pachymetric progression values. The latter, when combined with other parameters, including biomechanics ones, improve ectasia detection accuracy [18]. The pachymetry speed progression is a recent pachymetry progression map generated on the Galilei device. It displays the slope of the change in pachymetry, hence the speed, as opposed to the actual value, relative to the thinnest point on the map. It has the ability to detect early changes in a localized manner, avoiding data dilution which happens when all the meridians are averaged, or when all the points of a meridian or hemi-meridian are averaged (central to peripheral) (Fig. 2). Several indices are being developed around this new method to detect early keatoconus changes in a way independent of patient fixation [19].

3.3 Objective Indices to Diagnose Keratoconus Based on Anterior and Posterior Corneal Surfaces

There are several objective indices that make use of the information provided by the anterior and posterior corneal surfaces, the pachymetry map information, and many other parameters to accurately distinguish keratoconus eyes form normal eyes. The current challenge, however, is to identify keratoconus suspects or susceptible eyes, with enough sensitivity and specificity. This feature is vital for refractive surgery screening. The CLMI-X index on the Galilei system analyzes the anterior and posterior axial and instantaneous curvatures, pachymetry map, and posterior elevation map to accurately discriminate keratoconus from normal eyes. It has been found to be highly sensitive and specific for discriminating keratoconus from normal eyes [15]. The CLMI-X evaluates the highest values of search areas of a given diameter of curvature maps with its diametrically opposite counterparts, hence improving on the static infero-superior ratio (I:S ratio) that had been described long time ago for the anterior curvature. On the other hand, it uses a more or less conservative analysis of the posterior BFS, searching for the highest mean value of 0.5 mm area within 5 mm central zone (Fig. 3).

The support vector machine method, initially developed on the Sirius placido and scheimpflug tomographer (CSO, Florence, Italy) also makes use of the anterior, posterior, and pachymetry maps to accurately discriminate keatoconus, keratoconus suspects, normal, and operated eyes. It also uses symmetry indices for the anterior and posterior curvature (Symmetry Index of Front (SI_f) and Back Corneal Curvature (SI_b), anterior and posterior elevation data as decomposed into Zernike polynomials, and thickness index, all in a machine training model [20].

The Belin/Ambrósio Enhanced Ectasia display on the Pentacam presents evaluations of anterior corneal elevation, posterior corneal elevation, and pachymetric progression. The display shows graphical representations of the corneal thickness spatial profile (CTSP), as well as the percentage thickness increase (PTI) (Fig. 2a, b). In addition, it evaluates anterior/front and posterior/back elevations within the central 8.0 mm zone, and displays a comparison to the traditional best fit sphere, a comparison to an enhanced reference surface, and the difference between the two. The enhanced reference surface excludes the 3.0–4.0 mm centered on the thinnest point, and uses the patient's peripheral elevation data to generate a new, enhanced best fit sphere [21]. As such, the result is a flatter reference surface which, when compared to the patient's surface, will augment elevation abnormalities. The difference between the comparisons against the traditional BFS and the enhanced reference surface is likely to be minimal in normal corneas, which are expected to closely resemble the traditional BFS. However, in keratoconic or ectatic corneas, the comparison against the enhanced reference surface is likely to be flatter than the comparison against the traditional BFS, which would result in a tangible difference between the two. The main output parameters of the display are 6 D values, which represent deviation from normality: Df for front elevation, Db for back elevation, Dt for the thinnest point, Dp for pachymetric progression, Da for relational thickness, and a final BAD-D score. The BAD-D is derived from a regression analysis of the other D values, along with Kmax, anterior elevation at the thinnest point, posterior elevation at the thinnest point, and the Ambrósio relational thickness maximum (ARTmax). These D values represent the standard deviation from the normal average, with the value of 0 being the average of a normal population (Fig. 2a, b). Values that are at least 1.65 standard deviations away from the normal mean are highlighted in yellow and represent suspicious results, and values that are 2.69 standard deviations away from the mean are highlighted in red and represent abnormal results. Of the D scores presented in the display, the final BAD-D has been found to be effective at detecting keratoconus and ectasia [21–23], and can even detect, albeit to a much lesser extent, subclinical or forme fruste keratoconus [24–27].

4 Optical Coherence Tomography

OCT is the fastest growing diagnostic technology in the history of Ophthalmology. Even though it has become the leading imaging technology used by retina specialists, its adoption in the field of cornea and anterior degment has been slow. However, latest advances in resolution and measurement acquisition have suddenly made this technology the gold standard in corneal and anterior segment imaging. Just like with Scheimpflug technology, coupling with placido technology allowed for robust and powerful systems, although tomography and anterior segment imaging platforms using only OCT technology are now available. OCT platforms perform segmental tomography: imaging of the epithelium at every point of the cornea, Bowman's layer, stroma, and Descement's membrane, in addition to the anterior chamber structures. Abou Shousha et al. evaluated Bowman's Layer thickness maps and differential thickness between inferior and superior halves of the cornea and have found that they highly correlated with early diagnosis as well as the severity of keratoconus [28]. OCT also allows accurate evaluation of intracorneal landmarks, especially compared to scheimpflug technology, such as the demarcation line post corneal cross-linking [29], corneal haze [30], laser in situ keratomileusis flap interface, intrastromal corneal ring segments depth, and many others. Additionally, corneal pachymetry evaluation has been shown to be much more accurate than scheimpflug cameras when corneal scatter is present, especially in eyes after cross-linking [9, 10].

4.1 Epithelial Maps

Epithelial maps, along with Bowman's layer vertical maps, have been shown to be important in better diagnosing early keratoconus, as the epithelium is typically thinner over the area of impending cone [31–34]. Clinically, epithelial maps often help in ruling out keratoconus in cases with inferior anterior curvature steepening, due to marked epithelial discrepancy between the superior and inferior corneal hemispheres [35] (Fig. 4). Additionally, epithelial maps provide a great tool to treat Keratoconus eyes using customized transepithelial photorefractive keratectomy (TransPRK) and transepithelial phototherapeutic keratectomy (TransPTK) (Fig. 1d). Epithelial maps also help in better understanding processes and changes in the cornea, such as the the effect of intrastromal corneal ring segments in eyes with Keratoconus (Fig. 5).

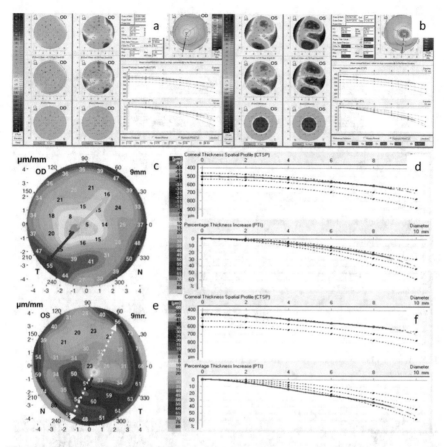

Fig. 2 a The Pentacam Belin/Ambrósio Enhanced Ectasia display with pachymetric progression of a "forme fruste" keratoconus eye. The fastest and slowest hemi-meridians are depicted without much detail is revealed within each hemi-meridien **b** The same display for the fellow eye shows clear keratoconus. **c** Corneal thickness speed progression map of the same forme fruste keratoconus eye on the Galilei, referenced to the thinnest point. The instantaneous speed of the pachymetry change (microns/mm) can be pinpointed at any given location of the cornea. The red arrow shows the fastest hemi-meridian (infero-temporal in this example), while the blue arrow depicts its diametrically opposite hemi-meridian, which is much slower. Instantaneous changes within the same hemi-meridian can be noted. For instance, the speed of pachymetry progression is highest about 2 mm infero-temporally, then it slows down towards the periphery. **d** The conventional corneal thickness spatial profile (CTSP), and the percentage thickness increase (PTI) of the "forme fruste" eye is an average of all meridians, which can dilute early focal changes in thickness or thickness speed. **e** Galilei thickness speed map of the fellow eye with keratoconus. The speed is largest at about 2 mm inferonasal from the thinnest point (red arrow), with slow progression of the opposite hemi-meridian (blue arrow). At the far periphery, the speed is about the same for both hemi-meridians (dotted white arrows). **f** Conventional thickness progression of the fellow keratoconus eye, with all the meridians averaged

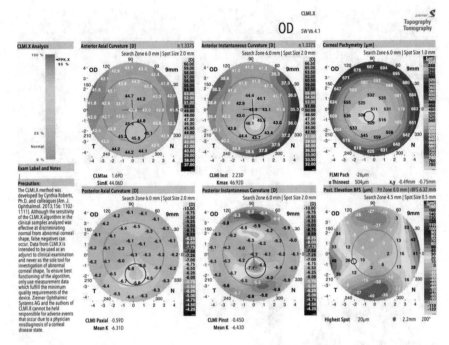

Fig. 3 The Galilei's Cone Location Magnitude Index (CLMI-X) report of an eye with early keratoconus

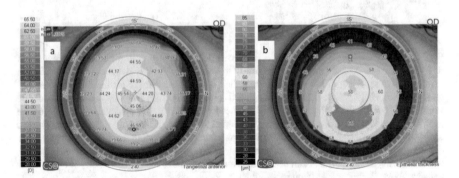

Fig. 4 a Anterior tangential corneal curvature map of an eye showing inferior steepening mimicking early keratoconus changes. **b** Corneal epithelial map of the same eye showing inferior epithelial thickening, which is responsible for the inferior steepening on the anterior curvature map. The posterior curvature and elevation maps are normal in this eye

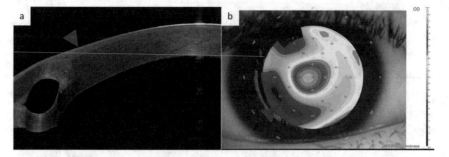

Fig. 5 **a** Anterior segment optical coherence tomography (OCT) of a cornea after intrastromal corneal ring segment insertion. Note the epithelial thickening proximal to the ring segment placement (red arrowhead). **b** Corneal epithelial map of the same eye showing the epithelial thickening (red arrowhead)

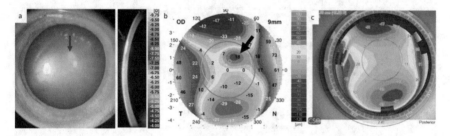

Fig. 6 **a** Slit-lamp photos showing a faint anterior corneal scar (red arrows). **b** Scheimpflug corneal tomography showing posterior elevation map derived from the best-fit sphere (BFS) mode showing artifactual nodular elevation underlying the exact site of the scar (black arrow). **c** Optical coherence tomography of the same eye showing posterior elevation BFS map with no artifact

4.2 Posterior Curvature and Aberrations

Another main advantage of OCT is its lower propensity to be affected by corneal scatter and haze (Fig. 6). Hence, especially in highly aberrated keratoconus eyes, the evaluation of the posterior curvature and pachymetry are much more reliable than Scheimpflug technology. This is especially important after corneal cross-linking, which generates corneal haze that leads to corneal pachymetry being significantly underestimated by Scheimpflug imaging [9, 10]. Hence, the measurement of posterior curvature higher order aberrations is much more accurate when using OCT technology in these aberrated eyes with stromal scatter and haze. As the posterior curvature of the cornea sits between stroma and aqueous, as opposed to the anterior one being between air and stroma, the posterior curvature power is negative. Posterior corneal aberrations therefore often negate anterior aberrations, and using both the anterior and posterior corneal aberrations is key in therapeutic laser refractive surgery in keratoconus, frequently generating an

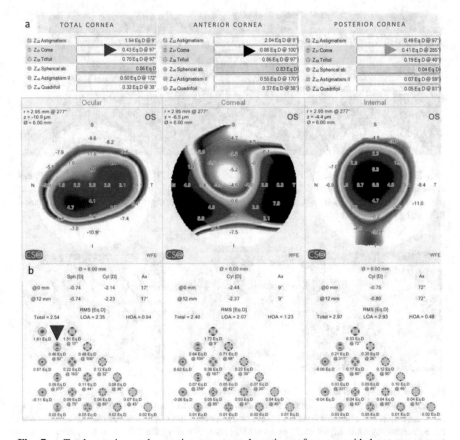

Fig. 7 a Total, anterior, and posterior curvature aberrations of an eye with keratoconus post corneal cross-linking and mild stromal haze, displayed by the MS-39 optical coherence tomography system (CSO, Florence, Italy). The coma of the anterior curvature (0.86@100) (black arrowhead) is partially offset by the coma of the posterior corneal surface which is diametrically opposite (0.41@285) (blue arrowhead). The resultant coma of the total cornea (red arrowhead) is 0.43@97. Topography-guided laser treatment would treat only the anterior cornea, leaving the posterior corneal coma unopposed, and the resultant coma would be around 0.40 D@285. **b** Pyramidal wavefront display of the same eye showing adequate capture the ocular wavefront. When combined with placido technology, (OSIRS or Peramis, CSO, Florence, Italy), it can display the ocular, the anterior corneal, and the internal wavefront (posterior curvature and intraocular). The total ocular coma (red arrowhead) is 0.46@92, which is strikingly similar to the coma of the total cornea (0.43@97). Therefore, in this example, it would be wise to proceed with ocular wavefront-guided ablation to address the right amount of coma. Future applications would enable the surgeon to treat using total corneal wavefront data

ablation pattern that is less tissue hungry than using the anterior curvature alone, as has been shown indirectly by comparing ocular wavefront-guided ablations to anterior corneal wavefront-guided ones [36] (Fig. 7). Finally, accurate measurement of the posterior curvature would also yield better total corneal power calculations for keratoconus eyes undergoing cataract surgery and needing intraocular lens power calculations.

5 Wavefront Sensing

Wavefront measurement of eyes with keratoconus has long been a controversial topic, especially in moderate to advanced stages. The main reason being that these eyes have large wavefront errors, while the aberrometers, mostly being Hartmann-shack or Tcherning, suffer from low dynamic range. These aberrometers are unable to represent a large wavefront error, even when equipped with large array of lenslets, without resultant aliasing. A way around this aliasing issue is to send one wavefront ray at a time, as in raytracing, available on the iTrace platform (Tracey Technologies, Houston, Texas). Recently, the advent of pyramidal aberrometers have dramatically improved the aliasing problem, with a fast wavefront capture, very large dynamic range, and very high resolution (up to 45,000 points on a 9 mm pupil, as opposed to a few hundreds to a few thousands in traditional aberrometers) [37, 38]. This has allowed the capture of ocular wavefront errors of advanced keratoconus, and paved the way for an additional customized laser therapeutic option in the surgeon's armamentarium for highly aberrated eyes with keratoconus, in addition to topography-guided and corneal wavefront-guided modalities [36]. This technology can be combined with videokeratography, among others, to analyze both the ocular and corneal wavefront, as well as the internal wavefront by automatic subtraction. An example of such machines is the OSIRIS or Peramis (CSO, Florence, Italy) (Fig. 7b).

6 Biomechanics

While significant technological advances have been made for the detection of morphologic markers of keratoconus, these findings are of later sequalae of the disease. Keratoconus is thought to begin with a focal biomechanical weakening of the cornea, followed by a cycle of decompensation resulting in corneal thinning and increased curvature [39, 40]. With the increasing number of corneal refractive surgeries being performed, the identification of the earliest form of the disease, before any morphologic changes have occurred, has become of paramount importance. This has led to efforts directed at measuring the in vivo biomechanical properties of the cornea.

6.1 The Ocular Response Analyzer

The Ocular Response Analyzer (ORA; Reichert Inc., Buffalo, NY, USA) was the first device used in clinical practice which measures corneal biomechanical parameters. Introduced in 2005, the ORA is a non-contact tonometer that provides a more accurate measure of intraocular pressure, by accounting for the biomechanical properties of the cornea. During a measurement, the device delivers a jet of air to the eye, causing the cornea to flatten and pass through a first applanation, and then continue to assume a slightly concave shape. The cornea then returns to its original convex form as the air jet is switched off, and in doing so passes through a second applanation. The deformation of the cornea is recorded by an infrared electro-optical system, and the pressure of the applied air at the first and second applanations is recorded (P1 and P2, respectively) (Fig. 8) [41]. The difference between the two pressures is what defines corneal hysteresis (CH), which is a measure of viscous damping, and is thus a reflection of the viscoelastic property of the cornea. Corneal resistance factor (CRF), is determined by the equation P1-kP2, where k is a constant determined from the relationship between P1 and P2, and the central corneal thickness. CRF is a measure of the overall resistance of the cornea [42]. Studies have shown that as compared to normal corneas, corneas with keratoconus have lower measures of CH and CRF [43]. While that difference is significant, a considerable degree of overlap exists between the two groups, particularly with mild keratoconus, and the sensitivity and specificity for diagnosis are low [43–46]. The ORA also provides a set of parameters that describe the waveform applanation response. These parameters, as well as several others derived from ORA data, have been analyzed and some have been found to be superior to the conventional CH and CRF in distinguishing between normal and keratoconus eyes [47, 48], and between normal and forme fruste keratoconus eyes [49]. In an attempt to further enhance diagnostic ability, ORA biomechanical parameters have been combined with Pentacam HR tomographic parameters based on a model of logistic regression, the result of which, while not perfect, has been better than that of any parameter alone, whether biomechanical or tomographic [50]. In addition, the ORA provides two parameters specifically related to keratoconus, the Keratoconus Match Index (KMI) and Keratoconus Match Probability (KMP). Both parameters have not been adequately studied, likely due to the emergence of newer technologies that assess corneal biomechanical properties.

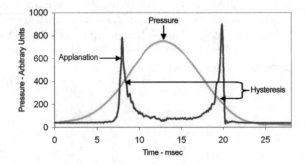

Fig. 8 The Ocular Response Analyzer (ORA; Reichert Inc., Buffalo, NY, USA) corneal deformation graph. The deformation of the cornea is recorded by an infrared electro-optical system, and the pressure of the applied air at the first and second applanations is recorded (P1 and P2, respectively)

6.2 The Corvis ST

The Corvis ST (Oculus Optikgeräte GmbH; Wetzlar, Germany) is the most recently introduced device used in clinical practice for the measurement of in vivo corneal biomechanical properties. Similar to the ORA, the Corvis ST is an important tool in the practice of glaucoma, as it is also capable of generating a more accurate measure of intraocular pressure, by accounting for the biomechanical properties of the cornea which it is measuring. The Corvis ST is a noncontact tonometer with an integrated ultra-high speed Scheimpflug camera. It uses an LED light source of a wavelength of 455 nm. The device first measures corneal thickness and then, similar to the ORA, the cornea is subjected to an air pulse with a maximum pressure of 25 kilopascals. In the following 31 ms, the camera captures 140 images of the central 8 mm of a single horizontal cross-sectional plane of the cornea, thereby tracking the cornea's biomechanical response at a speed of 4330 images per second [51]. As with the ORA, the cornea passes through two applanations; the first when the cornea is deformed by the air pulse to change from a convex to slightly concave shape, and the second when the cornea is recovering back to its original convex form. The Corvis measures several parameters of the corneal biomechanical deformation response (Table 1), many of which, such as applanation lengths, applanation velocities, and deflection amplitudes [22, 52], have been found to be significantly different between normal corneas and keratoconus corneas, and some of which, such as the DA Ratio [24, 25, 53], have been shown to be significantly different between normal and forme fruste, or keratoconus suspect corneas. The individual parameters however, are not sufficient for the purpose of diagnosis. Rather, the Corvis ST has been of particular utility in identifying corneas at risk of ectasia by means of indices that have developed integrating biomechanical parameters measured by the Corvis, and tomographic and topographic parameters measured by the Pentacam HR, a Scheimpflug tomographer to which the Corvis can be linked.

The Corneal Biomechanical Index (CBI) was developed to distinguish eyes with keratoconus from normal eyes. Using logistic regression, several biomechanical deformation parameters were combined with the Ambrósio Relational Thickness over the Hortizonal meridian (ARTh), which describes thickness progression in that meridian, relative to the thinnest point [54]. The biomechanical parameters that were included in the formulation of the CBI were SP-A1, A1 Velocity, DA Ratio 1 mm, DA Ratio 2 mm, and SD-Deformation Amplitude, which is the standard deviation of the deformation amplitude at highest concavity relative to the correlation of deformation amplitude with the bIOP [54]. The CBI ranges from 0 to 1.0, with values between 0 and 0.2 signifying a low risk for ectasia, values between 0.2 and 0.8 signifying a moderate risk for ectasia, and values above 0.8 signifying high risk for ectasia. The CBI has performed well for the purpose for which it was developed, which is discriminating keratoconus eyes from normal eyes (Fig. 9) [22, 54]. However, when its diagnostic ability was tested with forme fruste keratoconus eyes, it performed more poorly [24, 55, 56] particularly with such eyes that have strictly normal topographic and tomographic features [53, 57].

While the CBI can distinguish between normal and keratoconic corneas, it will also display an abnormal result for corneas that have undergone corneal refractive surgery. As such, it cannot be used to distinguish between stable corneas and ectatic corneas after surgery. This prompted the development of a newer version of the CBI, the CBI-LVC, which reflects biomechanical stability after laser vision correction (LVC). It is a purely biomechanical index which is useful for the early detection of post-LVC ectasia, for distinguishing ectasia from the regression of the effect of treatment, as well as determining whether the cornea is stable enough for a re-treatment. The newest Corvis ST software can automatically detect whether a cornea is a post-LVC cornea, and goes through a process of first distinguishing between normal corneas, and corneas that have keratoconus or have undergone LVC, then distinguishing between keratoconus corneas and post-LVC corneas, and finally distinguishing between stable post-LVC corneas and ectatic post-LVC corneas [58]. The examiner can also select the post-LVC option if it was missed by the software, and in such cases of post-LVC corneas, the CBI-LVC will be displayed instead of the CBI.

The Tomographic and Biomechanical Index (TBI) was also developed to identify eyes at risk for developing ectasia. The TBI incorporates both biomechanical parameters from the Corvis ST, including the CBI, as well as tomographic parameters from the Pentacam HR, including BAD-D. These parameters were combined using different methods of artificial intelligence, with the random forest, and leave-one-out cross-validation (LOOCV), resulting in the most accurate index, which was the TBI. The analysis included normal eyes, keratoconus eyes from patients with bilateral disease, keratoconus eyes from patients with very asymmetric ectasia, and the more normal eyes of patients with very asymmetric ectasia [56]. Thus, the index was designed to identify eyes with keratoconus, as well as suspect eyes that are at risk for developing ectasia. It is currently the best available index for these purposes [53, 55, 57]. For distinguishing between normal and keratoconic corneas, a cut-off of 0.79 had 100% sensitivity and 100% specificity. For distinguishing between normal and topographically normal corneas of patients with very asymmetric ectasia, a cut-off of 0.29 had 90.4% sensitivity and 96% specificity [56]. The TBI ranges from 0 to 1.0, and is interpreted as follows: values between 0 and 0.3 represent a low risk for ectasia, values between 0.3 and 0.75 represent moderate risk for ectasia, and values above 0.75 represent high risk for ectasia (Fig. 9).

The Stress–Strain Index (SSI) is the newest index developed to describe the biomechanical properties of the cornea. Using finite element numerical modeling of the eye, an algorithm was derived which estimates the stress–strain curve of the cornea, a reflection of its material stiffness [59]. The result of the algorithm was the SSI, which was clinically validated. It is based on Corvis biomechanical parameters, as well as bIOP and CCT, and is significantly correlated with age, but independent of both bIOP and CCT. An SSI value of 1 is indicative of a normal cornea, a value of less than 1 indicates a cornea that is less stiff and more prone to

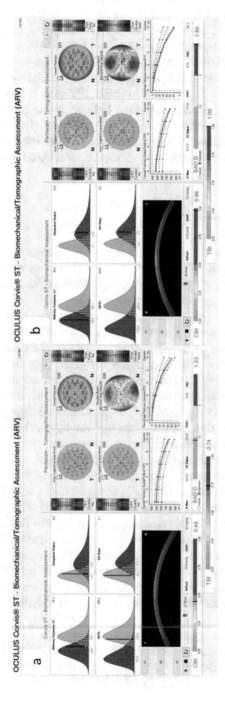

Fig. 9 **a** Corvis ST (Oculus, Wetzlar, Germany) display of a tomographically normal fellow right eye of a keratoconus patient. The BAD-D value is 1.23, but the Corneal Biomechanical Index (CBI) of 0.44, and the Tomographic and Biomechanical Index (TBI) of 0.74 are abnormal. The stiffness parameter at first applanation (SPA1) is also abnormal (78.3). **b** Corvis ST display of the ectatic left eye of the same patient, showing fully abnormal tomographical and biomechanical values

deformation, and a value of more than 1 indicates a stiffer cornea. In addition, the value of SSI has been shown to decrease with keratoconus disease severity. However, the measure of SSI as a single value is less meaningful than the change in SSI for an individual cornea, particularly since the material stiffness of the cornea varies substantially with age, and even among individuals of the same age [60]. The true utility of the SSI lies in its ability to detect keratoconus disease progression in individual patients, and more importantly, to detect increases in material stiffness, indicative of treatment success, following cross-linking, as has been demonstrated [61]. More recently, an improved version of the SSI, fSSI, was developed. The new algorithm takes into consideration the fluid–structure interaction of the Corvis air-puff with the cornea, and the results have also been validated clinically [62].

6.3   Brillouin Microscopy

Both the ORA and Corvis ST measure biomechanical properties of the entire cornea. However, keratoconus is thought to begin with a focal weakening of the cornea [39]. As such, a device that measures focal biomechanical properties, and detects asymmetries in the biomechanical profile of a cornea, is necessary to detect the earliest form of disease. The Brillouin microscope has been developed for just that purpose. It works by focusing a laser beam of a single frequency on the cornea with an objective lens, capturing the backscattering light from the cornea, coupling it to a single-mode fiber, and delivering it to a two-stage virtually imaged phase array (VIPA) spectrometer [63]. The technology is based on the principle of Brillouin scattering, which results from the interaction of incident light with the intrinsic acoustic phonons of the sample. The backscattered light experiences a frequency shift, or Brillouin shift, relative to the incident light. A material's acoustic phonons are related to its mechanical properties. As such, the shift in frequency that occurs is a measure of the mechanical properties of the sample, specifically related to its longitudinal elastic modulus [63]. Studies have been conducted, both ex-vivo and in vivo, and have demonstrated smaller Brillouin shifts in keratoconic corneas as compared to normal corneas, in the location of the cone [39, 40, 64]. The spatial distribution of Brillouin shifts within a keratoconic cornea was found to be highly asymmetrical, with the more "normal" portions of the cornea away from the cone displaying Brillouin shifts similar to those of normal healthy corneas [40, 65]. The significance of these findings is that keratoconic corneas exhibit a smaller elastic modulus, and thus a smaller resistance to deformation and are biomechanically weaker, specifically in the location of the cone. One of the challenges faced with using Brillouin microscopy, is that its measurements are highly influenced by the hydration state of the cornea [66]. However, a recent study determined that the Brillouin microscope can measure the solid, or stromal, mechanical properties of the cornea, independent of hydration. The contribution of hydration to the Brillouin shift was isolated, and it was found that cross-linking results in an increased

Brillouin shift due to changes in the solid mechanics of ex vivo porcine corneas [67].

7 Monitoring Keratoconus Progression

As opposed to the diagnosis of keratoconus, monitoring disease progression has still not made significant improvements, but our understanding of progression has improved markedly. The repeatability of measurements in eyes with keratoconus is still a concern [68–71], especially in moderate to advanced disease with kmax >50 D [72, 73]. Our group has shown that 3 and 4 mm zone averaging of data points centered on Kmax had significantly better repeatability than single point kmax [73]. The ABCD keratoconus grading system, initially described on the Pentacam by Belin [74], has also been proposed as a promising means by which to assess disease progression, even after cross-linking [75, 76]. The ABCD grading system comprises several corneal parameters, such as the 3 mm average anterior and posterior radii of axial curvature, centered on the point of thinnest corneal pachymetry, which is also a parameter, along with distance-corrected visual acuity. The accuracy and repeatability of the posterior radii as well as the thinnest corneal pachymetry is likely to be much better with OCT-based tomographers as compared to scheimp-flug, especially in post corneal cross-linking eyes. Another promising index to follow disease progression is the stress strain index [59–61], but more studies are expected in this area. Additionally, Brillouin microscopy, with its ability to detect focal shifts in biomechanical properties, might represent a very useful tool in the near future to detect early keratoconus progression. Finally, a multimodal index, combining all the above-mentioned parameters and technologies, and perhaps others, with the help of artificial intelligence, would probably be the next index to look at to determine disease evolution and decide on intervention such as corneal cross-linking.

8 Epilogue

We are witnessing a major revolution in both imaging technology and biome-chanical assessment, as well as data analysis and processing, the latter speared-headed by a dramatic evolution in artificial intelligence and deep learning. This should bring about a paradigm shift in disease diagnosis and treatment, and should greatly help in prevention, early detection, and early management. Notwithstanding, many challenges pertaining to the disease etiology, pathophysi-ology, and susceptibility remain unanswered and widely debated.

Table 1 Corvis biomechanical parameters

Parameter	Description
bIOP (mmHg)	Biomechanically-corrected intraocular pressure
A1 Time (ms)	Moment the first applanation occurs
A2 Time (ms)	Moment the second applanation occurs
HC Time (ms)	Moment of highest concavity of the cornea
A1 Length (mm)	Length of applanation at applanation 1
A2 Length (mm)	Length of applanation at applanation 2
A1 Velocity (m/s)	Velocity of corneal deformation during applanation 1
A2 Velocity (m/s)	Velocity of corneal deformation during applanation 2
Maximum Deformation (mm)	Maximum deformation of the cornea
Radius (mm)	Radius of curvature of the cornea at baseline
HC Radius (mm)	Radius of curvature of the cornea at highest concavity
Integrated Inverse Radius (mm^{-1})	Inverse of the radius of curvature during the concave phase of the deformation
Deformation Amplitude Ratio 1 mm	Deformation at the apex over the deformation 1 mm from the center
Deformation Amplitude Ratio 2 mm	Deformation at the apex over the deformation 2 mm from the center
SP-A1	Stiffness parameter at applanation 1
SP-HC	Stiffness parameter at highest concavity
WEMmax (mm)	Maximum whole eye movement
A1 Deflection Amplitude (mm)	Deflection amplitude at applanation 1
A2 Deflection Amplitude (mm)	Deflection amplitude at applanation 2
HC Deflection Amplitude (mm)	Deflection amplitude at highest concavity
Peak Distance (mm)	Distance between the two corneal peaks at highest concavity

References

1. Von Helmholtz H. Graefe's Archiv für Ophthalmologie. 1854;2:3.
2. Maeda N, Klyce SD, Smolek MK. Neural network classification of corneal topography. Preliminary demonstration. Invest Ophthalmol Vis Sci. 1995;36(7):1327–35.
3. Maeda N, et al. Automated keratoconus screening with corneal topography analysis. Invest Ophthalmol Vis Sci. 1994;35(6):2749–57.
4. Rabinowitz YS, Mcdonnell PJ. Computer-assisted corneal topography in keratoconus. Refract Cor Surg. 1988;5(6):400–8.
5. Rabinowitz YS. Videokeratographic indices to aid in screening for keratoconus. J Refract Surg. 1995;11(5):371.
6. Rabinowitz YS, Rasheed K. KISA% index: a quantitative videokeratography algorithm embodying minimal topographic criteria for diagnosing keratoconus. J Cataract Refract Surg. 1999;25(10):1327–35.

7. Mahmoud AM, et al. CLMI the cone location and magnitude index. Cornea. 2008;27(4):480.
8. Barsky BA, Klein SA, Garcia DD. Gaussian power with cylinder vector field representation for corneal topography maps. Optom Vis Sci. 1997;74(11):917–25.
9. Mencucci R, Paladini I, Virgili G, Giacomelli G, Menchini U. Corneal thickness measurements using time-domain anterior segment OCT, ultrasound, and Scheimpflug tomographer pachymetry before and after corneal cross-linking for keratoconus. J Refract Surg. 2012;28(8):562–6.
10. Antonios R, Abdul Fattah M, Maalouf F, Abiad B, Awwad ST. Central corneal thickness after cross-linking using high-definition optical coherence tomography, ultrasound, and dual scheimpflug tomography: a comparative study over one year. Am J Ophthalmol. 2016;2016 (167):38–47.
11. Belin MW, Khachikian SS. An introduction to understanding elevation-based topography: how elevation data are displayed a review. Clin Experiment Ophthalmol. 2009;1(37):14–29.
12. Arce C. Qualitative and quantitative analysis of aspheric symmetry and asymmetry on corneal surfaces. In: ASCRS symposium and congress. Boston, MA;2010.
13. Smadja D, Touboul D, Cohen A, Doveh E, Santhiago MR, et al. Detection of subclinical keratoconus using an automated decision tree classification. Am J Ophthalmol. 2013;156 (2):237–46.
14. Awwad ST, Yehyia M, Asroui L, Mehanna CJ. Comparative evaluation of corneal tomography symmetry based on centration: vertex versus geometric center of the cornea. In: ASCRS symposium and congress. Boston, MA;2020. www.ascrs.org.
15. Mahmoud AM, Nuñez MX, Blanco C, et al. Expanding the cone location and magnitude index to include corneal thickness and posterior surface information for the detection of keratoconus. Am J Ophthalmol. 2013;156(6):1102–11.
16. Ambrosio R Jr, Alonso RS, Luz A, Coca Velarde LG. Corneal-thickness spatial profile and corneal-volume distribution: tomographic indices to detect keratoconus. J Cataract Refract Surg. 2006;32:1851–9.
17. Luz A, Ursulio M, Castaneda D, Ambrosio R Jr. Corneal thickness progression from the thinnest point to the limbus: study based on a normal and a keratoconus population to create reference values. Arq Bras Oftalmol. 2006;69:579–83.
18. Ambrosio R Jr, Caiado AL, Guerra FP, et al. Novel pa- chymetric parameters based on corneal tomography for diagnosing keratoconus. J Refract Surg. 2011;27:753–8.
19. Mehanna CJ, Asroui L, Khalil J, El Zein L, Awwad ST. Sectorial thickness progression index: a fixation-independent parameter for the detection of keratoconus. In: ESCRS symposium and congress. Amsterdam, The Netherlands;2020. www.escrs.org.
20. Arbelaez MC, Versaci F, Vestri G, Barboni P, Savini G. Use of a support vector machine for keratoconus and subclinical keratoconus detection by topographic and tomographic data. Ophthalmology. 2012;119(11):2231–8.
21. Villavicencio OF, Gilani F, Henriquez MA, Izquierdo L, Ambrósio RR. Independent population validation of the Belin/Ambrósio enhanced ectasia display: implications for keratoconus studies and screening. Int J Keratoconus Ectatic Corneal Dis. 2014;3(1):1–8. https://doi.org/10.5005/jp-journals-10025-1069.
22. Sedaghat MR, Momeni-Moghaddam H, Ambrósio R, et al. Diagnostic ability of corneal shape and biomechanical parameters for detecting frank keratoconus. Cornea. 2018;37(8):1025–34. https://doi.org/10.1097/ICO.0000000000001639.
23. Chan TCY, Wang YM, Yu M, Jhanji V. Comparison of corneal dynamic parameters and tomographic measurements using Scheimpflug imaging in keratoconus. Br J Ophthalmol. 2018;102(1):42–7. https://doi.org/10.1136/bjophthalmol-2017-310355.
24. Wang YM, Chan TCY, Yu M, Jhanji V. Comparison of corneal dynamic and tomographic analysis in normal, forme fruste keratoconic, and keratoconic eyes. J Refract Surg. 2017;33 (9):632–8. https://doi.org/10.3928/1081597X-20170621-09.
25. Chan TCY, Meng Wang Y, Yu M, Jhanji V. Comparison of corneal tomography and a new combined tomographic biomechanical index in subclinical keratoconus. J Refract Surg. 2018;34(9):616–21. https://doi.org/10.3928/1081597X-20180705-02.

26. Ruiseñor Vázquez PR, Galletti JD, Minguez N, et al. Pentacam scheimpflug tomography findings in topographically normal patients and subclinical keratoconus cases. Am J Ophthalmol. 2014;158(1). https://doi.org/10.1016/j.ajo.2014.03.018.

27. Hashemi H, Beiranvand A, Yekta A, Maleki A, Yazdani N, Khabazkhoob M. Pentacam top indices for diagnosing subclinical and definite keratoconus. J Curr Ophthalmol. 2016;28 (1):21–6. https://doi.org/10.1016/j.joco.2016.01.009.

28. Abou Shousha M, Perez VL, Canto APFS, Vaddavalli PK, Sayyad FE, Cabot F, Feuer WJ, Wang J, Yoo SH. The use of Bowman's layer vertical topographic thickness map in the diagnosis of keratoconus. Ophthalmology. 2014;121(5):988–93.

29. Mazzotta C, Bagaglia SA, Vinciguerra R, Ferrise M, Vinciguerra P. Enhanced-fluence pulsed-light iontophoresis corneal cross-linking: 1-year morphological and clinical results. J Refract Surg. 2018;34(7):438–44.

30. Awwad ST, Chacra LM, Helwe C, Dhaini AR, Telvizian T, Torbey J, Abdul Fattah M, Torres-Netto EA, Hafezi F, Shetty R. Mitomycin C application after corneal cross-linking for keratoconus increases stromal haze. J Refract Surg. 2021;37(2):83–90.

31. Reinstein DZ, Archer TJ, Gobbe M. Corneal epithelial thickness profile in the diagnosis of keratoconus. Journal Refract Surg. 2009;25(7):604–10.

32. Li Y, Chamberlain W, Tan O, Brass R, Weiss JL, Huang D. Subclinical keratoconus detection by pattern analysis of corneal and epithelial thickness maps with optical coherence tomography. J Cataract Refract Surg. 2016;42:284–95.

33. Xu Z, Jiang J, Yang C, Huang S, Peng M, Li W, Cui L, Wang J, Lu F, Shen M. Value of corneal epithelial and Bowman's layer vertical thickness profiles generated by UHR-OCT for sub-clinical keratoconus diagnosis, vol. 6. In: Scientific Reports (Nature Publisher Group). London;2016. p. 31550.

34. Rocha KM, Perez-Straziota E, Stulting RD, Randleman JB. SD-OCT analysis of regional epithelial thickness profiles in keratoconus, postoperative corneal ectasia, and normal eyes. J Refract Surg. 2013;29(3):173–9.

35. El Wardani M, Hashemi K, Aliferis K, Kymionis G. Topographic changes simulating keratoconus in patients with irregular inferior epithelial thickening documented by anterior segment optical coherence tomography. Clin Ophthalmol. 2019;13:2103–10.

36. Gore DM, Leucci MT, Anand V, Cueto LF, Arba Mosquera S, Allan BD. Combined wavefront-guided transepithelial photorefractive keratectomy and corneal crosslinking for visual rehabilitation in moderate keratoconus. J Cataract Refract Surg. 2018;44(5):571–80.

37. Iglesias I, Ragazzoni R, Julien Y, Artal P. Extended source pyramid wave-front sensor for the human eye. Opt Express. 2002;10(9):419–28.

38. Plaza-Puche AB, Salerno LC, Versaci F, Romero D, Alio JL. Clinical evaluation of the repeatability of ocular aberrometry obtained with a new pyramid wavefront sensor. Eur J Ophthalmol. 2019;29(6):585–92.

39. Roberts CJ, Dupps WJ. Biomechanics of corneal ectasia and biomechanical treatments. J Cataract Refract Surg. 2014;40(6):991–8. https://doi.org/10.1016/j.jcrs.2014.04.013.

40. Scarcelli G, Besner S, Pineda R, Yun SH. Biomechanical characterization of keratoconus corneas ex vivo with brillouin microscopy. Investig Ophthalmol Vis Sci. 2014;55(7):4490–5. https://doi.org/10.1167/iovs.14-14450.

41. Luce DA. Determining in vivo biomechanical properties of the cornea with an ocular response analyzer. J Cataract Refract Surg. 2005;31(1):156–62. https://doi.org/10.1016/j.jcrs.2004.10.044.

42. Kaushik S, Pandav SS. Ocular response analyzer. J Curr Glaucoma Pract. 2012;2016(6):17–9.

43. Shah S, Laiquzzaman M, Bhojwani R, Mantry S, Cunliffe I. Assessment of the biomechanical properties of the cornea with the ocular response analyzer in normal and keratoconic eyes. Investig Ophthalmol Vis Sci. 2007;48(7):3026–31. https://doi.org/10.1167/iovs.04-0694.

44. Touboul D, Bénard A, Mahmoud AM, Gallois A, Colin J, Roberts CJ. Early biomechanical keratoconus pattern measured with an ocular response analyzer: Curve analysis. J Cataract Refract Surg. 2011;37(12):2144–50. https://doi.org/10.1016/j.jcrs.2011.06.029.

45. Fontes BM, Ambrósio R, Jardim D, Velarde GC, Nosé W. Corneal biomechanical metrics and anterior segment parameters in mild keratoconus. Ophthalmology. 2010;117(4):673–9. https://doi.org/10.1016/j.ophtha.2009.09.023.
46. Kirwan C, O'Malley D, O'Keefe M. Corneal hysteresis and corneal resistance factor in keratoectasia: findings using the Reichert ocular response analyzer. Ophthalmologica. 2008;222(5):334–7. https://doi.org/10.1159/000145333.
47. Hallahan KM, Sinha Roy A, Ambrosio R, Salomao M, Dupps WJ. Discriminant value of custom ocular response analyzer waveform derivatives in keratoconus. Ophthalmology. 2014;121(2):459–68. https://doi.org/10.1016/j.ophtha.2013.09.013.
48. Mikielewicz M, Kotliar K, Barraquer RI, Michael R. Air-pulse corneal applanation signal curve parameters for the characterisation of keratoconus. Br J Ophthalmol. 2011;95(6):793–8. https://doi.org/10.1136/bjo.2010.188300.
49. Luz A, Lopes B, Hallahan KM, et al. Discriminant value of custom ocular response analyzer waveform derivatives in forme fruste keratoconus. Am J Ophthalmol. 2016;164:14–21. https://doi.org/10.1016/j.ajo.2015.12.020.
50. Luz A, Lopes B, Hallahan KM, et al. Enhanced combined tomography and biomechanics data for distinguishing forme fruste keratoconus. J Refract Surg. 2016;32(7):479–85. https://doi.org/10.3928/1081597X-20160502-02.
51. OCULUS Optikgeräte GmbH. Corneal Biomechanics. https://www.corneal-biomechanics.com/en/biomechanics/.
52. Roberts CJ, Mahmoud AM, Bons JP, et al. Introduction of two novel stiffness parameters and interpretation of air puff-induced biomechanical deformation parameters with a dynamic Scheimpflug analyzer. J Refract Surg. 2017;33(4):266–73. https://doi.org/10.3928/1081597X-20161221-03.
53. Koc M, Aydemir E, Tekin K, Inanc M, Kosekahya P, Kiziltoprak H. Biomechanical analysis of subclinical keratoconus with normal topographic, topometric, and tomographic findings. J Refract Surg. 2019;35(4):247–52. https://doi.org/10.3928/1081597X-20190226-01.
54. Vinciguerra R, Ambrósio R, Elsheikh A, et al. Detection of keratoconus with a new biomechanical index. J Refract Surg. 2016;32(12):803–10. https://doi.org/10.3928/1081597X-20160629-01.
55. Ferreira-Mendes J, Lopes BT, Faria-Correia F, Salomão MQ, Rodrigues-Barros S, Ambrósio R. Enhanced ectasia detection using corneal tomography and biomechanics. Am J Ophthalmol. 2019;197:7–16. https://doi.org/10.1016/j.ajo.2018.08.054.
56. Ambrósio R, Lopes BT, Faria-Correia F, et al. Integration of scheimpflug-based corneal tomography and biomechanical assessments for enhancing ectasia detection. J Refract Surg. 2017;33(7):434–43. https://doi.org/10.3928/1081597X-20170426-02.
57. Kataria P, Padmanabhan P, Gopalakrishnan A, Padmanaban V, Mahadik S, Ambrósio R. Accuracy of Scheimpflug-derived corneal biomechanical and tomographic indices for detecting subclinical and mild keratectasia in a South Asian population. J Cataract Refract Surg. 2019;45(3):328–36. https://doi.org/10.1016/j.jcrs.2018.10.030.
58. OCULUS Optikgeräte GmbH. Biomechanical assessment post LASIK: The new CBI-LVC [Video]. YouTube. https://www.youtube.com/watch?v=SDoStHfqzUY. Accessed 25 Sep 2019.
59. Eliasy A, Chen K-J, Vinciguerra R, et al. Determination of corneal biomechanical behavior in-vivo for healthy eyes using CorVis ST tonometry: stress-strain index. Front Bioeng Biotechnol. 2019;7(May):1–10. https://doi.org/10.3389/fbioe.2019.00105.
60. Elsheikh A, Geraghty B, Rama P, Campanelli M, Meek KM. Characterization of age-related variation in corneal biomechanical properties. J R Soc Interface. 2010;7(51):1475–85. https://doi.org/10.1098/rsif.2010.0108.
61. Lopes B, Wang J, Eliasy A, Abass A. Early term results of the stress-strain index in patients with keratoconus submitted to corneal cross-linking;2019.
62. Maklad O, Eliasy A, Chen KJ, et al. Fluid-structure interaction based algorithms for IOP and corneal material behavior. Front Bioeng Biotechnol. 2020;8(August):1–11. https://doi.org/10.3389/fbioe.2020.00970.

63. Scarcelli G, Pineda R, Yun SH. Brillouin optical microscopy for corneal biomechanics. Investig Ophthalmol Vis Sci. 2012;53(1):185–90. https://doi.org/10.1167/iovs.11-8281.
64. Seiler TG, Shao P, Eltony A, Seiler T, Yun SH. Brillouin spectroscopy of normal and keratoconus corneas. Am J Ophthalmol. 2019;202:118–25. https://doi.org/10.1016/j.ajo.2019.02.010.
65. Shao P, Eltony AM, Seiler TG, et al. Spatially-resolved Brillouin spectroscopy reveals biomechanical abnormalities in mild to advanced keratoconus in vivo. Sci Rep. 2019;9(1):1–12. https://doi.org/10.1038/s41598-019-43811-5.
66. Shao P, Seiler TG, Eltony AM, et al. Effects of corneal hydration on brillouin microscopy in vivo. Investig Ophthalmol Vis Sci. 2018;59(7):3020–7. https://doi.org/10.1167/iovs.18-24228.
67. Webb JN, Zhang H, Roy AS, Randleman JB, Scarcelli G. Detecting mechanical anisotropy of the cornea using brillouin microscopy. Transl Vis Sci Technol. 2020;9(7):1–11. https://doi.org/10.1167/tvst.9.7.26.
68. Guber I, McAlinden C, Majo F, Bergin C. Identifying more reliable parameters for the detection of change during the follow-up of mild to moderate keratoconus patients. Eye Vis (London, England). 2017;4(1):24.
69. Prakash G, Philip R, Srivastava D, Bacero R. Evaluation of the robustness of current quantitative criteria for keratoconus progression and corneal cross-linking. J Refract Surg. 2016;32(7):465–72.
70. Guilbert E, Saad A, Elluard M, Grise-Dulac A, Rouger H, Gatinel D. Repeatability of keratometry measurements obtained with three topographers in keratoconic and normal corneas. J Refract Surg. 2016;32(3):187–92.
71. Flynn TH, Sharma DP, Bunce C, Wilkins MR. Differential precision of corneal Pentacam HR measurements in early and advanced keratoconus. Br J Ophthalmol. 2015. bjophthalmol-2015-307201.
72. Hashemi H, Yekta A, Khabazkhoob M. Effect of keratoconus grades on repeatability of keratometry readings: comparison of 5 devices. J Cataract Refract Surg. 2015;41(5):1065–72.
73. Asroui L, Mehanna CJ, Salloum A, Chalhoub RM, Roberts CJ, Awwad ST. Repeatability of zone averages compared to single point measurements of maximal curvature in keratoconus. Am J Ophthalmol. 2021;221(1):226–34.
74. Belin MW, Duncan JK. Keratoconus: the ABCD grading system. Klin Monbl Augenheilkd. 2016;233(6):701–7.
75. Duncan JK, Belin MW, Borgstrom M. Assessing progression of keratoconus: novel tomographic determinants. Eye Vis (London, England). 2016;3(1):6.
76. Belin MW, Alizadeh R, Torres-Netto E, Hafezi F, Ambrósio R, Pajic BP. Determining progression in ectatic corneal disease. Asia-Pacific J Ophthalmol . 2020;9(6):541–8.

Tear Film and Ocular Surface in Keratoconus

Samer Hamada and Artemis Matsou

1 Introduction

Keratoconus (KC) is an ectatic corneal disorder, characterised by progressive stromal thinning and structural weakening with apical cone-like protrusion, leading to progressive myopia, irregular astigmatism, scarring and decreased vision. It is a leading cause of corneal transplantation in the developed world. While keratoconus has been traditionally considered a predominantly degenerative, non-inflammatory disease of multivariate origin, the exact aetiology remains largely unknown. There is now evidence of genetic inheritance and possible association with systemic disease, as well as substantial evidence that certain environmental factors, such as ocular surface disease, atopy and contact lens wear, and behaviours, such as excessive eye rubbing, may play a key role. The factors that determine or affect the progression or stabilisation of the disease are not well characterised or understood.

A number of studies suggest a pivotal role of inflammation in the pathogenesis and progression of KC, contradicting the dogma that traditionally classified keratoconus as a non-inflammatory condition. Elevated levels of inflammatory mediators, such as pro-inflammatory cytokines, tumour necrosis factor, interleukins, cell adhesion molecules, and matrix metalloproteinases (MMPs) have been detected in keratoconic eyes compared to normal, implying that chronic inflammatory events are involved in the manifestation and progression of the disease. Many studies have attempted to investigate in depth the pathogenesis of keratoconus. And while it is widely accepted that complex interactions between genetic and environmental factors, both mechanical and biochemical, influence the development and course of

S. Hamada (✉) · A. Matsou
Department of Ophthalmology, Corneo-Plastic Unit, Queen Victoria Hospital NHS Trust, East Grinstead, UK

© The Author(s), under exclusive license to Springer Nature Switzerland AG 2022
A. Armia and C. Mazzotta (eds.), *Keratoconus*,
https://doi.org/10.1007/978-3-030-84506-3_2

the disease, discerning between a mere association versus a cause-effect relationship has proven challenging, possibly due to the wide variability in their expression and the presence of many confounding variables.

The potential role of ocular surface and tear film abnormalities in the pathophysiology and progression of keratoconus has been implied in many studies investigating the influence of various environmental and local factors on alterations of the tear film homeostasis in keratoconic patients, alluding to a powerful link between KC and these elements. It may be hypothesised that ocular surface abnormalities leading to a pro-inflammatory state, or local stimuli affecting the biomechanical properties of the cornea can trigger the degradation of corneal tissue, which is the hallmark of corneal ectatic disease. This occurs through secretion of inflammatory cytokines and degrading enzymes, which heighten the risk or even initiate the process for keratoconus onset and subsequent progression. An increased understanding of the role of ocular surface alterations and tear film composition in keratoconus, may shed more light and help elucidate the pathogenesis of this disorder. Furthermore, identifying potentially treatable risk factors for the onset or progression of keratoconus is of great importance and a field that merits further research.

2   Tear Film- What is Normal?

The tear film is the interface between the ocular surface epithelium and the environment. Under normal conditions, the ocular surface is maintained hydrated by a uniform, stable, three-layered tear film, which has protective and nutritional properties and bathes the ocular surface repeatedly through the blinking mechanism. A stable tear film is a prerequisite for maintenance of corneal smoothness, clarity and barrier function, which are crucial for comfort and high-resolution vision.

The tear film (TF) consists of:

   I. An aqueous layer, containing fluid and soluble factors produced by the lacrimal glands (main gland and accessory glands of Wolfring and Krause). The aqueous phase contains water, proteins and electrolytes, provides oxygen, nutrients and metabolites to maintain a transparent and avascular cornea, and helps in removal of epithelial debris and toxins.

  II. A mucin layer secreted by the conjunctival goblet cells with some transmembrane Outermucins also released from corneal epithelial cells. This mucinous layer has a high water-binding capacity, transforming the aqueous tears into a mucoaqueous gel, which represents the main volume of the preocular tear film and interacts directly with the glycocalyx of the epithelium. The mucins anchor to the epithelial cells and help stabilise the TF.

 III. Outer lipid layer produced by the Meibomian glands (meibomian lipid or meibum) located at the lid margin, which is spread onto the preocular tear film with each blink. It represents the anti-evaporation and pro-stabilising layer of the tear film, playing a protective role by preventing the cornea from drying and shielding against pathogens.

Although the estimated pre-corneal tear film thickness is 3 microns and volume 3 µl, it has a vital function to protect and lubricate the ocular surface, protecting it from desiccating stress through evaporation of tears. It has a highly complex composition containing water, electrolytes, mucins, an array of proteins, glyco-proteins and lipids which contribute to a stable, well-lubricated and smooth optical surface, but are also essential in promoting wound healing, defending against infection, suppressing inflammation and fighting free radicals. When the production or distribution of these factors is disrupted, the TF becomes unstable and insuffi-cient to meet the ocular surface demands, hence dry eye disease occurs.

The homeostatic mechanisms that protect the ocular surface through regulation of tear secretion, distribution and clearance are:

The Lacrimal functional unit (LFU)

Anatomically, this consists of the ocular surface (surface epithelium), its secretory appendages (main and accessory lacrimal glands, Meibomian glands, conjunctival goblet cells), eyelids and lacrimal drainage system, the glandular and mucosal immune system and the connecting innervation. The neural component of the LFU is complex and is known as the secretory reflex arc. This starts with the afferent limb of the feedback loop from the trigeminal innervation of the ocular surface epithelia, including the cornea, conjunctiva and lid margins, traveling to the central nervous system where central endings synapse with neurons in the superior salivary nucleus in the brain stem. The efferent pathway consists of parasympathetic secretomotor fibres that arise in the superior salivary nucleus and terminate within the main and accessory lacrimal glands, conjunctival goblet cells and the meibo-mian glands, regulating the secretion of all major components of the tear film to maintain a normal homeostatic tear composition. Dysfunction of the LFU leads to tear film instability, increased evaporation, inflammation, and visual degradation.

Corneal innervation

The cornea is a densely innervated tissue with most of the nerve fibres being sensory and largely originating from the ophthalmic branch of the trigeminal nerve. The trigeminal afferents from the cornea serve a range of sensory modalities which include pain, mechanoreception and temperature. Corneal nerves are key compo-nents of the physiological system that controls ocular surface and tear film home-ostasis. Sensory inputs generated by the ocular surface play an integral role in regulation of lacrimal gland secretion by a trigeminal–parasympathetic reflex and hence tear production, volume and composition. Corneal innervation stimulates reflex blinking and triggers the release of trophic substances such as neuropeptides, neurotrophins, and growth factors. Reduced corneal sensitivity through damaged corneal innervation is a recognised cause of dry eye disease and loss of ocular surface homeostasis. Disturbance to corneal innervation may occur in many ocular and systemic conditions and can be compromised after various ocular surgical procedures; diabetes, use of contact lenses, following refractive surgery (especially LASIK) and cataract surgery. Altered corneal sensation affects the corneal wound healing process, tear secretion, and the report of ocular symptoms.

The eyelid apparatus function-blink cycle

During a complete blink, several events take place that are important in maintaining tear film homeostasis. This includes the spreading of the tear film from the tear menisci reservoir across the ocular surface, the even distribution and regular refreshing of the TF. It also includes the release of meibum into the TF from the meibomian glands through the compressive effect of the orbicularis and muscle of Riolan. It also allows the upper and lower tear menisci to mix, thereby causing the even spread of the meibum and other TF components across the ocular surface. Another essential function of the blink is tear drainage. As the upper eyelid moves down and the lower nasally, tears are drawn towards the upper and lower puncti (mainly the lower), clearing cellular and other debris from the ocular surface.

The blink cycle consists of the blink itself and the interval in-between blinks during which evaporation of the tear film occurs. The blink rate is influenced by various environmental and ocular surface factors.

We can therefore appreciate that a number of factors can disrupt tear film homeostasis: eyelid and blink abnormalities, ocular surface irregularities, tear component deficiencies, and neurosensory abnormalities.

3   Ocular Surface and Tear Film in Keratoconus

A valid question is whether an impaired ocular surface microenvironment and disrupted tear film homeostasis can trigger corneal ectatic disease such as keratoconus. In other words, whether environmental and local factors that influence the ocular surface can indeed cause corneal ectasia, with or without a genetic predisposition.

This is an enigmatic topic that many investigators have been trying to answer over the years.

In fact, it is through this research that the conventional dogma of KC being a degenerative noninflammatory condition has been challenged, as evidence supporting the inflammatory nature of KC is growing. What has also come to light over the years, is the association of keratoconus with several ocular surface disorders, or systemic diseases with ocular surface implications, as well as the presence of strong links between KC and various environmental factors which were previously considered a coincidental correlation.

The published research to date corroborates that keratoconus is a multifactorial disease with both genetic and environmental components, with several biomechanical forces and inflammatory molecules and pathways implicated in its pathophysiology.

Looking at all the components that guarantee a healthy ocular surface and tear film homeostasis (corneal innervation, ocular surface irregularities, tear film alterations and eyelid/blink abnormalities), it becomes obvious that many of these factors are impaired in keratoconic patients either primarily or secondary to the disease presence.

- **Is Keratoconus an inflammatory disorder?**

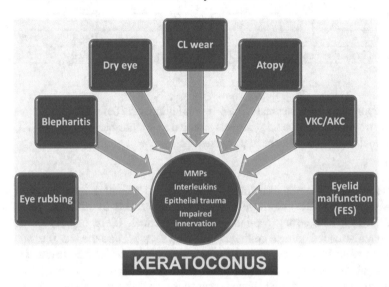

4   The Answer is in the Tear Film

On a molecular level, a number of pro-inflammatory molecules have been found elevated in keratoconic corneas such as interleukin-1 (IL-1), IL-6, matrix degrading enzymes (matrix metalloproteinases), transforming growth factor-beta (TGF-b), and tumour necrosis factor-alpha (TNF-a). A recent study [1] using cytokine antibody arrays, and scanning among 120 cytokines, unveiled that 23 of them showed significant elevation in keratoconic samples, while 15 were expressed in keratoconus only, suggesting that they can even be disease specific. The functions of these 23 cytokines included mediation of wound healing, neuroprotection, angiogenesis and inflammation pathways, while 8 cytokines were elevated as high as 1.7–42-fold (Table 1). And while the extent of the inflammatory contribution in keratoconus pathogenesis is uncertain, its involvement in the tissue degradation process seen in KC is becoming increasingly apparent. Environmental risk factors such as chronic eye rubbing, contact lens wear, atopic eye disease are all associated with alterations in the immunological corneal microenvironment, causing chronic epithelial injury,

Table 1 The 8 cytokines whose levels were distinctly elevated in keratoconic corneas compared to heterogenous group of non-keratoconic tissues, according to Loh et al. study [1]

IL-3 (interleukin-3)	×7.9
BDNF (brain-derived neurotrophic factor)	×15.2
BMP-4 (Bone morphogenetic protein 4)	×42.0
TNF-β (tumour necrosis factor-beta)	×11.7
TNF-α (tumour necrosis factor-alpha)	×5.8
Angiogenin	×1.7
Lymphotactin	×6.1
MIF (migration inhibition factor; macrophage inhibition factor)	×2.2

keratocyte apoptosis and stromal ECM remodelling. A defective reparative response in wounded keratoconic corneas compared to normal corneas or KC corneas without injury has also been suggested [2].

i. IL-1

The Interleukin 1 (IL-1) family of cytokines consists of 11 members, including IL-1 receptor antagonist (IL-1Ra) and two main agonists encoded by different genes (IL-1α and IL-1β), with strong pro-inflammatory potential. IL-1α and IL-1β are expressed by unwounded corneal epithelial cells and secreted into the tear film and corneal stroma after tissue damage. IL-1 holds a key role in modulating keratocyte apoptosis, regulation of corneal fibroblasts and myofibroblasts during corneal wound healing, leading to altered tissue organisation in KC patients [1–4]. IL-1α and IL-1β released by injured corneal epithelial cells, are involved in the promotion and chemotaxis of various pro-inflammatory molecules, up-regulation of chemokine production in keratocytes and corneal fibroblasts, activation of collagenases and MMPs, overexpression of IL-6 and growth factors that help restore epithelial structure and function. Evidently, the IL-1 cytokine-receptor system is a master regulator of many of the events involved in the corneal wound healing response linked to the complex cascade of stromal-epithelial interactions [1, 5]. Genetic polymorphisms involving the IL1RN (IL-1 receptor antagonist), IL-1A and B genes have been detected in several keratoconic populations (Japanese, Egyptian, Korean), suggesting the pivotal role of genetic susceptibility to inflammation through IL-1α and IL-1β overexpression that lead to the increased apoptotic activity in keratoconic corneal tissue [6–8].

IL-1α and IL-1β are both present in greater concentrations in keratoconic corneas, while stromal fibroblasts also display elevated expression of IL-1α receptors on their surface. IL-1α and IL-1β can induce apoptosis synergistically with tumour necrosis factor alpha (TNFα) via the production of reactive nitrogen species. Increased binding of IL-1 by keratoconic corneal fibroblasts facilitates induction of keratocyte apoptosis and enhanced tissue damage [9].

Loh et al. [1] demonstrated that IL-1α is expressed significantly more in keratoconic than non-keratoconic eyes with various corneal dystrophies, suggesting that

IL-1α is important in augmenting inflammation and abnormal wound healing in KC. The observed thinning and ectasia in KC suggests direct degradation of the corneal collagen by overexpression of MMPs, the activity of which is increased by IL-1 [10, 11]. Of note, IL-1α contributes to corneal oxidative damage exclusively in KC corneas by decreasing the production of superoxide scavenger SOD3 (extracellular-superoxide dismutase), stimulates overproduction of prostaglandin E2, while reducing collagen production [4, 10, 12].

Apparently, IL-1α and IL-1β can contribute to ectasia development and severity through their higher expression and defective action in genetically predisposed corneas.

ii. IL-6

Interleukin 6 (IL-6) is a pluripotent pro-inflammatory cytokine mainly produced and secreted by T helper 2 (Th2) cells and macrophages, affecting the pathogenesis of many autoimmune and inflammatory diseases, as well as processes involved in wound healing. IL-1 stimulates keratocyte production of IL-6 as part of the inflammatory and corneal wound repair cascade. Activated IL-6 binds to the IL-6 receptor or the soluble IL-6 receptor (sIL-6R) leading to wound healing events such as epithelial cell migration and vascularisation. The levels of IL-6 are increased in KC corneas compared to normal [4, 5, 11, 13] and notably, friction/trauma events such as eye rubbing and contact lens wear seem to augment IL-6 production in KC eyes. IL-6 has also been found elevated in eyes with vernal and atopic kerato-conjunctivitis, conditions also prevalent in the KC population [14–17]. A strong correlation between IL-6 and KC stage, keratometry, pachymetry and corneal hysteresis has also been reported [11, 14].

iii. TNF-alpha

TNF-alpha, also secreted by Th1 cells, is considered an important and potent pro-inflammatory mediator that plays a key role in systemic and corneal inflammation. In the cornea, TNF-alpha can be produced by all three major cell types: epithelial, stromal keratocytes and endothelial cells. TNF-alpha has been detected in significantly higher concentrations in the tear film and corneal samples of keratoconic eyes compared to normal in many studies [4, 5, 9, 10, 17, 18] and is one of the cytokines capable of upregulating the levels of IL-6 and synergistically modulating the expression of MMP-9 in human corneal epithelial cells [19]. Overexpression of TNF-α has a detrimental effect on the cornea. Environmental factors such as eye rubbing, CL wear and dry eye promote TNF-α production which can result in tissue damage. Upregulation of MMPs as a consequence of TNF-alpha over-activation can lead to corneal ectasia through degradation of stromal collagen. TNF-alpha has also been detected in early, subclinical stages of KC [15, 20]. It is therefore considered one of the pathogenic protagonists and principal mediators of the inflammatory component of keratoconus.

iv. IL-17

IL-17 is a pro-inflammatory cytokine associated with chronic tissue inflammation, and the principal cytokine produced by T helper 17 cells. IL-17 has been linked to autoimmune and inflammatory diseases and implicated in corneal inflammation by stimulating stromal cells to secrete other pro-inflammatory cytokines. These include IL-6, IL-8 and intercellular adhesion molecule 1 (ICAM-1), which mediates stromal interaction with inflammatory molecules and leukocytic infiltration. Increased levels of IL-17 have been detected in tear fluid samples of KC eyes [4, 13] in contrast to low levels in blood, thus confirming a dissociation between systemic and local inflammation [13]. Raised levels of IL-17 may contribute to the tissue degenerative processes observed in KC (stromal thinning-weakening) through activation of corneal fibroblasts and myofibroblasts and subsequent metalloproteinases production, and could even relate to disease severity [4].

v. Transforming Growth Factor- β

Transforming growth factor-β (TGFβ) with its 3 isoforms, TGFβ1, TGFβ2, and TGFβ3, is a family of pleiotropic cytokines involved in the restoration of tissue after injury by reorganisation of extracellular matrix, differentiation of keratocytes to myofibroblasts and induction of matrix-degrading enzymes. Each isoform has distinct effects on ECM, and unique characteristics in terms of potency, receptor affinity, and expression pattern, despite being structurally and functionally similar [21]. In the human cornea, ECM production by keratocytes is regulated amongst others by TGF-β signalling [17]. TGFβ secreted by epithelial cells diffuses into the stroma, particularly when the basement membrane is compromised, and binds to TGFβ receptors on keratocytes to enhance ECM secretion at injury sites. The TGFβ pathway can modulate cell proliferation and differentiation, stimulate MMP secretion and ECM production, leading to structural corneal changes seen in keratoconic eyes. A dysfunctional TGF-β axis has been implicated in the pathogenesis of keratoconus, either as a causative factor or a secondary abnormal wound healing response. Most of the studies have been performed on cultured corneal cells as the tear fluid may not be the optimal material to investigate this signalling pathway.

Elevated TGFβ2 levels have been detected in the aqueous humour of keratoconic eyes [5, 22], overexpressed in KC corneas, but also increased in the epithelium of severe keratoconus cases [21]. Although its role in KC is not fully elucidated, TGF-β2 could contribute to expression of inflammatory mediators that result in tissue damage. For example, TGF-β2 signalling can stimulate IL-6 expression by corneal epithelial cells, triggering the inflammatory cascade.

TGF-β3 is a multifunctional cytokine [1] mediating wound healing, and while it appears to modulate normal ECM formation in response to injury with an antifibrotic effect, it also seems to have pro-inflammatory and anti-inflammatory actions, with significantly elevated expression in KC corneas.

TGFβ1 is implicated in corneal fibrosis and scar formation via abnormal tissue repair. Keratocytes and corneal fibroblasts are especially sensitive to changes in TGF-β1 levels, and differentiate into myofibroblasts as a response to TGF-β1 stimulation. Aberrant TGF-β1 response has been noted in human keratoconic cells and can cause the corneal scarring observed in severe keratoconus. Dysregulation of this pathway has been associated with increased susceptibility of myofibroblasts to apoptosis mediated by IL-1. Imbalance of TGF-β1 (profibrotic actions) and TGF-β3 (antifibrotic action) can lead to pathological differentiation of corneal keratocytes in KC and accentuated fibrosis of corneal tissue [10, 17].

Accumulating evidence therefore supports a key role of the TGF-β family members to many of the pathogenic corneal changes in KC, such as overexpression of inflammatory mediators, the protease cascade of MMPs, and promotion of corneal fibrosis in KC. This evidence implies that control and regulation of the TGF-β pathway may be a treatment approach in KC [23]. Further investigation of the effect of blocking the TGFβ pathway with TGFβ receptor kinase inhibitors on Bowman membrane integrity, scar formation and other markers of keratoconus progression may provide useful insight on its role in the disease.

vi. Other Growth Factors

Other factors of interest that can influence cell proliferation-differentiation, mediate inflammatory response processes, wound healing and fibrosis (processes that are all altered in keratoconic eyes) include the vascular endothelial growth factor (VEGF), nerve growth factor (NGF), insulin-like growth factor (IGF) hepatocyte growth factor (HGF), keratinocyte growth factor (KGF) and epidermal growth factor (EGF) [24]. All these have been implicated in disrupted corneal homeostasis. The association of VEGF with KC is ambiguous, with some studies reporting lower levels in corneal samples [25] and others finding no difference in VEGF levels in tear fluid samples of KC patients vs controls [2, 26]. NGF and EGF are normal constituents of the tear film and contributors to the corneal wound healing response. NGF affects corneal epithelial cell proliferation and significant reduction in NGF expression has been detected in KC corneas as part of an imbalance in the NGF signalling pathway. A significant positive association between NGF and several topographic indices in keratoconic corneas has been detected, underscoring the potential key role of NGF in the pathophysiology of KC [11]. The exact effect of HGF and KGF on corneal stromal cells remains elusive due to inconclusive reported evidence [5].

5 MMP Levels in KC

Matrix metalloproteinases (MMPs) comprise a family of 24 zinc dependent proteases involved in processes of tissue remodelling, embryonic development, wound healing, angiogenesis and inflammation [27]. They include gelatinases (MMP-2, 9), collagenases (MMP-1, 8, 13), stromelysins (MMP-3, 10), and matrilysins (MMP-7, 26), although these groupings are increasingly considered overly simplistic, and perhaps inaccurate, as the range of potential targets for each enzyme has expanded since the original classification [28]. MMPs are synthesised by corneal epithelial cells, stromal cells and neutrophils as a response to stress, injury or disease and play a key role in extracellular matrix (ECM) degradation and remodelling. The ECM of human cornea is made up of 70% collagen (type I collagen principally found in the corneal stroma, type IV in the epithelial basement membrane and Descemet's membrane) as well as laminins, fibronectins, thrombospondins, proteoglycans and matrilins. MMPs have the ability to cleave all structural components of the ECM contributing to modification of tissue architecture, cell migration and adhesion [29]. The activity of MMPs is inhibited by four protease inhibitory proteins; the tissue inhibitors of matrix metalloproteinases (TIMP) -1, -2, -3, and -4. Disruption of the tight regulatory mechanisms of the corneal microenvironment may lead to an imbalance of enzyme activity with over-activation of MMPs and ECM degradation [27].

The corneal thinning and ectasia seen in KC is predominantly caused by increased ECM degradation, which progressively causes localised corneal thinning and weakening, eventually leading to change of corneal shape [30]. Considering that MMPs degrade ECM and undermine its structure and composition, several studies have investigated their role in KC pathogenesis. Elevated MMP levels have been detected in the tear film of keratoconic corneas compared to controls by many authors [31–34]. The more widely studied MMPs are MMP-9, MMP-2 and MMP-1.

- Matrix metalloproteinase-9 (MMP-9)

The association of MMP-9 (gelatinase B) with keratoconus seems to be the most comprehensively investigated so far. MMP-9 constitutes the primary matrix-degrading enzyme in the human cornea. MMP-9 activity is upregulated by epigenetic processes, cell–cell interactions and inflammatory cytokines (IL-6, TNF-alpha), with subsequent degradation of corneal collagen fibres. Mazzota et al. [35] demonstrated statistically significant progression of keratoconus in patients with concomitant allergies positive to MMP-9 point-of-care testing, compared to KC patients without allergies and negative to MMP-9. The first group (KC with allergies, positive to MMP-9) suffered a significant reduction in CDVA from baseline, an increase in Kmax, and reduction of minimum corneal thickness at 12 months follow-up. In a prospective case–control study, Lema et al. [36] also showed statistically significant increase in MMP-9 levels in patients with kerato-conus versus control subjects, while higher concentration of MMP-9 was associated with severe KC. No correlation was detected between eye rubbing and different concentrations of MMP-9. Pahuja et al. [37] discovered that MMP-9 levels were much higher in the stroma compared to epithelium in KC corneas, and higher in the epithelial and stromal cells of the cornea apex (the most ectatic zone) compared to the paired periphery, suggesting that altered corneal epithelial and stromal expression of specific genes at the corneal cone apex drives focal structural weakness in KC. In a randomised controlled trial, Shetty et al. [18] demonstrated that the mRNA expression levels of MMP-9 in the corneal epithelium as well as the MMP-9 protein levels in the tear film were indeed higher in KC patients compared with the control cohort, indicating that the corneal epithelium contributes to elevated MMP-9 and inflammatory cytokine expression in KC. Similarly, Mutlu et al. [38], showed that the tear MMP-9 enzyme levels were significantly higher in the keratoconus patients with or without seasonal allergic conjunctivitis when compared to the levels seen in healthy subjects. They also identified positive correlation between the severity of KC- MMP-9 levels and negative correlation between corneal pachymetry -MMP-9 levels, which indicates the importance of the protease enzymes in the pathogenesis of keratoconus. In 2009, Lema et al. studied MMP-9 levels in KC, subclinical KC and normal controls, and found raised levels in KC eyes compared to controls. However, MMP-9 levels between subclinical KC and controls were similar [15], while another study detected elevated MMP-9 protein in the tear film of 90% of KC eyes and 83% of subclinical disease, suggesting that MMP-9 may be a useful pre-symptomatic diagnostic marker in at-risk individuals [39]. A cross-sectional case–control study also showed significantly elevated MMP-9 levels in the blood serum of KC patients compared to normal controls [40]. The above studies support a key role for MMP-9 in the pathogenesis of keratoconus. With this in mind, Shetty et al. [18] investigated the use of topical cyclosporine A (CsA) to inhibit the inflammatory response in KC corneas by modulating transcript levels of MMP-9 and inflammatory cytokines. The authors demonstrated that treatment of KC patients with CsA for approximately 6 months reduced tear MMP-9 levels and led to local reduction in corneal curvatures as determined by corneal topography maps. The authors suggested that CsA might be a novel treatment strategy in KC patients by arresting disease progression.

- Matrix metalloproteinase-1 (MMP-1)

Significantly higher expression of MMP-1 has been detected in the tear film of keratoconic eyes compared to control and post corneal collagen cross-linking eyes in a study by Balasubramaniam et al. [41]. In this study a 1.9 times higher level of proteolytic activity and a combination of gelatinolytic (MMP-2,-9) and collagenolytic action (MMP -1,-8,-13) was detected in the tear film of KC subjects compared to the other groups. Seppala et al. showed augmented MMP-1 expression in epithelial cells of keratoconic corneas but also locally in a scattered manner in the stroma as compared to normal corneas where MMP-1 was only weakly expressed and restricted to epithelial cells [42]. Increased expression of matrix metalloproteinase-1 (MMP-1) was found in keratoconus subjects with and without gas permeable contact lenses by Pannebaker et al. [43], while only slight MMP-1 overexpression was detected in KC eyes in another study [44].

- Matrix metalloproteinase-2 (MMP-2)

MMP-2 (also known as gelatinase A, with interstitial collagenase activity) is the matrix metalloproteinase that will cleave Type IV basement membrane collagen, denatured Type I collagen (gelatin), Type V and VI collagen and elastin. MMP-2 is also the major protease secreted by corneal keratocytes, suggesting a possible role in the ECM degradation seen in KC. The evidence however on its role in KC are conflicting, with some studies showing increased MMP-2 activity in keratoconic keratocyte cultures compared to controls [45], while others reporting no differences in the amount of MMP-2 that could account for the increased gelatinolytic activity in KC cultures compared to normal [33], concluding that possibly it is the alteration in the interaction between MMP-2 and TIMP that causes the increased gelatinolytic activity seen in keratoconus tissues. Collier et al. [31] found that expression of MT1-MMP (the activator of MMP-2), but not MMP-2 directly, in the epithelium and stroma, was significantly elevated in keratoconus, compared to normal corneas, suggesting a possible role for MT1-MMP in the pathogenesis of KC. Another study demonstrated MMP-2 presence in keratoconic corneas, but only to the same extent as in the healthy control samples [44]. Similarly, a lack of difference in MMP-2 levels in tears of KC eyes and normal controls was identified by other authors [41, 43]. Finally, Ortak et al. detected reduced plasma levels of zinc and MMP-2 in patients with keratoconus compared with the healthy subjects [46].

- Other Matrix metalloproteinases (MMP-3, MMP-7, MMP-13)

Other MMPs have also been studied with regards to their role in the development and progression of keratoconus. Balasubramaniam et al. [16] detected significantly raised levels of MMP-3, -7, -13 in the tear film of keratoconic eyes compared to controls, but also raised levels of MMP-13 (collagenase 3) in normal corneas after 60 s of eye rubbing. Mackiewicz et al. [44] found only a moderate increase in MMP-13 in keratoconic corneas compared to weak expression in controls. Pannebaker et al. [43] found no significant upregulation of MMPs -3, -10, -13 in KC eyes except for a significant increase in MMP-1 levels in KC subjects with and without gas permeable contact lens wear. In contrast, Kolozsvari et al. [11] showed increased tear expression of MMP-13 in KC eyes and a strong positive correlation of MMP- 13 with the severity of the disease. No differences were found in the MMP-13 release between the KC group and control by Fodor et al. [47], while MMP-13 release increased in controls with RGP CL wear over time. This increase was significantly higher when compared with the KC group.

The role of MMPs in keratoconus development and progression has evidently been a topic of substantial interest for many years with speculation over their contribution to disease pathogenesis, as overexpression of MMPs or presence of active forms has not been consistent across different studies. The evidence presented above suggest that an imbalance and dysregulation of the proteolytic activity of MMPs can lead to tissue remodelling and degradation of ECM components, including collagen and elastin. In a chronic, slowly progressive disease, as is the case of keratoconus, even occasional transient upregulation of matrix degrading enzymes may be sufficient to cause damage. Raised levels of MMP-9 and MMP-1 in keratoconic eyes has been confirmed in multiple independent studies, however reports on upregulation of other MMPs in KC subjects has been conflicting. The use of MMPs (especially MMP-9) in early diagnosis, monitoring and potentially prevention of progression of KC by use of protease inhibitors merits further research, and could lead to a change and potentially innovative approach to corneal ectasia.

6 Corneal Innervation in Keratoconus

Traditionally, prominent corneal nerves are described as an early clinical sign of keratoconus, however the role of corneal innervation in KC is not well investigated. Corneal nerves play a crucial role in maintaining normal corneal structure, transparency and function via mediation of tear secretion and protective reflexes, while providing trophic support to epithelial and stromal corneal cells. Corneal sensitivity has been found significantly lower in eyes of subclinical and KC patients when compared with normal controls. This was the case across all corneal zones of keratoconic eyes, suggesting that decreased corneal sensation is associated with tear deficiency and corneal thinning [48, 49]. In addition, altered corneal nerve morphology, such as changes in tortuosity and orientation of nerve fiber bundles at the cone apex, reduced sun-basal nerve plexus density and thickening of stromal nerve fibres, especially within the area of the cone have been reported [50–53]. Stromal nerves within the cone area have shown a number of alterations of different severity, from mild looping and coiling to excessive tortuosity and overgrowth within the centre of the cone [50]. This evidence supports a possible involvement of impaired corneal innervation in the ocular surface changes that take place in KC, and a potential link to KC pathophysiology and disease progression.

- Could influencers of ocular surface homeostasis cause keratoconus?
- Atopy and allergic diseases

Atopy is defined as a genetic disposition to develop an exaggerated IgE-mediated immune response (type I hypersensitivity-immediate) following exposure to an antigen and involves the classic triad of atopic dermatitis (eczema), allergic rhinitis (hay fever) and asthma. All atopic disorders are type I hypersensitivity disorders. The terms atopy and allergy are often used interchangeably but are essentially different. The term allergy was originally coined to describe any exaggerated immune response to a foreign antigen regardless of the underlying mechanism, meaning that a hereditary component is not necessary, in contrast to atopy which was introduced in 1923 by Coca and Cooke to designate allergies of a familial or hereditary nature [54, 55]. Other types of IgE mediated allergic reactions, such as anaphylaxis to penicillin, are not considered atopic.

The increased incidence of atopy in keratoconus patients has been well represented in the literature since the beginning of the twentieth century, with the first reported case in 1937 by Hilgartner et al. [56] describing a case of keratoconus in an 18-year-old female patient with a long history of atopic eczema, other allergies and sensitivities to various foods. In 1955, Brunsting et al. published an observational study on 1,158 patients with atopic dermatitis, discovering only a low number of keratoconic patients amongst them (6 patients) [57]. Since then various reports have been published with conflicting evidence, making it unclear whether atopy itself or eye rubbing, the indirect consequence of atopy induced itch, is a causative factor of keratoconus. Harrison et al. found a positive association between atopy and keratoconus, but also observed that eye rubbing can strongly contribute to the aetiology of keratoconus, as unilateral keratoconus occurred more frequently on the side of the dominant hand [58]. In 2000, Bawazeer et al. attempted to study the atopy-KC association by conducting a case–control study while controlling for eye rubbing as an etiological factor [59]. Their results showed that while a history of atopy was significant in the univariate analysis, eye rubbing was the only risk factor that was significant in both the univariate and multivariate level, supporting their hypothesis that eye rubbing plays a critical part in keratoconus. The authors concluded that atopy may contribute to keratoconus, but most probably via the eye rubbing tendency that atopic individuals inevitably have from severe itching.

Without a doubt, there is a lot of speculation if the mechanical effect of eye-rubbing-related trauma alone can lead to the keratoconic deformation of the cornea, without necessarily the presence of other risk factors. Or whether a low-level subclinical, chronic inflammation associated with atopy provides an underlying inflammatory mechanism that triggers the onset and progression of KC in genetically predisposed individuals [29, 60]. In 1984, Coyle et al. reported the case of a young boy with paroxysmal atrial tachycardia (Wolf-Parkinson-White syndrome) since the age of 2, who discovered at the age of 5 that he could control the tachycardic episodes by vigorously massaging his left eye [61]. He was diagnosed with unilateral keratoconus at the age of 11 while having no other apparent risk factors for KC. At that point he was fitted with a hard contact lens to the left eye and was instructed to massage his carotid artery instead to control the tachycardic episodes, a measure that proved successful and eye rubbing was ceased. At the age of 20, his keratometric readings were unchanged, with no evidence of KC progression in the affected eye or KC development in the fellow eye. This led the authors to conclude that unilateral keratoconus is possible and may be mechanically induced.

In more recent years, Shajari et al. [62] conducted a retrospective study of 670 KC eyes, dividing them in 2 groups; a study group consisting of patients with known atopic syndrome and a control group of patients without known atopic disease, and compared the topographical changes in KC patients between groups. KC patients suffering from at least one atopic trait (asthma, eczema, allergic rhinitis) were significantly younger than non-atopic KC patients, however, no topographical changes except in corneal densitometry were detected, concluding that atopic syndrome is a factor that can trigger earlier manifestation of keratoconus.

What exactly links atopy to KC and whether there is indeed a true direct association remains unclear. It is estimated that approximately one out of three patients with KC has an underlying atopic disorder, although the prevalence of atopy varies between 1.8 and 57% amongst different studies [63, 64]. The conflicting evidence in the published literature may be due to different definitions of atopy/allergy and lack of standardised classification; some studies investigate the role of allergic keratoconjunctivitis (AKC) and vernal keratoconjunctivitis (VKC) only [65], others the association of the classic triad (eczema, asthma, allergic rhinitis) with KC [62, 66, 67], some evaluate only allergies and asthma but not eczema [68], some encompass a wider range of atopic and allergic conditions [69] and others only assess one symptom of atopy [70, 71]. The discrepancy may also stem from different methods of assessment as in most cases this is based on the patient's self-report of allergic symptoms.

To conclude, the correlation of atopy and keratoconus remains a controversial issue. The most evidence-based answer to this argument emerges from a large meta-analysis [72] on the prevalence and risk factors of KC in 50,358,341 cases. This study demonstrated a 3 times higher risk of KC onset in subjects with abnormal eye rubbing on a daily basis. Interestingly, although asthma, allergy, and eczema were all identified as effective risk factors for keratoconus, atopy per se did not increase the risk of the disease. As a result, atopy is a component of the KC causal pathway and an indirect cause of keratoconus. This statement needs to be interpreted with caution given the wide variation and inconsistency in the definition of atopy (Table 2).

- Vernal keratoconjunctivitis (VKC)/Atopic keratoconjunctivitis (AKC)

Atopic keratoconjunctivitis (AKC), vernal keratoconjunctivitis (VKC) and seasonal allergic conjunctivitis (SAC) are immune-mediated ocular allergic disorders, mainly triggered by environmental allergens [83]. The most severe form is AKC. Both AKC and VKC usually affect children and young adults with a higher

Table 2 Studies investigating the incidence of allergy, asthma, and eczema in Keratoconic patients

Study	Year	Country	Patients (n)	Allergy (%)	Asthma (%)	Eczema (%)
Zadnik et al. [73]	1998	USA	1209	52.9	14.9	8.4
Owens, Gamble [64]	2003	New Zealand	673	57	34	30
Assiri et al. [74]	2005	Saudi Arabia	125	39.2	13.2	6.6
Weed et al. [75]	2008	Scotland	200	30	23	14.9
Nemet et al. [68]	2010	Israel	426	17.6	8.2	ND
Agrawal [76]	2011	India	274	ND	11.3	26.6
Jordan et al. [77]	2011	New Zealand	266	25.5	26.2	22.4
Khor et al. [63]	2011	Singapore	116	1.8	26.3	18.4
Shneor et al. [78]	2012	Israel	244	34.4	13.3	6.6
Gordon- Shaag et al. [79]	2013	Israel	70	15.7	7.1	4.3
Naderan et al. [66]	2015	Iran	461	15.8	4.4	2.4
Gordon- Shaag et al. [80]	2015	Israel	219	19.2	8.1	ND
Naderan et al. [69]	2017	Iran	885	ND	5.3	3.6
Hashemi et al. [81]	2014	Iran	35	19.2	ND	ND
Woodward et al. [82]	2015	USA	16,053	28.3	14.3	ND

prevalence in hot, dry climates such as the Middle East, North Africa and some parts of South America. They are characterised by persistent ocular surface inflammation with eosinophilic infiltration, increased number of mast cells, basophils, neutrophils, macrophages, and type 2 (Th2) lymphocytes in the conjunctival tissues. They lead to intense ocular symptomatology with constant ocular irritation, severe eye itching and eye rubbing, photophobia, tearing, copious mucous discharge and eyelid changes [84–86]. The classification of VKC is based on the main site of the papillary reaction: limbal (fine papillae with circumferential gelatinous limbal infiltration and Horner-Trantas dots), palpebral (giant papillae of >1 mm on the superior tarsal conjunctiva) and mixed.

The first report of the VKC-KC association dates back to 1920 [87] and since then various studies reported a widely varying incidence of KC among VKC/AKC patients, ranging from 0.77 to 26.8% depending on geography and topographic parameters or methods used to diagnose KC [88, 89]. Umale et al. [90] reported a prevalence of 11.2% for keratoconus by the modified Rabinowitz-McDonnell criteria among VKC patients. The incidence of keratoconus in a series of 530 cases of VKC detected by videokeratography was 26.8%, while 8.5% were detected clinically and 18.3% by keratometry [91]. Gortzak et al. observed more abnormal corneal topographic patterns in VKC subjects compared to controls with 22.5% of keratoconus-like topography and 3.75% of the clinical keratoconus [92]. Barreto et al. [93] found 20% of VKC patients had keratoconus, and 14% had subclinical disease, after refining the diagnostic methods for KC evaluation, by analysing anterior and posterior corneal morphology of VKC patients versus an age-matched control group. The association of AKC with KC has been reported less frequently in the literature, however a recent large matched cohort study including 186.202 newly diagnosed AKC patients and 186.202 non-AKC age and sex-matched controls, concluded that the incidence rate of KC was 2.49 times higher in AKC than controls. Even after adjusting for potential confounders, AKC patients were 2.25 times more likely to develop KCN [85].

The role of eye-rubbing induced biomechanical corneal changes as an environmental trigger for keratoconus development and progression in predisposed individuals has been well known [94–96]. The chronic and vigorous eye rubbing as a common manifestation of severe ocular allergic states like AKC/ VCK is therefore a clear risk factor for keratoconus development and progression and as such, KC in association with AKC/VKC is a commonly reported finding in the literature. Environmental allergens bind to immunoglobulin E (IgE) molecules on the surface of mast cells of the conjunctiva, triggering histamine release, while also stimulating a number of inflammatory cytokines. A number of studies report the strong link between VCK/AKC and KC, while also highlighting that keratoconus in association with VKC tends to begin at a much younger age, progress at a rapid rate, escalate to a more advanced stage, while acute corneal hydrops is also more common in this group of patients [91].

Cingu et al. [65] reported that patients with VKC had more severe KC than patients with keratoconus alone or keratoconus and simple allergic conjunctivitis (AC) and that KC tended to present at a younger age in this group of patients. They defined simple allergic conjunctivitis as presence/history of itching during spring/ summer, serous conjunctival discharge-hyperaemia, mild papillae on upper tarsal conjunctiva, while VKC was defined as severe and intractable itching, giant papillae on the upper eyelid, Horner-Tranta's dots, ropy discharge and infiltration in the limbus. Grade 4 KC was significantly higher in patients with VKC than that of the other two groups, as was the presence of acute hydrops as presenting symptom (11.8% in KC + VKC vs. 4.9% in KC + AC vs. 4.2% in KC alone). Naderan et al. [69] also demonstrated that patients with VKC or AC (prevalence of 21.4% and 16.6% respectively among 885 KC patients) had significantly thinner and steeper corneas in comparison with non-allergic KC patients. For this reason and due to the higher risk of more advanced, severe KC, these patients should be closely followed up and intensively treated.

Except for the mechanical stress caused by chronic eye-rubbing related cornea trauma in allergic states, a number of inflammatory cytokines, MMPs and lyso-somal enzymes have been found elevated in the tear film of patients with AKC/ VKC, not only at the time of active symptomatic phases, but also during asymp-tomatic, clinically quiescent periods. The corneal complications seen are thought to be the result of the epitheliotoxic effects of proteins and enzymes released by activated eosinophils [97]. Eosinophils and Th2 lymphocytes produce mediators such as the eosinophil-derived granule proteins, MMP-9, and Th2 cytokines which compromise the epithelial barrier and expose corneal fibroblasts to inflammatory mediators. T cells also express or regulate MMPs [83]. The conjunctival and cor-neal remodelling of the extracellular matrix (ECM) that take place in VKC/AKC lead to formation of giant papillae, sub-epithelial fibrosis, chronic cellular infiltrate, epithelial thickening, plaque formation, mucous metaplasia, neovascularisation and scarring. Altered homeostasis leads to degradation of ECM in addition to synthesis and deposition of new matrix. Increased levels of matrix metalloproteinase MMP-1, MMP-2, MMP-3, MMP-8, MMP-9, and MMP-10 have been reported in VKC patients [97], as well as tumour necrosis factor (TNF)-α and IL-6 [16]. Active forms of MMP-9 and MMP-2 have been detected in the tear film of nearly all VKC subjects and none of healthy controls in a study by Kumagai et al. [98]. Since the structure and function of the corneal epithelium depends on the underlying base-ment membrane (mainly formed of type IV collagen and laminin), the presence of high levels of proteolytic enzymes especially MMP-2 and MMP-9 in the tear film of VKC patients may further explain the high prevalence of KC in VKC, but also the higher severity of KC in these cases [99].

There is evidently a vicious cycle triggered by conjunctival inflammation, atopic-related and keratoconus-related ocular irritation, leading to eye rubbing and corneal complications, with a potential to either cause corneal deformation and ectasia or induce faster and more severe progression.

The combination of frequent and intense eye rubbing that characterises VCK/ AKC along with the chronic tissue degradation and corneal stromal cell apoptosis from constant exposure to inflammatory cytokines, may lead to the development of keratoconus in genetically predisposed individuals. The association between cor-neal ectasia and VKC highlights the importance of obtaining annual (or more frequent according to keratometry values) corneal topography in subjects with long-standing AKC/VKC, especially in severe forms, in the presence of an already high/suspicious refractive error or in the event of suboptimal vision in order to achieve an early detection of keratoconus and assume appropriate treatment strategy and follow-up.

- Eye rubbing

Intense and prolonged eye rubbing has been recognized as an independent important risk factor for the development and progression of KC according to many epidemiological studies, with abundant clinical evidence that vigorous eye-rubbing can lead to de novo development of KC [59–61, 100]. The prevalence of eye rubbing in keratoconic patients ranges in the literature from 66 to 73% [101–103]. Rabinowitz [104] and Naderan et al. [66] have conducted case–control studies demonstrating that KC patients rub their eyes more often than normal controls (80% and 83% versus 58% and 52% respectively).

A history of eye rubbing is usually defined as rubbing of the eye for any reason including ocular disease, dry eye syndrome, bacterial or viral conjunctivitis, trichiasis, blepharitis, allergic eye disease (AKC, VKC), dermatological conditions (rosacea, periocular eczema, atopic dermatitis), "removal relief" in contact lens wearers [105]. Behavioural repetitive and prolonged eye rubbing can also be observed in a number of conditions such as developmental disorders, mental retardation (oculo-digital sign), Down's Syndrome, Lebers' congenital amaurosis, or psychiatric affections (obsessive–compulsive eye rubbing) [106, 107].

Directed history taking regarding eye rubbing should include not only questioning whether or not the patient rubs their eyes, but also in what way the eyes are rubbed as patients rub their eyes in a number of different ways; with the pulp of their fingertips, their fingernails or their knuckles. Hafezi et al. conducted a prospective study to assess the average forces typically applied to the globe during eye rubbing in 57 patients with keratoconus [108], where patients were asked to perform their individual eye rubbing movement and then repeat the same movement on a surface of a high-precision balance. At the same time the authors observed which part of the finger came into contact with the eyelids every time an eye-rubbing movement was performed, while hand dominance was also recorded. The authors found that knuckle eye rubbing exerts the greatest force on the globe, being 2.2 and 3.7 times greater when compared to fingertip or fingernail eye-rubbing respectively.

The question whether the mechanical effect of eye rubbing alone can lead or contribute to KC onset and progression has long been a subject of debate [95], since the detection of a strong association between an environmental factor and a disease is undeniably a prerequisite, but not a sufficient condition for establishing a causal role. A controlled multivariate analysis by Bawazeer et al. [59] identified eye rubbing as the single most important predictor of KC development, while the association between atopy and KC was attributed to the itching tendency experienced by atopic individuals. A number of case reports on unilaterally occurring keratoconus in patients with a corresponding unilateral habit of intense and repetitive eye rubbing, supports the concept that even normal corneas can become ectatic in response to rubbing-related corneal trauma [61, 109–114] (Table 3). However, observational case reports can only provide low level of evidence to infer a causative link.

Repetitive mechanical trauma caused by vigorous and frequent eye rubbing can lead to biochemical and biomechanical corneal alterations, with subsequent corneal weakening through increased keratocyte apoptosis and oxidative damage due to cyclic shear stress on corneal microstructures [101, 102]. Various mechanisms have been suggested to explain the link between eye rubbing and corneal remodelling with a potential for keratoconus onset/progression. These include:

- Increased intraocular pressure (IOP) [95, 101, 115–117]:

Corneal tissue behaves viscoelastically with an ability to almost instantaneous deformation in response to a mechanical force, and vice versa; instantaneous recovery of deformation when mechanical stress is removed. Nevertheless, distending intraocular pressure (IOP) forces that are in excess of the corneal resistance to them is a known mechanism of permanent corneal deformation and keratectasia with cone formation [101]. These forces are accentuated during eye rubbing. Thus many studies suggest that the acute IOP elevation taking place during eye rubbing

Table 3 Cases of apparent unilateral/highly asymmetric keratoconus related to eye rubbing	**Unilateral Keratoconus after Chronic Eye Rubbing by the Nondominant Hand** Bral N, Termote K. Case Rep Ophthalmol. 2017 Dec 14;8 (3):558–561
	Keratoconus and eye rubbing Coyle JT. Am J Ophthalmol. 1984;97: 527–528
	Unilateral keratoconus in a child with chronic and persistent eye rubbing Ioannidis AS, Speedwell L, Nischal KK. Am J Ophthalmol. 2005 Feb;139(2):356–7
	Incorrect sleeping position and eye rubbing in patients with unilateral or highly asymmetric keratoconus: a case–control study Mazharian A, Panthier C, Courtin R, Jung C, Rampat R, Saad A, Gatinel D. Graefes Arch Clin Exp Ophthalmol. 2020 Nov;258(11):2431–2439
	Asymmetric keratoconus attributed to eye rubbing Jafri B, Lichter H, Stulting RD. Cornea 2004;23:560–564
	Keratoconus associated with continual eye rubbing due to punctal agenesis Lindsay RG, Bruce AS, Gutteridge IF. Cornea. 2000 Jul;19 (4):567–9
	Eye Rubbing and Transient Corneal Ectasia Detected by Topography in a Pediatric Patient Scotto R, Vagge A, Traverso CE. Cornea. 2021 Feb 1;40 (2):251–253

and the associated mechanical strain on the cornea may lead to alterations at the cellular level [118]. In 2019, Turner et al. [116] conducted an experimental study to determine the magnitude of IOP elevation associated with eye rubbing in vivo in non-human primates, showing that IOP increased as much as 310 mmHg due to eye rubbing. Mean IOP elevations of 80–150 mmHg above baseline were elicited for 3–4 s during eye rubbing, with peak IOP elevations reaching 205–310 mmHg. A prior study showed that the mean compressive globe indentation force in subjects with keratoconus generated during eye rubbing was 10 times greater than the mean force observed in non-KC patients [119]. The corneal apex is the location exposed to the highest compressive forces.

- Micro-trauma and friction between palpebral conjunctiva and corneal epithelium [95, 101, 120]:

The corneal epithelium sustains a number of intrinsic and extrinsic forces in vivo, such as the intraocular pressure, eyelid movement, tear film motion, contact lens use and eye rubbing. Eye rubbing seems to have considerable effects on corneal topography and epithelial thickness profile. Even passive upper lid forces have been shown to cause topographic changes to the corneal surface. McMonnies et al. demonstrated a significant epithelial thickness reduction up to 18.4% centrally and mid-peripherally in response to compressive and shearing forces produced by 15 s of circular pattern rubbing over the cornea [120]. Rubbing related epithelial thinning may include cell flattening, as well as displacement from the rubbed area of epithelial cells/extracellular fluid/cytoplasm from burst cells/mucin. Significant increase in surface regularity index and a small amount (0.5 diopter) of induced astigmatism has also been observed immediately after 60 s of experimental eye rubbing [121]. These findings suggest the significant epithelial trauma resulting from cyclic shear stress caused by eye rubbing and the biomechanical fatigue, which can lead to corneal thinning, loss of rigidity, tissue weakening and cone-shaped bulging.

- Elevated corneal epithelial temperature [95, 101, 122]

The corneal surface (epithelial) temperature increases during eyelid closure due to i) inhibition of heat loss through evaporation from the ocular surface and ii) the proximity of the cornea to the palpebral conjunctival vasculature (blood temperature of 38.8 °C). This temperature rise is intensified during eye rubbing, especially during prolonged and vigorous rubbing, due to conjunctival hyperaemia [101]. The biomechanical properties of corneal collagen depend on temperature. Increased enzyme activity and enzyme denaturation occurs as temperature rises, and can be associated with upregulation of collagenase activity. As a result, rubbing-related temperature spikes render a susceptible cornea more prone to deformation through matrix degradation [122].

- Release of inflammatory mediators [16, 36, 95, 123]

As previously discussed, several studies have demonstrated increased levels of proteolytic enzymes and inflammatory molecules in the tear film and cornea of keratoconic patients. These include MMP-1, MMP3, MMP-7, MMP-13, interleukin (IL)-4, -5, -6, -8, tumour necrosis factor (TNF)-α, -β [30–32]. Balasubramanian et al. [16] investigated the influence of eye rubbing on MMP-13, IL-6 and TNF-α in the tear film of normal volunteers before and after 60 s of experimental eye rubbing. MMP-12, IL-6 and TNF-α levels were significantly increased from baseline after 60 s of eye rubbing in non keratoconic eyes. This inflammatory insult may be exacerbated after persistent and forceful eye rubbing. Any imbalance in the expression and activity of collagenolytic and pro-inflammatory molecules in the corneal tissue as a consequence of an epigenetic factor like eye rubbing, may lead to progressive corneal weakening and KC manifestation [27].

- Contact lens wear

Contact lens (CL) wear, and specifically rigid gas permeable (RGP) CLs, is one of the environmental risk factors that has been implicated in the development and progression of keratoconus, although its role remains controversial and has been termed as a "circumstantial association" without a direct cause-effect relationship proven [75, 124–127]. Ironically, a significant number of KC patients will require contact lenses for adequate sight restoration and visual functioning (soft contact lenses/RGPs/hybrid/scleral etc. according to severity of keratoconus), which have been the cornerstone of visual rehabilitation for keratoconic eyes, nevertheless exposing them to this external pressure trigger implicated in KC onset and progression.

Contact lens wear has been reported to interfere with normal corneal physiology in a number of ways and across all corneal layers; squamous metaplasia and decreased goblet cell density in conjunctival impression cytology, decreased central corneal thickness-CCT (with hard CLs causing a greater reduction than soft CLs), increase of corneal curvature and surface irregularity, keratocyte apoptosis, increased endothelial polymegathism and pleomorphism [128, 129].

McMonnies [130] studied the role of CL insertion, wear and removal in triggering eye rubbing, the prevalence of 'removal-relief' rubbing in CL wearers and its potential consequences. In this study, CL wearing patients (with/without KC) reported significantly more rubbing before CL insertion compared to non-CL wearers. Eye rubbing after CL removal ('removal-relief' rubbing) was found to be significantly more prevalent among CL-wearing keratoconic patients compared to CL-wearing non-keratoconic patients. 'Removal-relief' rubbing can be more harmful and potentially cause greater corneal trauma, since the corneal epithelium and stroma is already compromised immediately after contact lens wear.

In addition to provoking an eye rubbing tendency, prolonged CL wear may induce mechanical micro-trauma on the corneal epithelium, thus stimulating the release of apoptotic cytokines such as interleukin 1 (IL-1), contributing to decrease in keratocyte cell density via apoptosis. A link between upregulation of degrading enzymes that have been directly linked to oxidative stress and degradation of the corneal collagen (MMP-9 and MMP-13), has been shown in keratoconic eyes with CL use (RGPs and scleral CLs) [27, 47, 131]. Decreased anterior keratocyte density has been detected with confocal microscopy in patients with keratoconus who wear contact lenses, significantly more so than those who do not [132, 133]. Similarly, increased levels of pro-inflammatory mediators have also been described in tears of RGP contact lens wearers, as has increased tear osmolarity [134, 135]. As known, contact lens wear is a risk factor for dry eye syndrome, the inflammatory implications of which on keratoconic corneas, or corneas predisposed to ectasia are evident. Tear film inflammatory molecules are, as already mentioned, elevated in keratoconic eyes, eyes with contact lens wear, eyes following eye rubbing, but also in dry eye syndrome, meaning that the presence of all these risk factors further increases the risk for ectasia, as these patients are at a constant state of subclinical inflammation.

Overall, current evidence suggests that contact lens wear modifies the surface of the cornea through mechanical stimulation of the epithelial cells and favouring a pro-inflammatory and matrix-degrading environment with keratocyte apoptosis, ECM remodelling. It can therefore predispose to keratoconus development and/or progression in susceptible individuals. The anoxic environment produced by CLs may also inhibit cell proliferation in the central cornea after prolonged wear and delay in the migratory capacity of epithelial cells, as well as adhesion between the lens and the cornea and corneal warpage [136–138].

On the other hand, ongoing progression of KC occurs in patients not wearing contact lenses after the age of 30 years old [139], which makes it challenging indeed to draw a conclusion as to the causative Vs coincidental nature of contact lens wear in KC onset/progression. As environmental risk factors play a significant role in the development of keratoconus in genetically predisposed individuals, controlling them may reduce the risk of developing keratoconus, however no strong evidence exists at this stage to suggest that contact lens wear should be avoided.

• Dry eye

A number of studies report increased prevalence and greater severity of signs and symptoms of dry eye in keratoconus patients when compared to non-KC control groups [140–142]. KC patients suffer greater tear film instability, as indicated by significantly lower tear film break-up time (TFBUT), higher fluorescein and Rose Bengal corneal staining scores, primarily due to decreased mucin production. Clinical experience substantiates this claim, as the majority of KC patients report dry eye disease (DED) symptoms (as indicated by higher scores on Ocular Surface Disease Index-OSDI-questionnaire). It is common to observe clinical signs of DED.

The strong link between dry eye and keratoconus has been reported in many studies [140–144]. Disruption of tear film stability in KC eyes can be the consequence of:

(a) *Corneal irregularities*

An abnormal corneal curvature with irregular steepening can lead to tear film disruption. The conical elevation of the cornea may disturb the tear film, by inducing a focal discontinuity in the precorneal tear film due to thinning and stretching of the tear film thickness over the elevated area, similarly as a rock would tower above the sea level. This interrupted continuity can give rise to local tear film defect and inadequate coating, with a repeatedly dry underlying corneal tissue after every blink. The sites that would be expectedly more affected are the more elevated-steep, such as the apex of the cone. In addition, more mechanical friction between the cone apex and the palpebral conjunctiva during blinking is expected. In such a manner, even with intact homeostatic mechanisms, keratoconic eyes may demonstrate tear film instability and dry eye symptomatology as commonly encountered in this group of patients.

Vice versa, an unstable tear film may result in an irregular corneal surface and disruption of topographic measurements. As such, inferior steepening is a common result of dry eye due to chronic desiccation and epithelial dehydration, to the extent that can even mimic keratoconus [145]. Topographic irregularity indices correlate significantly with the severity of dry eye, while treatment of dry eye can reverse the topographic changes to normal.

(b) *Reduced corneal sensitivity*

The cornea is a densely innervated tissue, by sensory fibres from the ophthalmic branch of the trigeminal nerve. Impaired corneal innervation has been reported in KC, characterised by reduced density and abnormal morphology of the corneal sub-basal and stromal nerves (detected by confocal microscopy and histological examinations) affecting primarily the region of the cone [48, 146]. This can compromise the function of the reflex arc responsible for the tearing reflexes that maintain tear film homeostasis [145]. Patients with KC have a higher threshold for detection of mechanical, chemical and thermal stimuli that would normally trigger the tear reflexes and tear production in normal non-KC eyes. This sensory impairment leading to corneal hypoesthesia (measured with Cochet-Bonnet esthesiometer) manifests early in the development of KC, accounting for the early onset of abnormal tear secretion and is considered a strong indicator of corneal epithelial and stromal disease.

(c) *Squamous metaplasia with reduction in goblet cell density*

Goblet cells are important for mucin production and maintenance of ocular surface integrity. Reduced goblet cell density has been detected in KC eyes on impression cytology, while the extent of goblet cell loss is related to the severity of KC [140, 143]. Furthermore, KC goblet cells produced less mucin, as indicated by a lower goblet cell layer thickness (CLT) in scanning laser confocal microscopy, thus secreting less mucin into the tears as suggested by a lower mucin cloud height (MCH) [140]. At the same time, goblet cell loss is also associated with contact lens wear-especially rigid gas permeable-which patients with advanced KC are more likely to wear, making it difficult to separate the effect of the RGP wear on ocular surface changes [129, 148]. Squamous metaplasia of the conjunctiva has also been demonstrated in conjunctival impression cytology of KC eyes [129, 140, 143] in bulbar conjunctiva, an area that does not come in direct contact with RGPs, but can be affected indirectly by the pro-inflammatory cytokines released from the impaired corneal and conjunctival epithelium in KC. It would therefore be worth saying that in keratoconus there is a diffuse ocular surface epitheliopathy, not limited to the corneal epithelium only, hence treatments targeted to improving ocular surface epithelium and increase mucin secretion have been suggested. Amongst these suggestions is the use of topical retinoids which are chemical derivatives or synthetic compounds of vitamin A. As known, vitamin A deficiency can cause epithelial squamous metaplasia and glandular atrophy, with studies showing reversal of squamous metaplasia or keratinisation on impression cytology in eyes with dry eye states (keratoconjunctivitis sicca, Stevens-Johnson syndrome, mucous membrane pemphigoid). Similarly, treatment with topical formulations of vitamin A could be considered in KC eyes where squamous metaplasia of the conjunctiva has been reported. However, as alterations in retinoid metabolism in the conjunctival cells may exist, a retinoid toxicity hypothesis has also been suggested where vitamin A might adversely affect the ocular surface due to accumulation and toxicity [149]. Further studies on the role of topical retinoids in keratoconus could shed more light into this field.

(d) *Release of inflammatory mediators*

Dry eye is characterised by subclinical ocular surface inflammation, as demonstrated by increased expression of immune activation markers, such as inflammatory cytokines (IL-1, -6, -8, TNF-a) and MMPs (MMP-9), as detected in the tear film of patients with keratoconjunctivitis sicca (KCS) and Sjogren's syndrome (SS) when compared to normal subjects [15, 150–153]. At the same time, various proteomic studies reveal disease-specific alterations in the tear fluid elements in eyes with KC and subclinical KC, with higher levels of multiple inflammatory mediators and proteolytic enzymes when compared to controls, similar to those found in dry eye states. This observation suggests that the tear film may be a vehicle of some of the pathogenic protagonists of keratoconus, such as IL-6, TNF-a or MMP-9, the action of which could be accentuated by the concurrent dry eye inflammatory contribution. Whether the dry eye inflammatory microenvironment can stimulate de novo keratoconus development or in reverse, whether the pro-inflammatory state of keratoconus induces dry eye, is an ongoing matter of discussion.

Evidently keratoconic eyes have an impaired ocular surface sustaining the consequences of inadequate tear and mucin production, flawed corneal innervation, prominent squamous metaplasia, goblet cell loss and aberrant proteome alterations that lead to tear fluid instability and poor quality.

The presence and severity of dry eye syndrome in keratoconic eyes could be further accentuated by co-existing environmental factors such as atopic eye disease, contact lens wear, blepharitis, and behavioural or secondary eye rubbing tendency.

Whether these factors lead to high prevalence of dry eye in KC eyes, or vice versa (dry eye causes KC) remains unknown. It seems however that tear function disturbance and ocular surface disease evolve in close proximity with the extent of KC progression [144, 145], while similar findings of tear film instability have been encountered in subclinical keratoconic corneas [144].

- Blepharitis

Blepharitis, anterior or posterior (meibomian gland dysfunction-MGD) is one of the most commonly encountered conditions in ophthalmic practice, with MGD considered the main cause of evaporative dry eye disease [154]. Epidemiological investigation of MGD has been limited from lack of consensus on definition and lack of a standardised way of clinical assessment, however some studies report a prevalence as high as 60% in certain populations. Chronic blepharitis is a common cause of ocular irritation, discomfort and eye rubbing, the mechanical impact of which leads to corneal sheer strength reduction and possibly conical deformation. In addition, the mechanical stimulation of epithelial cells during eye rubbing triggers the release of inflammatory molecules, such as interleukins and tumour necrosis factor. High concentrations of the degrading enzymes matrix metalloproteinases have also been reported in tears of subjects with MGD [140, 150]. The association of blepharitis and MGD with keratoconus has not been widely investigated.

Mohamed et al. [155] demonstrated that keratoconic eyes with no clinical signs of blepharitis, showed a higher dropout in meibomian glands when compared to a control group of non-KC eyes, while OSDI scores were also much higher in the KC group and more advanced stages of KC showed significantly worse gland distortion (abnormal gland to tarsus ratio, tortuous glands) and gland shortening (glands not extending from the eyelid margin to the opposite edge of the tarsal plate). Another study showed an increased prevalence of signs and symptoms of blepharitis and dry-eye syndrome in keratoconic eyes when compared to control group [141], suggesting that micro-trauma from chronic mechanical rubbing, a characteristic feature of chronic blepharitis, may be a factor in the pathogenesis of keratoconus. The chronic inflammation and inflammatory mediators, present in subjects with blepharitis may also play a key role, since these inflammatory molecules have been implicated in the pathophysiology of keratoconus. Keratoconus-like topography (pseudokeratoconus) has been reported in a patient with ocular rosacea and attributed possibly to chronic inflammation and exposure to matrix degrading enzymes, such as MMP-9, in the inferior tear meniscus.

Obviously, not all patients with blepharitis will go on to develop keratoconus, which further verifies the multifactorial nature of the disease and the genetic predisposition to ectasia that these patients manifest.

The reasons why blepharitis holds an important role in KC onset-progression and management are as follows:

 i. Prompt and effective management of blepharitis can help in achieving optimum symptom control, thereby reducing ocular irritation and eye rubbing in predisposed or already keratoconic patients early on. In such a way, the mechanical stress on the already vulnerable corneas is alleviated, reducing the risk or rate of progression and improving quality of vision.

ii. The treatment of meibomian gland dysfunction frequently involves application of warm compresses and eyelid massage to promote lipid secretion from obstructed glands. However, massaging of the eyelids and globe entails the same risks of chronic habitual eye rubbing, which is the development of corneal deformation and keratoconus in apparently normal eyes, or progression of the disease in already ectatic corneas [122]. McMonnies et al. [122] reported a case of 24-year old patient with normal corneal topography at presentation, who following treatment of blepharitis with warm compresses and eyelid massage developed abnormal keratoconic-like topography after a few weeks, which was then reversed at cessation of topical treatment. The combination of warm compresses and (excessive) eyelid massage frequency and/or force can lead to increased corneal temperature, epithelial thinning, increased concentrations of inflammatory mediators in the precorneal tear film, increased enzymatic activity, and slippage between collagen fibrils at the corneal apex. Using the distal end of the index finger during gentle experimental eye rubbing in a horizontal direction for 1 min (as patients with MGD are usually instructed) and without the application of warm compresses resulted in the induction of 0.50–0.75D of astigmatism, which however was transient and may be explained by transient regional changes in epithelial thickness [121]. This however shows how predisposed patients with chronic blepharitis who apply daily eyelid massage may develop ectatic corneal disease.

iii. It is known that raised temperature (generated by warm compresses/eyelid massage) increases enzyme activity, while denaturing of enzymes starts at temperatures above 40 [156]. Dysregulation of enzyme function in susceptible corneas may increase the risk for deformation in addition to the mechanical effect of eye rubbing, especially after prolonged and recurrent episodes in the context of blepharitis treatment. It is therefore worth considering alternative strategies for MGD management in cases of high risk for ectasia/KC suspects/established KC patients (amongst whom MGD had a high prevalence) [141], while aiming to control ocular irritation to avoid eye rubbing.

iv. Both keratoconic eyes and eyes with MGD share the common feature of inflammatory cytokine overexpression (IL1, IL6, IL8, TNF-alpha) and high levels of degradation enzymes (MMP9) [41, 150]. Chronic exposure of the inferior cornea to an amplified pool of inflammatory mediators and matrix-degrading factors in the inferior tear meniscus of MGD eyes in addition to the already higher concentrations of these molecules in KC eyes, can have a significant impact on disease onset, progression and severity [157]. Similarly, inverted keratoconus with superior steepening, a less frequently encountered entity, can be the consequence of corneal tissue exposure to upper tear meniscus inflammatory mediators. This association may also warrant a more tailored anti-inflammatory therapy approach with a two-fold benefit on MGD management and possibly keratoconus control.

7 Floppy Eyelid Syndrome

Floppy eyelid syndrome (FES) is characterised by a thin, rubbery upper tarsus that can be folded upon itself and easily everted with upward traction due to abnormal eyelid and tarsal laxity, accompanied by diffuse reactive palpebral papillary conjunctivitis with or without the presence of symptoms of ocular surface inflammation [158]. It can lead to significant ocular irritation and its coexistence with keratoconus has been well reported in the literature [159–161]. Many studies have found a significantly higher level of FES in KC patients (up to 71%) [161, 162]. The mechanism, though, behind its contribution to the pathogenesis/progression of keratoconus remains unknown. Upregulation of Matrix metalloproteinase 9 (MMP-9) may be the underlying connecting link between the two conditions, as MMP-9 levels have been found elevated in the ocular surface and skin samples of FES subjects, and are also increased in the tear film of patients with keratoconus [163–165]. Based on this theory of MMP involvement, the mechanical trauma sustained by the ocular surface in FES patients triggers an inflammatory cascade in the eyelid tissue, with release of cytokines and immune molecules where MMP-9 has a predominant role, and is responsible for matrix degradation and structural changes of elastin.

In addition, FES is associated with dry eye disease with symptoms that tend to be chronic, worse in the morning and refractory to dry eye treatments. Objective tools for dry eye evaluation have been found decreased in people with eyelid hyperlaxity, including tear film break-up time, increased corneal staining, increased Meibomian gland dropout, abnormal meibum quality and decreased Schirmer test scores [161].

Due to the strong association between keratoconus and FES, it would be recommended to investigate these individuals for keratoconus by means of retinoscopy, keratometry, or corneal tomography, especially when considering these patients for refractive surgery.

8 Managing Keratoconus by Modifying the Ocular Surface

Despite the nearly 160 years that have passed since keratoconus was first identified as an entity, its exact pathophysiology remains enigmatic. Thanks to newer molecular, genetic, biomechanical and immunochemistry research strategies, some aspects of KC pathophysiology are gradually becoming clearer. The involvement of ocular surface inflammatory pathways in the disease process are now evolving into indisputable evidence, raising the possibility of beneficial anti-inflammatory interventions in controlling disease manifestation or progression. Likewise, environmental factors such as eye rubbing, contact lens wear, dry eye disease, blepharitis, atopy, AKC/VKC, all of which can affect the ocular surface homeostasis, have all been firmly linked to keratoconus. Currently there are no topical applications that are available to control the disease progression, hence necessitating surgical intervention with corneal collagen cross-linking or corneal transplantation.

Exploring non-invasive ways to arrest progression or even manifestation of KC through manipulation of environmental factors or local ocular surface influencers, presents an attractive alternative which could have a profound impact on the future approach in keratoconus management.

- Various proteomic studies have unveiled disease-specific alterations in the tear film molecules of KC patients. Dysregulation and abnormal levels of proteins, proteinases and cytokines have all been described in KC, all of which are factors associated with an imbalance of both ocular surface and collagen homeostasis. The tear fluid may be the vehicle of some of the inflammatory protagonists of KC. Higher expression of proteolytic enzymes such as MMPs in KC eyes compared to controls has been described in numerous studies, with MMP-9 being the predominant degrading enzyme.
- Matrix metalloproteinase 9 typically is measured in the laboratory by enzyme-linked immunosorbent assay, multi-plex bead analysis, proteomic technology, or a combination thereof.
- Tear fluid MMP-9 can be easily measured in the clinic office, as detection devices are commercially available in the market such as the point-of-care InflammaDry (Rapid Pathogen Screening Inc., Sarasota, FL, USA). This is a non-invasive, disposable, relatively inexpensive, easy-to-use, single-use assay that provides a result in 10 minutes, allowing MMP-9 testing in the office. It measures both active and latent MMP-9 and produces positive results when MMP-9 levels exceed 40 ng/ml. It has a sensitivity of 85% and specificity of 94%.
- Considering the high frequency at which MMP-9 is found elevated in keratoconic eyes, it would be worth considering performing this test in all KC patients as part of the standard evaluation along with keratometry and corneal tomography. A positive MMP-9 test is an indication of ocular surface inflammation, nevertheless, it is not specific to keratoconus. Several studies have reported increased levels of MMP-9 in the tear film and conjunctival epithelial cells of patients with dry eye disease, ocular allergies, blepharitis and it has been found that increased positivity is linked to increased severity of dry eye clinical signs.
- For that reason, MMP-9 testing in KC becomes more meaningful when the above ocular conditions are not present or when they are adequately managed, as that would further confirm the inflammatory status of KC and signify the need for anti-inflammatory treatment. Indeed, KC eyes do not typically show clinical signs of inflammation (redness, oedema, conjunctival reaction, neovascularisation) and therefore presence of inflammation is not assumed. Positive MMP-9 results could be helpful in stratifying KC patients between those who will need and will profit from anti-inflammatory treatment and those who will not.
- Topical application of Cyclosporine A (CSA) is an already approved treatment for inflammatory dry eye disease. It has been proven effective in reducing

inflammatory markers, including MMP-9, at the ocular surface of patients with DED in several studies. It has recently been demonstrated that the administration of cyclosporine A strongly reduces the inflammatory stimulation and expression of MMP-9 in tears of KC eyes. Moreover, it has been suggested that there may be progression-freezing effect of CSA use as MMP-9 levels drop, which if further validated in larger and longer follow-up studies, makes the use of topical CSA a very promising, novel treatment modality in possibly halting KC progression.

- Therefore, point of care MMP-9 testing is recommended when available and if positive, it would be justified to proceed with topical cyclosporine A or other anti-inflammatory treatment even in the absence of clinical signs of inflammation.

- In the same notion of battling the inflammatory component which drives matrix degradation in keratoconus, other options could include systemic tetracyclines. Tetracyclines are known for their anti-inflammatory and anti-collagenase properties, protecting the cornea against proteolytic degradation and commonly used in corneal ulcerations, corneal melt and chemical injuries. Systemically administered doxycycline has been reported to reduce expression and activity of MMP-9 in the ocular surface of dry eye patients, reduce symptoms of dry eye syndrome, increase tear film stability, decrease the severity of ocular surface disease in patients with ocular rosacea and inhibit collagenolytic degradation of the cornea in ulcers. There are no studies to date investigating the role of tetracyclines in keratoconus management, however, they appear to be a reasonable choice for KC patients with positive indices for ocular surface inflammation.

- Tacrolimus, also known as FK 506, is a macrolide derivative with anti-inflammatory and immunomodulatory activity. It is a steroid-sparing agent similar to CsA in its mode of action. It suppresses T cell activation and interleukin-2 production by binding to an immunophilin and inhibiting the enzymatic activity of calcineurin. The use of Tacrolimus in ophthalmology is off-label. Available formulations are 0.03 and 0.1%, and have been found to be safe and well tolerated for the treatment of giant papillary conjunctivitis and other chronic allergic conjunctivitis cases, including VKC. Lower dose topical formulations (0.01 and 0.005%), have also been used for refractory VKC with good results and it has been found more effective in cases refractory to topical CsA. Although there are no studies available on its use in keratoconus, it is considered a powerful tool in paediatric VKC treatment. Considering the lack of FDA approval though and that no studies have evaluated its long term safety as an ophthalmic preparation, it is not recommended as a first line treatment of ocular allergic inflammation and VKC and many ophthalmologists reserve it in cases of recalcitrant VKC or when all other modalities fail.

- Autologous or allogenic serum eye drops are an effective treatment method in a significant number of ocular surface diseases such as dry eye, recurrent epithelial erosions, persistent epithelial defects, neurotrophic keratopathy, limbal stem cell deficiency, following laser corneal refractive surgery and even after corneal collagen cross-linking. They are rich in epitheliotrophic growth factors, fibronectin, immunoglobulins, and vitamins. Keratoconus is not currently an indication for treatment with autologous serum eye drops and their application in corneal ectasia has not been studied. The favourable effects of blood-derived products on corneal epithelial cell proliferation, vitality and migration have been well documented by both in vitro and in vivo experimental studies. They could therefore prove a valuable treatment in keratoconus to reduce the irritation of corneal epithelium by local or systemic factors which then leads to the inflammatory sequelae. They are currently a third line treatment approach for dry eye disease, but usually reserved for more severe cases due to the limited accessibility and substantial cost.

Taking all into consideration and based on the current level of knowledge we have on this corneal ectatic disorder, one can argue that the management approach should be very tailored to keratoconic patients, it should start very early in the disease process and it may necessitate more aggressive strategies to be employed in order to break the vicious cycle of ocular surface inflammation.

Recommendations in summary are:

- Actively assess for ocular surface inflammation even in the absence of clinical signs (MMP-9 point of care test) If results are positive consider early introduction of topical or systemic anti-inflammatory treatments.
- In the presence of Meibomian gland dysfunction, warm compresses and eyelid massage (usually recommended as a first line treatment) should be avoided in patients with keratoconus. Tea-tree oil application/manual expression of Meibomian glands or Intense Pulsed Light (IPL) treatment may be offered instead, in order to avoid the rubbing effect of massaging on the corneal surface, as well as the increase in temperature from warm compresses.
- There is no strong evidence at this stage to suggest that contact lens wear should be avoided in patients in keratoconus. However, considering the evident contribution of CL wear in ocular surface inflammation and epithelial biomechanical stress, other typed of visual rehabilitation should be offered to KC patients. These could include intracorneal ring segments (ICRS) or implantable collamer lenses (ICL).
- Ocular allergic disease (AKC/VKC) should be treated promptly and effectively with topical anti-inflammatories, immunomodulators or systemic treatment. Treatment should be reviewed in frequent intervals to ensure appropriate escalation to effectively control the disease. Patients with VCK/AKC should be screened early for the presence of keratoconus with corneal tomography.
- Eye rubbing should be particularly and extensively investigated as a behavioural habit or consequence of ocular surface irritation and patients thoroughly counselled about the detrimental effects on disease progression. Video demonstration of the deforming forces applied on the cornea during eye rubbing could be part of the counselling process for effective patient education.

- Management of dry eye disease by breaking the chronic inflammatory circle would have positive impact on stopping or slowing keratoconus progression. Optimising the ocular surface environment will result in modulating the biochemical and mechanical triggers of keratoconus.
- Eyelid malpositions (Floppy eyelid syndrome or other) should also be specifically looked for, and appropriate surgical correction offered if significant. Patients with FES should also be screened for keratoconus with corneal tomography.
- Future studies on targeted, specific anti-cytokine therapies are needed as a number of cytokines have been proven to be markedly elevated in keratoconic eyes and have been linked to disease progression. It would be interesting to see studies on the effects of TGFβ pathway blockage, or IL-1α and IL-1β inhibitors in arresting progression of KC.

References

1. Loh IP, Sherwin T. Is keratoconus an inflammatory disease? The implication of inflammatory pathways. Ocul Immunol Inflamm. 2020;13:1–10.
2. Cheung IM, McGhee CNj, Sherwin T. Deficient repair regulatory response to injury in keratoconic stromal cells. Clin Exp Optom. 2014;97(3):234–9.
3. Wilson SE, Esposito A. Focus on molecules: interleukin-1: a master regulator of the corneal response to injury. Exp Eye Res. 2009;89(2):124–5.
4. Wisse RP, Kuiper JJ, Gans R, Imhof S, Radstake TR, Van der Lelij A. Cytokine expression in keratoconus and its corneal microenvironment: a systematic review. Ocul Surf. 2015;13 (4):272–83.
5. Volatier TLA, Figueiredo FC, Connon CJ. Keratoconus at a molecular level: a review. Anat Rec (Hoboken). 2020;303(6):1680–8.
6. Nabil KM, Elhady GM, Morsy H. The association between interleukin 1 beta promoter polymorphisms and keratoconus incidence and severity in an Egyptian population. Clin Ophthalmol. 2019;14(13):2217–23.
7. Mikami T, Meguro A, Teshigawara T, et al. Interleukin 1 beta promoter polymorphism is associated with keratoconus in a Japanese population. Mol Vis. 2013;19:845–51.
8. Kim SH, Mok JW, Kim HS, Joo CK. Association of -31T>C and -511 C>T polymorphisms in the interleukin 1 beta (IL1B) promoter in korean keratoconus patients. Mol Vis. 2008;14:2109–16.
9. Fabre EJ, Bureau J, Pouliquen Y, Lorans G. Binding sites for human interleukin 1 alpha, gamma interferon and tumor necrosis factor on cultured fibroblasts of normal cornea and keratoconus. Curr Eye Res. 1991;10:585–92.
10. Ionescu C, Corbu CG, Tanase C, Jonescu-Cuypers C, Nicula C, Dascalescu D, Cristea M, Voinea LM. Inflammatory biomarkers profile as microenvironmental expression in keratoconus. Dis Markers. 2016;2016:1243819.
11. Kolozsvári BL, Petrovski G, Gogolák P, Rajnavölgyi É, Tóth F, Berta A, Fodor M. Association between mediators in the tear fluid and the severity of keratoconus. Ophthalmic Res. 2014;51(1):46–51.
12. Olofsson EM, Marklund SL, Pedrosa-Domellof F, Behndig A. Interleukin-1 alpha downregulates extracellular-superoxide dismutase in human corneal keratoconus stromal cells. Mol Vis. 2007;13:1285–90.

13. Jun AS, Cope L, Speck C, Feng X, Lee S, Meng H, Hamad A, Chakravarti S. Subnormal cytokine profile in the tear fluid of keratoconus patients. PLoS One. 2011;6(1):e16437.
14. Ionescu IC, Corbu CG, Tanase C, Ionita G, Nicula C, Coviltir V, Potop V, Constantin M, Codrici E, Mihai S, Popescu ID, Enciu AM, Dascalescu D, Burcel M, Ciuluvica R, Voinea LM. Overexpression of tear inflammatory cytokines as additional finding in keratoconus patients and their first degree family members. Mediators Inflamm. 2018;2 (2018):4285268.
15. Lema I, Sobrino T, Durán JA, Brea D, Díez-Feijoo E. Subclinical keratoconus and inflammatory molecules from tears. Br J Ophthalmol. 2009;93(6):820–4.
16. Balasubramanian SA, Pye DC, Willcox MD. Effects of eye rubbing on the levels of protease, protease activity and cytokines in tears: relevance in keratoconus. Clin Exp Optom. 2013;96:214–8.
17. Soiberman U, Foster JW, Jun AS, Chakravarti S. Pathophysiology of keratoconus: what do we know today. Open Ophthalmol J. 2017;31(11):252–61.
18. Shetty R, Ghosh A, Lim RR, Subramani M, Mihir K, Reshma AR, Ranganath A, Nagaraj S, Nuijts RM, Beuerman R, Shetty R, Das D, Chaurasia SS, Sinha-Roy A, Ghosh A. Elevated expression of matrix metalloproteinase-9 and inflammatory cytokines in keratoconus patients is inhibited by cyclosporine A. Invest Ophthalmol Vis Sci. 2015;56(2):738–50.
19. Du G, Liu C, Li X, Chen W, He R, Wang X, Feng P, Lan W. Induction of matrix metalloproteinase-1 by tumor necrosis factor-α is mediated by interleukin-6 in cultured fibroblasts of keratoconus. Exp Biol Med (Maywood). 2016;241(18):2033–41.
20. Arbab M, Tahir S, Niazi MK, Ishaq M, Hussain A, Siddique PM, Saeed S, Khan WA, Qamar R, Butt AM, Azam M. TNF-α genetic predisposition and higher expression of inflammatory pathway components in keratoconus. Invest Ophthalmol Vis Sci. 2017;58 (9):3481–7.
21. Engler C, Chakravarti S, Doyle J, et al. Transforming growth factor-beta signaling pathway activation in keratoconus. Am J Ophthalmol. 2011;151:752-759.e2.
22. Maier P, Broszinski A, Heizmann U, et al. Active transforming growth factor-beta2 is increased in the aqueous humor of keratoconus patients. Mol Vis. 2007;13:1198–202.
23. Priyadarsini S, McKay TB, Sarker-Nag A, Karamichos D. Keratoconus in vitro and the key players of the TGF-β pathway. Mol Vis. 2015;21:577–88.
24. Shetty R, Deshmukh R, Ghosh A, Sethu S, Jayadev C. Altered tear inflammatory profile in Indian keratoconus patients—The 2015 Col Rangachari Award paper. Indian J Ophthalmol. 2017;65(11):1105–8.
25. Saghizadeh M, Chwa M, Aoki A, Lin B, Pirouzmanesh A, Brown DJ, Ljubimov AV, Kenney MC. Altered expression of growth factors and cytokines in keratoconus, bullous keratopathy and diabetic human corneas. Exp Eye Res. 2001;73(2):179–89.
26. Lambiase A, Merlo D, Mollinari C, Bonini P, Rinaldi AM, D' Amato M, Micera A, Coassin M, Rama P, Bonini S, Garaci E. Molecular basis for keratoconus: lack of TrkA expression and its transcriptional repression by Sp3. Proc Natl Acad Sci U S A. 2005;102 (46):16795–800.
27. di Martino E, Ali M, Inglehearn CF. Matrix metalloproteinases in keratoconus—too much of a good thing? Exp Eye Res. 2019;182:137–43.
28. Sivak JM, Fini ME. MMPs in the eye: emerging roles for matrix metalloproteinases in ocular physiology. Prog Retin Eye Res. 2002;21(1):1–14.
29. Galvis V, Sherwin T, Tello A, Merayo J, Barrera R, Acera A. Keratoconus: an inflammatory disorder? Eye (Lond). 2015;29:843–59.
30. Balasubramanian SA, Pye DC, Willcox MD. Are proteinases the reason for keratoconus? Curr Eye Res. 2010;35(3):185–91.
31. Collier SA, Madigan MC, Penfold PL. Expression of membrane-type 1 matrix metalloproteinase (MT1-MMP) and MMP-2 in normal and keratoconus corneas. Curr Eye Res. 2000;21(2):662–8.
32. Fini ME, Yue BY, Sugar J. Collagenolytic/gelatinolytic metalloproteinases in normal and keratoconus corneas. Curr Eye Res. 1992;11(9):849–62.

33. Kenney MC, Chwa M, Opbroek AJ, Brown DJ. Increased gelatinolytic activity in keratoconus keratocyte cultures. A correlation to an altered matrix metalloproteinase-2/tissue inhibitor of metalloproteinase ratio. Cornea. 1994;13(2):114–24.
34. Smith VA, Easty DL. Matrix metalloproteinase 2: involvement in keratoconus. Eur J Ophthalmol. 2000;10(3):215–26.
35. Mazzotta C, Traversi C, Mellace P, Bagaglia SA, Zuccarini S, Mencucci R, Jacob S. Keratoconus progression in patients with allergy and elevated surface matrix metalloproteinase 9 point-of-care test. Eye Contact Lens. 2018;44(Suppl 2):S48–53.
36. Lema I, Durán JA. Inflammatory molecules in the tears of patients with keratoconus. Ophthalmology. 2005;112(4):654–9.
37. Pahuja N, Kumar NR, Shroff R, Shetty R, Nuijts RM, Ghosh A, Sinha-Roy A, Chaurasia SS, Mohan RR, Ghosh A. Differential molecular expression of extracellular matrix and inflammatory genes at the corneal cone apex drives focal weakening in keratoconus. Invest Ophthalmol Vis Sci. 2016;57(13):5372–82.
38. Mutlu M, Sarac O, Cağıl N, Avcıoğlu G. Relationship between tear eotaxin-2 and MMP-9 with ocular allergy and corneal topography in keratoconus patients. Int Ophthalmol. 2020;40 (1):51–7.
39. Zilfyan A, Abovyan A. A new approach to keratoconus diagnostics using matrix metalloproteinase-9 marker. Georgian Med News. 2017;270:20–4.
40. Sobrino T, Regueiro U, Malfeito M, Vieites-Prado A, Pérez-Mato M, Campos F, Lema I. Higher expression of toll-like receptors 2 and 4 in blood cells of keratoconus patients. Sci Rep. 2017;7(1):12975.
41. Balasubramanian SA, Mohan S, Pye DC, Willcox MD. Proteases, proteolysis and inflammatory molecules in the tears of people with keratoconus. Acta Ophthalmol. 2012;90(4):e303–9.
42. Seppala HP, Maatta M, Rautia M, Mackiewicz Z, Tuisku I, Tervo T, Konttinen YT. EMMPRIN and MMP-1 in keratoconus. Cornea. 2006;25:325–30.
43. Pannebaker C, Chandler HL, Nichols JJ. Tear proteomics in keratoconus. Mol Vis. 2010;16:1949–57.
44. Mackiewicz Z, Määttä M, Stenman M, Konttinen L, Tervo T, Konttinen YT. Collagenolytic proteinases in keratoconus. Cornea. 2006;25(5):603–10.
45. Smith VA, Rishmawi H, Hussein H, Easty DL. Tear film MMP accumulation and corneal disease. Br J Ophthalmol. 2001;85:147–53.
46. Ortak H, Söğüt E, Taş U, Mesci C, Mendil D. The relation between keratoconus and plasma levels of MMP-2, zinc, and SOD. Cornea. 2012;31(9):1048–51.
47. Fodor M, Kolozsvári BL, Petrovski G, Kettesy BA, Gogolák P, Rajnavölgyi É, Ujhelyi B, Módis L, Petrovski BÉ, Szima GZ, Berta A, Facskó A. Effect of contact lens wear on the release of tear mediators in keratoconus. Eye Contact Lens. 2013;39(2):147–52.
48. Cho KJ, Mok JW, Choi MY, Kim JY, Joo CK. Changes in corneal sensation and ocular surface in patients with asymmetrical keratoconus. Cornea. 2013;32(2):205–10.
49. Zabala M, Archila EA. Corneal sensitivity and topogometry in keratoconus. CLAO J. 1988;14:210–2.
50. Al-Aqaba MA, Dhillon VK, Mohammed I, Said DG, Dua HS. Corneal nerves in health and disease. Prog Retin Eye Res. 2019;73:100762.
51. Spadea L, Salvatore S, Vingolo EM. Corneal sensitivity in keratoconus: a review of the literature. Sci World J. 2013;2013:683090.
52. Mandathara PS, Stapleton FJ, Kokkinakis J, Willcox MD. Pilot study of corneal sensitivity and its association in keratoconus. Cornea. 2017;36(2):163–8.
53. Brookes NH, Loh IP, Clover GM, Poole CA, Sherwin T. Involvement of corneal nerves in the progression of keratoconus. Exp Eye Res. 2003;77(4):515–24.
54. Igea JM. The history of the idea of allergy. Allergy. 2013;68(8):966–73.
55. Coca AF, Cooke RA. On the classification of the phenomena of hypersensitiveness. J Immunol. 1923;8:163.

56. Hilgartner HL, Hilgartner HL Jr. Gilbert JT A preliminary report of a case of keratoconus successfully treated with organotherapy, radium and shortwave diathermy. Am J Ophthalmol. 1937;20:1032–9.
57. Brunsting LA, Reed WB, Blair HL. Occurrence of cataract and keratoconus with atopic dermatitis. Arch Dermatol. 1955;72:237–41.
58. Harrison RJ, Klouda PT, Easty DL, et al. Association between keratoconus and atopy. Br J Ophthalmol. 1989;73:816–22.
59. Bawazeer AM, Hodge WG, Lorimer B. Atopy and keratoconus: a multivariate analysis. Br J Ophthalmol. 2000;84(8):834–6.
60. Galvis V, Tello A, Carreño NI, Berrospi RD, Niño CA. Risk factors for keratoconus: atopy and eye rubbing. Cornea. 2017;36(1):e1.
61. Coyle JT. Keratoconus and eye rubbing. Am J Ophthalmol. 1984;97:527–8.
62. Shajari M, Eberhardt E, Müller M, Al Khateeb G, Friderich S, Remy M. Kohnen T effects of atopic syndrome on keratoconus. Cornea. 2016;35(11):1416–20.
63. Khor WB, Wei RH, Lim L, Chan CM, Tan DT. Keratoconus in Asians: demographics, clinical characteristics and visual function in a hospital-based population. Clin Exp Ophthalmol. 2011;39:299–307.
64. Owens H, Gamble G. A profile of keratoconus in New Zealand. Cornea. 2003;22:122–5.
65. Cingu AK, Cinar Y, Turkcu FM, et al. Effects of vernal and allergic conjunctivitis on severity of keratoconus. Int J Ophthalmol. 2013;6:370–4.
66. Naderan M, Shoar S, Rezagholizadeh F, et al. Characteristics and associations of keratoconus patients. Cont Lens Anterior Eye. 2015;38:199–205.
67. Merdler I, Hassidim A, Sorkin N, et al. Keratoconus and allergic diseases among Israeli adolescents between 2005 and 2013. Cornea. 2015;34:525–9.
68. Nemet AY, Vinker S, Bahar I, et al. The association of keratoconus with immune disorders. Cornea. 2010;29:1261–4.
69. Naderan M, Rajabi MT, Zarrinbakhsh P, Bakhshi A. Effect of allergic diseases on keratoconus severity. Ocul Immunol Inflamm. 2017;25(3):418–23.
70. Mcmonnies CW, Boneham GC. Keratoconus, allergy, itch, eye-rubbing and hand-dominance. Clin Exp Optom. 2003;86(6):376–84.
71. Rabinowitz YS. The genetics of keratoconus. Ophthalmol Clin North Am. 2003;16(4):607–20.
72. Hashemi H, Heydarian S, Hooshmand E, Saatchi M, Yekta A, Aghamirsalim M, Valadkhan M, Mortazavi M, Hashemi A. Khabazkhoob M the prevalence and risk factors for keratoconus: a systematic review and meta-analysis. Cornea. 2020;39(2):263–70.
73. Zadnik K, Barr JT, Edrington TB, et al. Baseline findings in the collaborative longitudinal evaluation of keratoconus (CLEK) study. Invest Ophthalmol Vis Sci. 1998;39:2537–46.
74. Assiri AA, Yousuf BI, Quantock AJ, et al. Incidence and severity of keratoconus in Asir province, Saudi Arabia. Br J Ophthalmol. 2005;89:1403–6.
75. Weed KH, MacEwen CJ, Giles T, et al. The Dundee University Scottish Keratoconus study: demographics, corneal signs, associated diseases, and eye rubbing. Eye (Lond). 2008;22:534–41.
76. Agrawal VB. Characteristics of keratoconus patients at a tertiary eye center in India. J Ophthalmic Vis Res. 2011;6:87–91.
77. Jordan CA, Zamri A, Wheeldon C, et al. Computerized corneal tomography and associated features in a large New Zealand keratoconic population. J Cataract Refract Surg. 2011;37:1493–501.
78. Shneor E, Millodot M, Blumberg S, et al. Characteristics of 244 patients with keratoconus seen in an optometric contact lens practice. Clin Exp Optom. 2013;96:219–24.
79. Gordon-Shaag A, Millodot M, Essa M, et al. Is consanguinity a risk factor for keratoconus? Optom Vis Sci. 2013;90:448–54.
80. Gordon-Shaag A, Millodot M, Kaiserman I, et al. Risk factors for keratoconus in Israel: a case-control study. Ophthalmic Physiol Opt. 2015;35:673–81.

81. Hashemi H, Khabazkhoob M, Yazdani N, et al. The prevalence of keratoconus in a young population in Mashhad, Iran. Ophthalmic Physiol Opt. 2014;34:519–27.
82. Woodward MA, Blachley TS, Stein JD. The association between sociodemographic factors, common systemic diseases, and keratoconus: an analysis of a Nationwide heath care claims database. Ophthalmology. 2016;123:457–65 e2.
83. Solomon A. Corneal complications of vernal keratoconjunctivitis. Curr Opin Allergy Clin Immunol. 2015;15(5):489–94.
84. Al-Akily SA, Bamashmus MA. Ocular complications of severe vernal keratoconjunctivitis (VKC) in Yemen. Saudi J Ophthalmol. 2011;25(3):291–4.
85. Weng SF, Jan RL, Wang JJ, Tseng SH, Chang YS. Association between atopic keratoconjunctivitis and the risk of keratoconus. Acta Ophthalmol. 2021;99(1):e54–61.
86. Gautam V, Chaudhary M, Sharma AK, Shrestha GS, Rai PG. Topographic corneal changes in children with vernal keratoconjunctivitis: a report from Kathmandu, Nepal. Cont Lens Anterior Eye. 2015;38(6):461–5.
87. Gonzalez J de J. Keratoconus consecutive to vernal conjunctivitis. Am J Ophthalmol. 1920;3:127–8.
88. Feizi S, Javadi MA, Alemzadeh-Ansari M, Arabi A, Shahraki T, Kheirkhah A. Management of corneal complications in vernal keratoconjunctivitis: a review. Ocul Surf. 2021;19:282–9.
89. Caputo R, Versaci F, Pucci N, de Libero C, Danti G, De Masi S, Mencucci R, Novembre E, Jeng BH. Very low prevalence of keratoconus in a large series of vernal keratoconjunctivitis patients. Am J Ophthalmol. 2016;172:64–71.
90. Umale RH, Khan MA, Moulick PS, Gupta S, Shankar S, Sati A. A clinical study to describe the corneal topographic pattern and estimation of the prevalence of keratoconus among diagnosed cases of vernal keratoconjunctivitis. Med J Armed Forces India. 2019;75(4):424–8.
91. Totan Y, Hepşen IF, Cekiç O, Gündüz A, Aydin E. Incidence of keratoconus in subjects with vernal keratoconjunctivitis: a videokeratographic study. Ophthalmology. 2001;108(4):824–7.
92. Lapid-Gortzak R, Rosen S, Weitzman S, Lifshitz T. Videokeratography findings in children with vernal keratoconjunctivitis versus those of healthy children. Ophthalmology. 2002;109(11):2018–23.
93. Barreto J Jr, Netto MV, Santo RM, Jose NK, Bechara SJ. Slit-scanning topography in vernal keratoconjunctivitis. Am J Ophthalmol. 2007;143(2):250–4.
94. Taneja M, Ashar JN, Mathur A, Vaddavalli PK, Rathi V, Sangwan V, Murthy S. Measure of keratoconus progression in patients with vernal keratoconjunctivitis using scanning slit topography. Cont Lens Anterior Eye. 2013;36(1):41–4.
95. Ben-Eli H, Erdinest N, Solomon A. Pathogenesis and complications of chronic eye rubbing in ocular allergy. Curr Opin Allergy Clin Immunol. 2019;19(5):526–34.
96. Dantas PE, Alves MR, Nishiwaki-Dantas MC. Topographic corneal changes in patients with vernal keratoconjunctivitis. Arq Bras Oftalmol. 2005;68(5):593–8.
97. Leonardi A, Sathe S, Bortolotti M, Beaton A, Sack R. Cytokines, matrix metalloproteases, angiogenic and growth factors in tears of normal subjects and vernal keratoconjunctivitis patients. Allergy. 2009;64(5):710–7.
98. Kumagai N, Yamamoto K, Fukuda K, Nakamura Y, Fujitsu Y, Nuno Y, Nishida T. Active matrix metalloproteinases in the tear fluid of individuals with vernal keratoconjunctivitis. J Allergy Clin Immunol. 2002;110(3):489–91.
99. Leonardi A, Brun P, Abatangelo G, Plebani M, Secchi AG. Tear levels and activity of matrix metalloproteinase (MMP)-1 and MMP-9 in vernal keratoconjunctivitis. Invest Ophthalmol Vis Sci. 2003;44(7):3052–8.
100. Najmi H, Mobarki Y, Mania K, Altowairqi B, Basehi M, Mahfouz MS. Elmahdy M the correlation between keratoconus and eye rubbing: a review. Int J Ophthalmol. 2019;12(11):1775–81.
101. McMonnies CW. Mechanisms of rubbing-related corneal trauma in keratoconus. Cornea. 2009;28:607–15.

102. Norouzpour A, Mehdizadeh A. A novel insight into keratoconus: mechanical fatigue of the cornea. Med Hypothesis Discov Innov Ophthalmol. 2012;1(1):14–7.
103. Kennedy RH, BourneWM DJA. A 48-year clinical and epidemiological study of keratoconus. Am J Ophthalmol. 1986;101:267–73.
104. Rabinowitz YS. Keratoconus. Surv Ophthalmol. 1998;42:297–319.
105. McMonnies CW. Eye rubbing type and prevalence including contact lens 'removal-relief' rubbing. Clin Exp Optom. 2016;99(4):366–72.
106. Mashor RS, Kumar NL, Ritenour RJ, Rootman DS. Keratoconus caused by eye rubbing in patients with Tourette syndrome. Can J Ophthalmol. 2011;46(1):83–6.
107. Panikkar K, Manayath G, Rajaraman R, Saravanan V. Progressive keratoconus, retinal detachment, and intracorneal silicone oil with obsessive-compulsive eye rubbing. Oman J Ophthalmol. 2016;9(3):170–3.
108. Hafezi F, Hafezi NL, Pajic B, Gilardoni F, Randleman JB, Gomes JAP, Kollros L, Hillen M, Torres-Netto EA. Assessment of the mechanical forces applied during eye rubbing. BMC Ophthalmol. 2020;20(1):301.
109. Bral N, Termote K. Unilateral Keratoconus after Chronic Eye Rubbing by the Nondominant Hand. Case Rep Ophthalmol. 2017;8(3):558–61.
110. Ioannidis AS, Speedwell L, Nischal KK. Unilateral keratoconus in a child with chronic and persistent eye rubbing. Am J Ophthalmol. 2005;139(2):356–7.
111. Jafri B, Lichter H, Stulting RD. Asymmetric keratoconus attributed to eye rubbing. Cornea. 2004;23:560–4.
112. Mazharian A, Panthier C, Courtin R, Jung C, Rampat R, Saad A, Gatinel D. Incorrect sleeping position and eye rubbing in patients with unilateral or highly asymmetric keratoconus: a case-control study. Graefes Arch Clin Exp Ophthalmol. 2020;258(11):2431–9.
113. Lindsay RG, Bruce AS, Gutteridge IF. Keratoconus associated with continual eye rubbing due to punctal agenesis. Cornea. 2000;19(4):567–9.
114. Scotto R, Vagge A. Traverso CE eye rubbing and transient corneal ectasia detected by topography in a pediatric patient. Cornea. 2021;40(2):251–3.
115. Osuagwu UL, Alanazi SA. Eye rubbing-induced changes in intraocular pressure and corneal thickness measured at five locations, in subjects with ocular allergy. Int J Ophthalmol. 2015;8:81–8.
116. Turner DC, Girkin CA, Downs JC. The magnitude of intraocular pressure elevation associated with eye rubbing. Ophthalmology. 2019;126:171–2.
117. McMonnies CW. Management of chronic habits of abnormal eye rubbing. Cont Lens Anterior Eye. 2008;31:95–102.
118. McMonnies CW, Boneham GC. Corneal responses to intraocular pressure elevations in keratoconus. Cornea. 2010;29:764–70.
119. Korb DR, Leahy CD, Greiner JV. Prevalence and characteristics of eye rubbing for keratoconic and non-keratoconic subjects. Invest Ophthalmol Vis Sci. 1991;32(Suppl):884.
120. McMonnies CW, Alharbi A, Boneham GC. Epithithelial responses to rubbing-related mechanical forces. Cornea. 2010;29:1223–31.
121. Mansour AM, Haddad RS. Corneal topography after ocular rubbing. Cornea. 2002;21:756–8.
122. McMonnies CW, Korb DR, Blackie CA. The role of heat in rubbing and massage-related corneal deformation. Cont Lens Anterior Eye. 2012;35(4):148–54.
123. Kao WW, Vergnes JP, Ebert J, Sundar-Raj CV, Brown SI. Increased collagenase and gelatinase activities in keratoconus. Biochem Biophys Res Commun. 1982;107:929–36.
124. Gasset AR, Houde WL, Garcia-Bengochea M. Hard contact lens wear as an environmental risk in keratoconus. Am J Ophthalmol. 1978;85(3):339–41.
125. Macsai MS, Varley GA, Krachmer JH. Development of keratoconus after contact lens wear. Patient characteristics. Arch Ophthalmol. 1990;108(4):534–8.
126. Phillips CI. Contact lenses and corneal deformation: cause, correlate or co-incidence? Acta Ophthalmol (Copenh). 1990;68(6):661–8.

127. Kalogeropoulos G, Chang S, Bolton T, Jalbert I. The effects of short-term lens wear and eye rubbing on the corneal epithelium. Eye Contact Lens. 2009;35(5):255–9.
128. Liu Z, Pflugfelder SC. The effects of long-term contact lens wear on corneal thickness, curvature, and surface regularity. Ophthalmology. 2000;107:105–11.
129. Moon JW, Shin KC, Lee HJ, et al. The effect of contact lens wear on the ocular surface changes in keratoconus. Eye Contact Lens. 2006;32:96–101.
130. McMonnies C. Eye rubbing type and prevalence including contact lens 'removal-relief' rubbing. Clin Exp Optom. 2016;99:366–72.
131. Carracedo G, Blanco MS, Martin-Gil A, Zicheng W, Alvarez JC, Pintor J. Short-term effect of scleral lens on the dry eye biomarkers in keratoconus. Optom Vis Sci. 2016;93(2):150–7.
132. Ghosh S, Mutalib HA, Sharanjeet K, et al. Effects of contact lens wearing on keratoconus: a confocal microscopy observation. Int J Ophthalmol. 2017;10:228–34.
133. Bitirgen G, Ozkagnici A, Malik RA, et al. Evaluation of contact lens induced changes in keratoconic corneas using in vivo confocal microscopy. Invest Ophthalmol Vis Sci. 2013;54:5385–91.
134. Lema I, Dura'n JA, Ruiz C, Di'ez-Feijoo E, Acera A, Merayo J. Inflammatory response to contact lenses in patients with keratoconus compared with myopic subjects. Cornea. 2008;27:758Y63.
135. Schultz CL, Kunert KS. Interleukin-6 levels in tears of contact lens wearers. J Interferon Cytokine Res. 2000;20(3):309–10.
136. Ferdi AC, Nguyen V, Gore DM, et al. Keratoconus natural progression: a systematic review and meta-analysis of 11 529 eyes. Ophthalmology. 2019;126:935–45.
137. Crawford AZ, Zhang J, Gokul A, McGhee CNJ, Ormonde SE. The enigma of environmental factors in keratoconus. Asia Pac J Ophthalmol (Phila). 2020;9(6):549–56.
138. McMonnies CW. The biomechanics of keratoconus and rigid contact lenses. Eye Contact Lens. 2005;31(2):80–92.
139. Gokul A, Patel DV, Watters GA, et al. The natural history of corneal topographic progression of keratoconus after age 30 years in non-contact lens wearers. Br J Ophthalmol. 2017;101:839–44.
140. Carracedo G, Recchioni A, Alejandre-Alba N, et al. Signs and symptoms of dry eye in keratoconus patients: a pilot study. Curr Eye Res. 2014;1–7.
141. Mostovoy D, Vinker S, Mimouni M, Goldich Y, Levartovsky S, Kaiserman I. The association of keratoconus with blepharitis. Clin Exp Optom. 2018;101(3):339–44.
142. Rattan SA, Anwar DS. Comparison of corneal epithelial thickness profile in dry eye patients, keratoconus suspect, and healthy eyes. Eur J Ophthalmol. 2020;30(6):1506–11.
143. Dogru M, Karakaya H, Ozçetin H, Ertürk H, Yücel A, Ozmen A, Baykara M, Tsubota K. Tear function and ocular surface changes in keratoconus. Ophthalmology. 2003;110 (6):1110–8.
144. Moran S, Gomez L, Zuber K, Gatinel D. A case-control study of keratoconus risk factors. Cornea. 2020;39(6):697–701.
145. De Paiva CS, Harris LD, Pflugfelder SC. Keratoconus-like topographic changes in keratoconjunctivitis sicca. Cornea. 2003;22(1):22–4.
146. Dienes L, Kiss HJ, Perényi K, Nagy ZZ, Acosta MC, Gallar J, Kovács I. Corneal sensitivity and dry eye symptoms in patients with keratoconus. PLoS One. 2015;10(10):e 0141621.
147. Zemova E, Eppig T, Seitz B, Toropygin S, Arnold S, Langenbucher A, Gräber S, Szentmáry N. Interaction between topographic/tomographic parameters and dry eye disease in keratoconus patients. Curr Eye Res. 2014;39(1):1–8.
148. Uysal BS, Yaman D, Kalkan Akcay E, Kilicarslan A, Sarac O, Cagil N. Evaluation of corneal topography, tear film function and conjunctival impression cytology after long-term scleral contact lens wear in keratoconus patients. Semin Ophthalmol. 2021;27:1–7.
149. Shanbhag SS, Basu S. Controversial role of retinoids in ocular surface disease. Br J Ophthalmol. 2019;103(8):1013–4.

150. Solomon A, Dursun D, Liu Z, Xie Y, Macri A, Pflugfelder SC. Pro- and anti-inflammatory forms of interleukin-1 in the tear fluid and conjunctiva of patients with dry-eye disease. Invest Ophthalmol Vis Sci. 2001;42(10):2283–92.
151. Lema I, Brea D, Rodriguez-Gonzalez R, et al. Proteomic analysis of the tear film in patients with keratoconus. Mol Vis. 2010;16:2055–61.
152. Meloni M, De Servi B, Marasco D, Del Prete S. Molecular mechanism of ocular surface damage: application to an in vitro dry eye model on human corneal epithelium. Mol Vis. 2011;17:113–26.
153. Balasubramanian SA, Pye DC, Willcox MD. Levels of lactoferrin, secretory IgA and serum albumin in the tear film of people with keratoconus. Exp Eye Res. 2012;96:132–7.
154. Nichols KK, Foulks GN, Bron AJ, et al. The international workshop on meibomian gland dysfunction: executive summary. Invest Ophthalmol Vis Sci. 2011;52(4):1922–29. Accessed 30 Mar 2011.
155. Mohamed Mostafa E, Abdellah MM, Elhawary AM, Mounir A. Noncontact meibography in patients with keratoconus. J Ophthalmol. 2019;2(2019):2965872.
156. Peterson ME, Daniel RM, Danson MJ, Eisenthal R. The dependence of enzyme activity on temperature: determination and validation of parameters. Biochem J. 2007;402:331–7.
157. Dursun D, Piniella AM, Pflugfelder SC. Pseudokeratoconus caused by rosacea. Cornea. 2001;20:668Y9.
158. Salinas R, Puig M, Fry CL, Johnson DA, Kheirkhah A. Floppy eyelid syndrome: a comprehensive review. Ocul Surf. 2020;18(1):31–9.
159. Donnenfeld ED, Perry HD, Gibralter RP, Ingraham HJ, Udell IJ. Keratoconus associated with floppy eyelid syndrome. Ophthalmology. 1991;98(11):1674–8.
160. Negris R. Floppy eyelid syndrome associated with keratoconus. J Am Optom Assoc. 1992;63(5):316–9.
161. Naderan M, Jahanrad A, Farjadnia M. Prevalence of eyelid laxity and its association with ophthalmic findings and disease severity in patients with keratoconus. Eur J Ophthalmol. 2017;27:670–4.
162. Ines Tran, J. Harquel, A. Sauer, D. Gaucher, C. Speeg-Schatz, P. Bourgin, T. Bourcier; atopy, floppy eyelid syndrome, obstructive sleep apnea syndrome, eye rubbing and keratoconus. Invest Ophthalmol Vis Sci. 2012;53(14):6818.
163. Ezra DG, Beaconsfield M, Sira M, Bunce C, Wormald R, Collin R. The associations of floppy eyelid syndrome: a case control study. Ophthalmology. 2010;117:831–8.
164. Kymionis GD, Grentzelos MA, Liakopoulos DA, Kontadakis GA, Stojanovic N. Corneal collagen crosslinking failure in a patient with floppy eyelid syndrome. J Cataract Refract Surg. 2014;40:1558–60.
165. Schlotzer-Schrehardt U, Stojkovic M, Hofmann-Rummelt C, Cursiefen C, Kruse FE, Holbach LM. The pathogenesis of floppy eyelid syndrome: involvement of matrix metalloproteinases in elastic fiber degradation. Ophthalmology. 2005;112:694–704.

The Role of Biomarkers in Keratoconus Pathogenesis and Diagnosis

Sharon D'Souza, Mor M. Dickman, and Rohit Shetty

1 Introduction

Keratoconus(KC) is a condition characterized by varying degrees of corneal thinning and ectasia [1]. The estimated global prevalence of 1.38 cases per 1000 population [2] or higher in certain ethnic groups [3] and the significant visual morbidity associated in advanced cases, makes it important to direct efforts to understand the disease etiopathogenesis and find new targets for treatment.

KC can be stable in some cases but progressive in others and the resultant irregular astigmatism, keratometric changes and even corneal scarring can cause severe visual disturbances [1]. Clinical features include scissoring reflex on retinoscopy, features like fleischers ring, vogt's striae and ectasia on slitlamp examination and munson's sign in advanced cases. The diagnosis of keratoconus is confirmed both by clinical features and specific changes on the corneal topography or tomography which are also used to grade the severity of the disease [4].

Changes in the ultrastructure and molecular features are believed to trigger the focal changes of thinning and ectasia classic to the disease [5]. Keratoconus is believed to be a polygenic disease in which the pathogenesis and progression is influenced by environmental and genetic factors. Various factors like eye rubbing, allergy and ocular surface inflammation among others have been found to be risk factors for progression in KC [6, 7]. However the exact pathogenesis is still unknown in many cases [5, 8].

Keratoconus management depends on disease severity, progression and the need for visual rehabilitation. The treatment options for this condition range from spectacles and contact lens for visual rehabilitation, collagen crosslinking to halt

S. D'Souza · R. Shetty (✉)
Department of Cornea and Refractive Surgery, Narayana Nethralaya, Bangalore, India

M. M. Dickman
University Eye Clinic Maastricht, Maastricht University Medical Center, Maastricht, The Netherlands

© The Author(s), under exclusive license to Springer Nature Switzerland AG 2022   61
A. Armia and C. Mazzotta (eds.), *Keratoconus*,
https://doi.org/10.1007/978-3-030-84506-3_3

progression, adjunctive therapies like intracorneal ring segments or topoguided regularisation of the corneal surface to improve visual outcomes and corneal transplants in most severe cases [9]. Despite the advancements in treatment, there are still lacunae in our understanding of the disease outcomes and ability to predict possible progression. Adequate management of KC would require a thorough understanding of the etiopathogenesis and the associated biomarkers and factors which need to be controlled.

Keratoconus eyes show microstructural changes in almost all layers of the cornea including epithelium, bowmans layer and stroma. The tear film, aqueous humour, serum and even saliva of KC patients have also been studied and found to have changes in composition compared to normals. However, the contribution of the various inflammatory and ultrastructural changes in the development of the classical clinical features and biomechanical changes is yet to be determined. Since the disease can range from very mild to advanced ectasia it is important to understand the importance of specific biomarkers which could affect the disease and its progression [5, 10].

This chapter gives an overview of the various biomarkers of keratoconus associated with disease pathogenesis, diagnosis and progression.

2   Keratoconus Biomarkers

2.1   Inflammatory factors

An inflammatory link to KC has been demonstrated in various studies even though the classic clinical signs of inflammation are not seen in this condition [11, 12]. ECM remodelling is a key feature in keratoconus development driven by inflammatory molecules like cytokines, chemokines, cell adhesion molecules and matrix metalloproteinases [13]. Various interleukins (IL), tumor necrosis factor (TNF) α and β, matrix metalloproteinases (MMP) 1, 3, 7,9, 13, are elevated in tears from KC patients [11].

Increased levels of IL1a/b [15–17], IL-6 [15, 20], IL-8, [15] IL-17 family including IL-17A, IL-21, and IL-23 have been reported in KC tears [16]. IL-17 is known to induce MMP9, thus making it key to KC pathogenesis as well. Corneal tissue in KC showed higher levels of IL1a/b, IL6 [20]. It was found that IL-6 expression was higher in the epithelium of the ectatic part of the cornea compared to the periphery further linking it to the disease pathology [7].

TNF-a has been found to higher in tears, serum and cornea of KC patients [14, 15] with good association with clinical and topographical markers of KC [7, 16] and more in patients with Bowman's layer breaks demonstrated on anterior segment optical coherence tomography imaging [7]. Patients with associated ocular allergy and eye rubbing also had higher levels of IL-6 and TNF-a [11]. KC patients may not always have clinically evident ocular allergy but cytokines like IL-4, IL-5, and

IL-13 which are commonly associated with allergy are also elevated in KC tears. Elevated serum and tear fluid IgE levels have been found in KC patients even without atopy or obvious clinical allergy. This could be due to an underlying molecular association between the conditions [6]. Increased interferon γ (IFN-γ) level in KC tears was strongly associated with disease severity and progression [14, 17].

Thus inflammatory mediators could be important factors in the pathogenesis, progression and outcomes of this disease. Many of these factors are deregulated in the cornea, tears and even serum in KC patients. This further validates their role in the disease.

2.2 ECM-Related Factors

Ultrastructural studies on the KC cornea have revealed disruption in the organization of collagen fibrils [18, 19], decrease in total collagen in the area affected and decreased linkages between collagen fibres [20, 21]. These changes are seen across different layers of the cornea with decreased expression of collagen I, III, IV, V, VI, and XII levels in the stroma and collagen I, VI, VII, XII, and XIII in the epithelium of KC corneas [22, 23]. There is also a difference in expressions of collagen I and IV between ectatic and nonectatic regions [7]. It has been found that the expression of ECM proteins in KC varies based on grade and type of disease. Correlating these changes with clinical features can help better understand the disease.

Imbalance in proteolytic enzymes such as matrix metalloproteinases (MMP), cathepsin, collagenase, gelatinase, can result in structural changes seen in KC. MMP9 was found to be increased in the cornea, tears and serum of KC patients [16, 24, 25]. It has been shown to increase with worsening grade of KC [13, 26, 27] and has been demonstrated to be higher in the ectatic region of the cornea [7]. KC patients with associated ocular and systemic allergy also showed higher levels of MMP9 in tears [26]. These findings point towards an important role of MMP9 in the etiopathogenesis of the disease. MMP2 and MMP13 levels in KC corneas [28, 29] and MMP13 level in the tears of KC patients were elevated in associated with disease severity and progression [30, 31]˙ Levels of proteinase inhibitors like alpha 1-proteinase inhibitor [32], and tissue inhibitor of matrix metalloproteinase-1 [33] which regulate proteolytic enzymes were significantly lower in KC.

Expression of proteoglycans and glycosaminoglycans are altered in KC [23, 34]. As they interact with collagen fibrils, they have an important role in the biomechanical properties of the cornea [18, 35].

The collagen crosslinkages which are key to the corneal biomechanical strength are decreased in KC corneas [36]. Endogenous cross-linking enzyme lysyl oxidase (LOX) is decreased in KC and shows an inverse relation with KC grade [22]. The levels were especially reduced in the ectatic region of the cornea [7, 37, 38]. These observations clearly emphasize the relevance of endogenous cross-linking enzyme in KC pathogenesis.

2.3   Genetic Risk Factors/Markers of Keratoconus

There has been a lot of research into the genetics of KC and an underlying genetic link has been found in some patients [39]. Understanding this aspect of disease etiology could aid in easy screening and early diagnosis of patients and family members. However, the heterogenous nature of the genetic involvement have made it difficult to make clear associations with KC. Genetic studies by GWLS (Genes identified through genome-wide linkage studies) and GWAS (Genome-wide association studies) have identified many genetic variations associated with keratoconus. Single nucleotide polymorphisms (SNPs) associated with various genes have been found, however not all have a confirmed role in KC. The pathogenesis of KC probably involves a number of different interlinked biochemical pathways in which altered gene expression also has a role to play [40]. The identification of polymorphisms in the LOX (collagen crosslinking enzyme lysyl oxidase) gene is an important development in our understanding of the disease and is a promising KC candidate gene [41].

SNPs in lysyl oxidase (LOX), collagen type XXVII A1 (COL27A1), hepatocyte growth factor RAB 3 GTP-ase activating protein 1 (RAB3GAP1), interleukin 1β (IL1B) and cadherin 11 (CDH11),) were identified by genome wide association studies (GWAS) as risk factors for keratoconus [42]. Dysregulations of LOX and collagen I alpha 1 (COLIA1) and collagen IV alpha 1 (COLIVA1) was found in KC corneal epithelium by differential gene expression analysis [22, 43]. These were associated with elevated IL-6 in the tears and corneal epithelium in KC. The clinical relevance of this is seen in the inverse correlation of the collagen expression and grade of KC [22]. A novel finding noted was the decreased levels of secreted-frizzled related protein 1 (SFRP1), a protein associated with the WNT signaling pathway in tears from KC patients [44].

TGFBI (Transforming growth factor beta induced) gene was one the most common transcript found in the cDNA data evaluated in KC corneas [45]. Altered TGFβ signaling can have a role in the progression of keratoconus however it was not found to be associated in all KC patients [46]. Other genes found to be associated are CAST (encoding calpastatin), DOCK9 (Dedicator of cytokinesis 9), HGF (hepatocyte growth factor), ZNF469(zinc finger protein 469), ZEB1 (zinc finger E-box binding homeobox 1), VSX1 (visual system homeobox 1), collagen related genes—COL5A1, COL4A3, COL4A4, FNDC3B, FOXO1, SOD1 (superoxide dismutase 1) and miR184 (microRNA184) [40] (Fig. 1). Given the multifactorial etiopathogenesis of the disease it is important to understand the genetic, epigenetic and molecular factors changes associated.

Figure 1 lists the different biomarkers of Keratoconus across blood, tears and cornea.

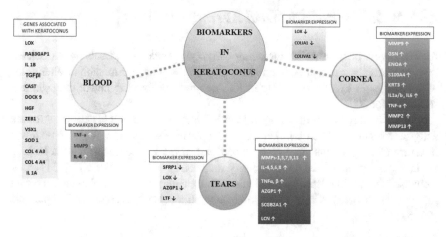

Fig. 1 Biomarkers in Keratoconus. The schematic summarizes the various biomarkers available in keratoconus patients. The factors have been grouped into those altered in tears, cornea and/or blood of keratoconus patients. Where relevant, there are arrows to indicate if the biomarker expression is increased or decreased. *LOX*—Lysyl oxidase, RAB3GAP1—Rab GTPase activating protein IL1A—Interleukin 1alpha, IL1B- Interleukin 1beta *TGFβI*—Transforming growth factor beta induced, CAST—Calpain/calpastatin, DOCK9—Dedicator of cytokinesis 9, HGF—Hepatocyte growth factor, *COL5A1*—Collagen type V, alpha-1 chain, ZEB1—Zinc finger E-box binding homeobox 1, SOD1—Superoxide dismutase 1, COL4A3—Collagen type IV, alpha-3 chain, COL4A4—Collagen type IV, alpha-4 chain, VSX1—Visual system homeobox 1, alpha enolase (ENOA), S100A4 and cytokeratin3 (KRT3), mammoglobin B (SGB2A1), lipocalin (LCN), lactoferrin (LTF), zinc-α2- glycoprotein (AZGP1)

2.4 Hormones

Hormonal changes in the body are known to influence KC pathogenesis and progression. Thyroid related disease and other hormonal disorders can be associated with KC [47]. Hormonal changes during pregnancy can lead to biomechanical changes in the cornea and progression of keratoconus [48]. Hormone replacement therapy using estrogen/ progesterone is also known to be associated with KC [49]. Significantly increased levels of dehydroepiandrosterone sulfate (DHEA-S) and reduced estrone levels have been found in saliva of KC patients [50]. There is no direct correlation between hormonal changes and KC severity, however estrogens have a role in modulating pro-inflammatory cytokine expression, including IL-6 and TNF-α in corneal epithelial cells [50]. Hence it is possible that hormone levels modulate the stromal microenvironment like inflammatory factors and cellular metabolism which can affect KC [51]. Deficiency of Vitamin D which is a steroid hormone has also been associated with increased predisposition to KC in some studies probably due to its role as an inflammatory modulator and stress response [52].

2.5   Metabolic and Chemical Alterations

Altered levels of metabolites including carboxylic acids and sterols are associated with oxidative stress and inflammation [53]. Evaluating the metabolic alterations with changes in ECM remodeling in KC, can help in forming newer management strategies for KC.

Copper could play an important role in KC pathogenesis as it is necessary for the activity of endogenous crosslinker LOX. Copper levels have been found to be lower in serum of KC patients and in the weaker part of the KC cornea as well [54]. This could result in decreased LOX activity and act as a trigger for KC [55] Other elemental factors like Iron, zinc, selenium and magnesium which play an important role in cellular balance have also showed altered levels in the serum of KC patients [56, 57].

3   Emerging Perspectives from Biomarker Studies

Potential applications for biomarkers for diagnostics

The goal of identifying biomarkers is not only to understand the molecular basis of the disease, but also to apply that knowledge for disease stratification, predicting disease progression and treatment response. Since KC is a disease of the cornea with underlying surface inflammation, the potential for using a tear based diagnostic test has obvious importance [58]. Tear based factors that have demonstrated associations with increasing disease severity such as increase in MMP or reduction in LOX have potential for being used as diagnostic tests [22]. In fact, it has been demonstrated [59] that patients with considerably reduced LOX levels in their tears have sub-optimal results post collagen crosslinking for KC. Metabolites such as DHEA or estrone may similarly have utility as saliva based diagnostic tests [50]. DNA based genetic tests form another layer of diagnostic test possibility, particularly applicable in families where one or both parents have KC [39, 60]. Similar to corneal dystrophy panels, a KC genetic panel constituting the list of genes where mutations have been described may prove to have applications for diagnosing the disease early or informing those at risk. These tests are also critical in the context of refractive surgery, where those at risk of developing KC may be advised against undergoing the procedure to avoid post surgical ectasia [61]. As more such factors are studied for their correlation with clinical outcomes, it may be possible to establish simple diagnostic tests to establish the best treatment regimen for each KC patient.

Pathways for therapeutic targeting:

An important application of the knowledge base created by profiling molecular factors in KC has been the identification of possible mechanistic pathways amenable to therapeutic intervention. Inflammatory pathways have been shown by multiple studies to drive KC. Using cyclosporine-A eye drops to reduce MMP9 in KC patients was shown to reduce disease progression and even induce flattening in a small subset of patients [16]. Since oxidative stress has been shown to also be of critical importance in driving KC pathology [53], it is possible that antioxidant eye drops may be useful for treatment. The antioxidant activity recently demonstrated for trehalose eye drops, may have significance in KC as well. The key pathological feature of KC is the loss of biomechanical stiffness, which is due to altered collagen organisation and decrease in crosslinking enzymes. Therefore, another potential method for KC treatment would be to enhance the function of LOX in the corneal stroma. LOX requires copper as a co-activator and hence an approach to activate stromal LOX by using copper sulphate eye drops [62] to achieve stromal strengthening. Many more such pathways are being validated by various research studies, raising the hope for topical treatments for early stage KC.

Lacunae in KC biomarker studies:

While a vast amount of information has emerged from the biomarker studies, only a small group of biomarkers have shown the potential to have clinical applications for diagnostics or therapeutics. A primary reason for the same is the lack of in depth longitudinal studies to associate the molecular factors with disease progression. Since such studies require a great amount of resources and time, these are typically challenging to conduct, yet that leaves an important lacunae in our classification of biomarkers as causative or consequential. In addition, the disease is asymmetric and focal in nature and associated with local changes to the biomarkers as well [7]. This necessitates a thorough investigation of these local factors longitudinally to try and identify the molecular initiators of disease. Although microtrauma induced break of Bowman's membrane has been proposed [7, 63], it still needs to be validated. Finally, detailed correlation of biomarkers with corneal biomechanical and curvature parameters needs to be done extensively to select the right biomarkers for clinical applications and therapeutics.

4 Conclusion

There has been a lot of advancement in our understanding of keratoconus pathogenesis. Environmental influences, atopy, ocular allergy and eye rubbing, systemic and syndromic associations are all important aspects to be evaluated when we are treating these patients. Inflammation and oxidative stress leading to changes in the extracellular matrix has been found to be one of the key underlying mechanisms. However, as inflammation is a feature of many ocular surface diseases, the molecular factor changes in keratoconus are not very specific to it and can show an overlap with these diseases. The alteration in these factors like MMP9 or IL-6 need to interpreted in tandem with other molecular, inflammatory, oxidative and clinical features. There are still gaps in our understanding of the changes in keratoconus, however applying an integrated approach using biomarkers from imaging, molecular profile and genetics have provided newer potential treatment options. Ongoing research in this field is directed along these lines in the hope of better treatment outcomes and prevention of disease progression by least invasive methods.

References

1. Rabinowitz YS. Keratoconus. Surv Ophthalmol. 1998;42(4):297–319.
2. Hashemi H, Heydarian S, Hooshmand E, Saatchi M, Yekta A, Aghamirsalim M, et al. The prevalence and risk factors for keratoconus: a systematic review and meta-analysis. Cornea. 2020;39(2):263–70.
3. Ferrari G, Rama P. The keratoconus enigma: a review with emphasis on pathogenesis. Ocul Surf. 2020;18(3):363–73.
4. Matalia H, Swarup R. Imaging modalities in keratoconus. Indian J Ophthalmol. 2013;61(8):394–400.
5. Shetty R, D'Souza S, Khamar P, Ghosh A, Nuijts R, Sethu S. Biochemical markers and alterations in keratoconus. Asia Pac J Ophthalmol (Phila). 2020;9(6):533–40.
6. Ahuja P, Dadachanji Z, Shetty R, Nagarajan SA, Khamar P, Sethu S, et al. Relevance of IgE, allergy and eye rubbing in the pathogenesis and management of keratoconus. Indian J Ophthalmol. 2020;68(10):2067–74.
7. Pahuja N, Kumar NR, Shroff R, Shetty R, Nuijts RM, Ghosh A, et al. Differential molecular expression of extracellular matrix and inflammatory genes at the corneal cone apex drives focal weakening in keratoconus. Invest Ophthalmol Vis Sci. 2016;57(13):5372–82.
8. Wentz-Hunter K, Cheng EL, Ueda J, Sugar J, Yue BY. Keratocan expression is increased in the stroma of keratoconus corneas. Mol Med. 2001;7(7):470–7.
9. Shetty R, Kaweri L, Pahuja N, Nagaraja H, Wadia K, Jayadev C, et al. Current review and a simplified "five-point management algorithm" for keratoconus. Indian J Ophthalmol. 2015;63(1):46–53.
10. Blackburn BJ, Jenkins MW, Rollins AM, Dupps WJ. A review of structural and biomechanical changes in the cornea in aging, disease, and photochemical crosslinking. Front Bioeng Biotechnol. 2019;7:66.
11. Balasubramanian SA, Pye DC, Willcox MD. Effects of eye rubbing on the levels of protease, protease activity and cytokines in tears: relevance in keratoconus. Clin Exp Optom. 2013;96(2):214–8.
12. Lema I, Duran JA, Ruiz C, Diez-Feijoo E, Acera A, Merayo J. Inflammatory response to contact lenses in patients with keratoconus compared with myopic subjects. Cornea. 2008;27(7):758–63.
13. Lema I, Duran JA. Inflammatory molecules in the tears of patients with keratoconus. Ophthalmology. 2005;112(4):654–9.
14. Ionescu IC, Corbu CG, Tanase C, Ionita G, Nicula C, Coviltir V, et al. Overexpression of tear inflammatory cytokines as additional finding in keratoconus patients and their first degree family members. Mediators Inflamm. 2018;2018:4285268.
15. Arbab M, Tahir S, Niazi MK, Ishaq M, Hussain A, Siddique PM, et al. TNF-alpha genetic predisposition and higher expression of inflammatory pathway components in keratoconus. Invest Ophthalmol Vis Sci. 2017;58(9):3481–7.
16. Shetty R, Ghosh A, Lim RR, Subramani M, Mihir K, Reshma AR, et al. Elevated expression of matrix metalloproteinase-9 and inflammatory cytokines in keratoconus patients is inhibited by cyclosporine A. Invest Ophthalmol Vis Sci. 2015;56(2):738–50.
17. Fodor M, Vitalyos G, Losonczy G, Hassan Z, Pasztor D, Gogolak P, et al. Tear mediators NGF along with IL-13 predict keratoconus progression. Ocul Immunol Inflamm. 2020:1–12.

18. Fullwood NJ, Tuft SJ, Malik NS, Meek KM, Ridgway AE, Harrison RJ. Synchrotron x-ray diffraction studies of keratoconus corneal stroma. Invest Ophthalmol Vis Sci. 1992;33 (5):1734–41.

19. Meek KM, Tuft SJ, Huang Y, Gill PS, Hayes S, Newton RH, et al. Changes in collagen orientation and distribution in keratoconus corneas. Invest Ophthalmol Vis Sci. 2005;46 (6):1948–56.

20. Quantock AJ, Young RD. Development of the corneal stroma, and the collagen-proteoglycan associations that help define its structure and function. Dev Dyn. 2008;237(10):2607–21.

21. Radner W, Zehetmayer M, Skorpik C, Mallinger R. Altered organization of collagen in the apex of keratoconus corneas. Ophthalmic Res. 1998;30(5):327–32.

22. Shetty R, Sathyanarayanamoorthy A, Ramachandra RA, Arora V, Ghosh A, Srivatsa PR, et al. Attenuation of lysyl oxidase and collagen gene expression in keratoconus patient corneal epithelium corresponds to disease severity. Mol Vis. 2015;21:12–25.

23. Chaerkady R, Shao H, Scott SG, Pandey A, Jun AS, Chakravarti S. The keratoconus corneal proteome: loss of epithelial integrity and stromal degeneration. J Proteomics. 2013;87:122–31.

24. Sobrino T, Regueiro U, Malfeito M, Vieites-Prado A, Perez-Mato M, Campos F, et al. Higher expression of toll-like receptors 2 and 4 in blood cells of keratoconus patiens. Sci Rep. 2017;7 (1):12975.

25. Smith VA, Rishmawi H, Hussein H, Easty DL. Tear film MMP accumulation and corneal disease. Br J Ophthalmol. 2001;85(2):147–53.

26. Mazzotta C, Traversi C, Mellace P, Bagaglia SA, Zuccarini S, Mencucci R, et al. Keratoconus progression in patients with allergy and elevated surface matrix metalloproteinase 9 point-of-care test. Eye Contact Lens. 2018;44(Suppl 2):S48–53.

27. Mutlu M, Sarac O, Cagil N, Avcioglu G. Relationship between tear eotaxin-2 and MMP-9 with ocular allergy and corneal topography in keratoconus patients. Int Ophthalmol. 2020;40 (1):51–7.

28. Smith VA, Matthews FJ, Majid MA, Cook SD. Keratoconus: matrix metalloproteinase-2 activation and TIMP modulation. Biochim Biophys Acta. 2006;1762(4):431–9.

29. Kolozsvari BL, Berta A, Petrovski G, Mihaltz K, Gogolak P, Rajnavolgyi E, et al. Alterations of tear mediators in patients with keratoconus after corneal crosslinking associate with corneal changes. PLoS One. 2013;8(10):e76333.

30. Balasubramanian SA, Mohan S, Pye DC, Willcox MD. Proteases, proteolysis and inflammatory molecules in the tears of people with keratoconus. Acta Ophthalmol. 2012;90 (4):e303–9.

31. Kolozsvari BL, Petrovski G, Gogolak P, Rajnavolgyi E, Toth F, Berta A, et al. Association between mediators in the tear fluid and the severity of keratoconus. Ophthalmic Res. 2014;51 (1):46–51.

32. Whitelock RB, Fukuchi T, Zhou L, Twining SS, Sugar J, Feder RS, et al. Cathepsin G, acid phosphatase, and alpha 1-proteinase inhibitor messenger RNA levels in keratoconus corneas. Invest Ophthalmol Vis Sci. 1997;38(2):529–34.

33. Kenney MC, Chwa M, Atilano SR, Tran A, Carballo M, Saghizadeh M, et al. Increased levels of catalase and cathepsin V/L2 but decreased TIMP-1 in keratoconus corneas: evidence that oxidative stress plays a role in this disorder. Invest Ophthalmol Vis Sci. 2005;46(3):823–32.

34. Sharif R, Fowler B, Karamichos D. Collagen cross-linking impact on keratoconus extracellular matrix. PLoS One. 2018;13(7):e0200704.

35. Fullwood NJ, Meek KM, Malik NS, Tuft SJ. A comparison of proteoglycan arrangement in normal and keratoconus human corneas. Biochem Soc Trans. 1990;18(5):961–2.

36. Takaoka A, Babar N, Hogan J, Kim M, Price MO, Price FW Jr, et al. An evaluation of Lysyl oxidase-derived cross-linking in keratoconus by liquid chromatography/mass spectrometry. Invest Ophthalmol Vis Sci. 2016;57(1):126–36.

37. Dudakova L, Liskova P, Trojek T, Palos M, Kalasova S, Jirsova K. Changes in Lysyl oxidase (LOX) distribution and its decreased activity in keratoconus corneas. Exp Eye Res. 2012;104:74–81.

38. Dudakova L, Sasaki T, Liskova P, Palos M, Jirsova K. The presence of Lysyl oxidase-like enzymes in human control and keratoconic corneas. Histol Histopathol. 2016;31(1):63–71.
39. Jeyabalan N, Shetty R, Ghosh A, Anandula VR, Ghosh AS, Kumaramanickavel G. Genetic and genomic perspective to understand the molecular pathogenesis of keratoconus. Indian J Ophthalmol. 2013;61(8):384–8.
40. Bykhovskaya Y, Margines B, Rabinowitz YS. Genetics in keratoconus: where are we? Eye Vis (Lond). 2016;3:16.
41. Li X, Rabinowitz YS, Tang YG, Picornell Y, Taylor KD, Hu M, et al. Two-stage genome-wide linkage scan in keratoconus sib pair families. Invest Ophthalmol Vis Sci. 2006;47(9):3791–5.
42. Manolio TA. Genomewide association studies and assessment of the risk of disease. N Engl J Med. 2010;363(2):166–76.
43. Ghosh A, Zhou L, Ghosh A, Shetty R, Beuerman R. Proteomic and gene expression patterns of keratoconus. Indian J Ophthalmol. 2013;61(8):389–91.
44. You J, Hodge C, Wen L, McAvoy JW, Madigan MC, Sutton G. Tear levels of SFRP1 are significantly reduced in keratoconus patients. Mol Vis. 2013;19:509–xxx.
45. Rabinowitz YS, Dong L, Wistow G. Gene expression profile studies of human keratoconus cornea for NEIBank: a novel cornea-expressed gene and the absence of transcripts for aquaporin 5. Invest Ophthalmol Vis Sci. 2005;46(4):1239–46.
46. Priyadarsini S, McKay TB, Sarker-Nag A, Karamichos D. Keratoconus in vitro and the key players of the TGF-beta pathway. Mol Vis. 2015;21:577–88.
47. El-Massry A, Doheim MF, Iqbal M, Fawzy O, Said OM, Yousif MO, et al. Association between keratoconus and thyroid gland dysfunction: a cross-sectional case-control study. J Refract Surg. 2020;36(4):253–7.
48. Bilgihan K, Hondur A, Sul S, Ozturk S. Pregnancy-induced progression of keratoconus. Cornea. 2011;30(9):991–4.
49. Coco G, Kheirkhah A, Foulsham W, Dana R, Ciolino JB. Keratoconus progression associated with hormone replacement therapy. Am J Ophthalmol Case Rep. 2019;15:100519.
50. Suzuki T, Sullivan DA. Estrogen stimulation of proinflammatory cytokine and matrix metalloproteinase gene expression in human corneal epithelial cells. Cornea. 2005;24(8):1004–9.
51. McKay TB, Hjortdal J, Sejersen H, Asara JM, Wu J, Karamichos D. Endocrine and metabolic pathways linked to keratoconus: implications for the role of hormones in the stromal microenvironment. Sci Rep. 2016;6:25534.
52. Akkaya S, Ulusoy DM. Serum Vitamin D levels in patients with keratoconus. Ocul Immunol Inflamm. 2020;28(3):348–53.
53. Wojakowska A, Pietrowska M, Widlak P, Dobrowolski D, Wylegala E, Tarnawska D. Metabolomic signature discriminates normal human cornea from keratoconus-A pilot GC/MS study. Molecules. 2020;25(12).
54. Zarei-Ghanavati S, Yahaghi B, Hassanzadeh S, Mobarhan MG, Hakimi HR, Eghbali P. Serum 25-Hydroxyvitamin D, Selenium, Zinc and Copper in patients with keratoconus. J Curr Ophthalmol. 2020;32(1):26–31.
55. Avetisov SE, Mamikonian VR, Novikov IA. The role of tear acidity and Cu-cofactor of Lysyl oxidase activity in the pathogenesis of keratoconus. Vestn Oftalmol. 2011;127(2):3–8.
56. Ortak H, Sogut E, Tas U, Mesci C, Mendil D. The relation between keratoconus and plasma levels of MMP-2, zinc, and SOD. Cornea. 2012;31(9):1048–51.
57. Bamdad S, Owji N, Bolkheir A. Association between advanced keratoconus and serum levels of Zinc, Calcium, Magnesium, Iron, Copper, and Selenium. Cornea. 2018;37(10):1306–10.
58. Nishtala K, Pahuja N, Shetty R, Nuijts RM, Ghosh A. Tear biomarkers for keratoconus. Eye Vis (Lond). 2016;3:19.
59. Shetty R, Rajiv Kumar N, Pahuja N, Deshmukh R, Vunnava K, Abilash VG, et al. Outcomes of corneal cross-linking correlate with cone-specific Lysyl oxidase expression in patients with keratoconus. Cornea. 2018;37(3):369–74.

60. Wheeler J, Hauser MA, Afshari NA, Allingham RR, Liu Y. The genetics of keratoconus: a review. Reprod Syst Sex Disord. 2012(Suppl 6).
61. Giri P, Azar DT. Risk profiles of ectasia after keratorefractive surgery. Curr Opin Ophthalmol. 2017;28(4):337–42.
62. Molokhia S, Muddana SK, Hauritz H, Qiu Y, Burr M, Chayet A, et al. IVMED 80 eye drops for treatment of keratoconus in patients -Phase 1/2a. Invest Ophthalmol Vis Sci. 2020;61 (7):2587.
63. Tuori AJ, Virtanen I, Aine E, Kalluri R, Miner JH, Uusitalo HM. The immunohistochemical composition of corneal basement membrane in keratoconus. Curr Eye Res. 1997;16(8):792–801.

The Potential Roles of Genetic Testing and Biomechanical Evaluation in Keratoconus

Abby Wilson, Larry DeDionisio, John Marshall, and Tara Moore

1 Introduction

The advent of laser refractive surgery has stimulated a huge interest in diseases of the cornea whereby the mechanical properties of the tissue are altered either by genetics or behaviour. Foremost among such diseases is keratoconus and a pre-knowledge of such a condition will help the surgeon avoid enhancing the disease process by removal of tissue and further exacerbating the loss of mechanical integrity. Huge advances have been made in both determining risk factors associated with genes with potential involvement in causing keratoconus, and diagnosis of such genetic defects via the introduction of simple techniques as buccal swabs or finger prick blood studies. Complimentary advances have also been made in non-invasive measuring techniques allowing assessment of the biomechanical properties of suspect eyes. The present chapter reviews both the genetic advances in understanding and diagnosing high risk factors in keratoconus and current and future methods to determine changes in biomechanical properties associated with the disease.

A. Wilson
Manufacturing and Electrical Engineering, Wolfson School of Mechanical, Loughborough University, Loughborough, UK

L. DeDionisio
Avellino Labs, CA, USA

J. Marshall (✉)
Department of Genetics, Institute of Ophthalmology, University College London, London, UK

T. Moore
School of Biomedical Sciences, Ulster University, Belfast, NI, UK

2   Genetics of Keratoconus

Keratoconus (KC) is recognized as a complex, genetically heterogeneous, multi-factorial degenerative disorder. KC together with pellucid marginal degeneration (PMD), which develops by the same basic disease process but results in a different clinical presentation is classified as a corneal ectatic disorder (ECD) [1]. Prevalence, largely based on a study conducted in the United States from 1935 to 1982 was believed to be 54.5 per 100,000 (1 in 1835 or 0.05%) with an incidence of 2 per 100,000 per year [2, 3]. Subsequent studies found the prevalence to be higher in different parts of the world. A study conducted on a population of Caucasian patients compared to patients of primarily of Northern Pakistani origin found the incidence of KC to be significantly higher in the Asian population: 25 per 100,000 compared to 3.3 per 100,000 in the white population [4]. Another study carried out on children and adolescents ranging from 6 to 21 years of age in Riyadh, Saudi Arabia found the prevalence of KC to be 4.79% in that region of the world [5]. A study that utilized health records within the Netherlands found the prevalence of KC to be 265 cases per 100,000 (1 in 375) [6], a 5 to tenfold difference from what was reported by Kennedy et al. in 1986 [2]. It is recognized that the incidence will continue to rise due to advances in, and access to imaging technology in the clinical diagnosis of KC [7]. These studies and others also reveal there to be a genetic predisposition for KC and estimates of heritability range between 5 and 23% [8]. Furthermore, the genes associated with KC interact with environmental, and/or other factors. Thus, it is important to understand the role that familial KC plays for individuals considering refractive surgery or other corneal treatments.

3   Genome and Exome Studies

In recent years, there have been multiple studies conducted and papers published that explore the genetic aspects of KC [9–13]. Much of this work focused on well-defined population groups and is based on either genome wide association studies (GWAS) that utilized microarray chip technology or whole exome sequencing (WES) conducted with the next generation sequencing (NGS) platform. In general, these studies revealed a vast heterogeneity and rather than focus a genetic link to a well-defined locus or gene, they instead widened the genetic complexity of the disease. One possibility is that the disease has an ethnic component where different ethnicities in different parts of the world result in a different set of variants within genes pointing to differences in prevalence or severity [4, 5, 14–16]. Genetics do play a larger role in the aetiology of the disease in regions where consanguineous marriages are socially acceptable since this practice serves to propagate potentially pathogenic genetic variants within the population; consequently, these regions of the world do show a higher prevalence than other parts of the world where consanguineous marriages are less frequent. Consanguinity does not, however explain the wide diversity of genomic loci linked to KC within these regions, and the fact remains that even though multiple loci within the human genome have been identified, no single causative mutation in any gene has been definitively identified [8]. The results of family-based studies have proven valuable in revealing the breadth of possible genetic association to KC. Table 1 contains a representative list of studies linking KC to at least 23 different loci in the human genome. The research into the genetics of KC is on-going, and a recently published multi-ethnic GWAS for KC, consisting of 4669 cases and 116,547 controls identified 31 loci that had never before been identified [17].

3.1 Central Corneal Thickness (CCT)

CCT is recognized as a highly heritable trait and is often associated with KC [18]. CCT is a measurable and therefore a quantifiable facet of the KC phenotype. Ultrasound pachymetry and topographical mapping with instruments such as the Orbscan II (Bausch and Lomb, Rochester, NY, USA) are commonly used to measure CCT [19]. In 2013, Lu et al. conducted a meta-analysis GWAS linking CCT to KC. The cohort consisted of more than 20,000 individuals of European and Asian populations [20]. The study identified 16 loci associated with CCT, and in 2020, a study found 41 new loci associated with CCT in a multi-ethnic genome-wide analysis of 44,039 individuals [21]. Although much of the data involving the heritability of CCT from a diverse range of ethnicities show clear ethnic-related differences [22], the study conducted by Lu, et al. identified CCT-associated loci that were shared between European and Asian populations [20].

Variants within collagen genes known to play a role in CCT such as *COL4A1, COL4A2, COL4A3, COL4A4, COL5A1*, and *COL5A2* are believed to contribute towards a higher risk for KC [28, 41–43]. Utilizing genome SNP and gene expression chip arrays, additional research has uncovered links between CCT and KC within such genes as *ZNF469, AKAP13*, and *PRMD5* [20, 44–49]. *ZNF469* is a gene that has been implicated within multiple population studies as well as focused case studies of KC patients [12, 40, 50–54].

The results of focused research into a specific gene or group of genes often do not find evidence of a genetic correlation to KC, or in the case of family studies, rare variants found in members of a family who suffer from the disease are also found in members who do not display the phenotype. Consequently, rare variants do not always segregate within family groups in a predictable manner. This phenomenon brings about questions concerning known environmental factors that can bring on KC, such as habitual eye rubbing, secondary inflammation resulting from allergies and even climatic conditions, which has been suggested for why the prevalence is higher in India and in the Middle East [15, 55]. Another consideration that studies on the genetics suggest however, is that the disease could be brought on

Table 1 Family based studies

Gene/loci	Study participants	Geographic location	Reference
Various loci: 5q32-q33; 5q21.2; 14q11.2; 15q2.32	133 individuals from 25 families	Southern Italy	Bisceglia et al. [23]
MIR184 15q25.1	familial KC with cataracts	Northern Ireland; Galicia, Spain	Hughes et al. [24] Bykhovskaya et al. [25]
COL4A1,COL4A2 13q34;	15 families	Ecuador	Czugala et al. [26] Gajecka et al. [27] Karolak et al. [28]
DOCK9 13q32.3	23 individuals from one family	Ecuador	Karolak et al. [29]
COL5A1 9q34.3	3 generation family	South India	Lin et al. [30]
Locus 16q22.3-q23.1	20 families	Northern Finland	Tyynismaa et al. [31]
Locus 3p14-q13	2 generation family	Italy	Brancati et al. [32]
Locus 5q14.3-q21.1	4 generation Caucasian family	United States	Tang et al. [33, 34]
PPIP5K2 5q21.1	A four-generation family	United States	Khaled et al. [35]
LOX 5q23.1	146 KC patients from 70 families	United States	Bykhovskaya et al. [36]
Loci 1p36.23–36.21; 8q13.1-q21.11	A large Australian pedigree	Australia	Burdon et al. [37]
14q24.3	Multi ethnic study from 6 families	England	Liskova et al. [38]
Various loci in Chromosomes 4, 5, 9, 12, 14, 17	Multi ethnic study—351 individuals from 67 sib pair families	United States	Li et al. [39]
ZNF469 16q24.2	11 families with KC	United Kingdom; United Arab Emirates; Saudi Arabia	Davidson et al. [40]

by multiple genetic factors within various genes and loci that act in cooperation among interconnected molecular pathways. Diseases that are caused by multiple genetic components are often referred to as polygenic disorders.

3.2 Polygenic Risk Scores (PRS)

For inherited diseases driven by multiple variants of unknown penetrance the exact boundary between having and not having the disease blurs. Veritably, the genetics of KC presents the possibility of a disease based on an additive effect of underlying variants identified on a patient-by-patient basis. If KC is a polygenic disorder, it may be more apt to define this disease within a spectrum quantified on a continuous scale of 'risk' based on a PRS. Risk scores has been used to better understand genetic factors leading to common diseases like cardiovascular disorders, but it has also been successfully applied to eye disorders such as age related macular degeneration (AMD) [56]. Consequently, studies have demonstrated the utility of a PRS in assessing treatment therapies for patients with AMD [57], and a PRS was used to classify patients with primary open-angle glaucoma (POAG) for different treatment therapies [58]. Bykhovskaya and Rabinowitz outline an approach to risk scoring for KC that combines a genetic KC phenotype with clinical variables such as videokeratography (VK), Pentacam Scheimpflug HR Tomography (PST), and optical coherence tomography (OCT) (Fig. 1) [9]. For individuals considering refractive surgery or for KC patients who may want corneal collagen cross-linking (CXL) therapy, a PRS could better predict outcome and minimize adverse effects.

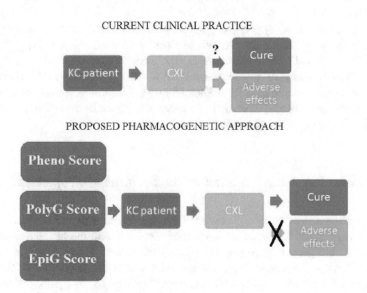

Fig. 1 A combined prediction model based on imaging (Pheno Score), polygenic modeling (PolyG score), and epigenetics/CpG methylation (EpiG score). Corneal cross-linking (CXL) is a therapy often used to treat keratoconus Bykhovskaya and Rabinowitz. [9]

4 Biomechanical Properties Determined by Current Clinical Devices, Corneal Hysteresis (CH) and Corneal Resistance Factor (CRF)

All current clinical devices have significant shortcomings in terms of measuring mechanical properties of the cornea but several studies have shown some correlation between current clinical measurements and defective genes. These clinical/ genetic correlations will now be discussed but reference should be made to future biomechanical devices later in the chapter.

Similar to CCT, there is evidence that corneal biomechanical properties such as CH and CRF are inherited, and understanding the genetics behind these properties may tell us more regarding the aetiology of KC [13]. CH is measured with a high-speed air-puff which is then quantified to give a measure of corneal deformation and recovery, and CRF measures the overall elastic resistance of the cornea. In eyes affected with KC, both the CH and CRF are lower, and this attribute has been correlated to severity KC severity [59].

In 2020, Simcoe et al. published the results from a GWAS that identified over 200 loci associated with either or both CH and CRF [12]. In this study, it was found that many loci known to be associated with corneal diseases, including KC were strongly associated with both traits. Specifically, the genes that were linked to CH and CRF and likewise, to KC were *FNDC3B, ZNF469, MPDZ* and *FOXO1* [54]. The evidence provided by this group supports the hypothesis that CH and CRF are etiologically and genetically linked to corneal disease in general [12, 13]. Combining CH and CRF measurements with clinical imaging obtained with VK, PDT or OCT would give a better understand to the nuances of the KC phenotype and provide quantitative data for a Pheno Score (Fig. 1), which along with a PRS based on the genetics of KC, could give higher confidence in the ability to predict a risk for developing KC or a related corneal ectasia.

4.1 Gene Expression Linked to Biomechanical Properties

Gene expression studies in KC corneas have uncovered serious alterations in the expression of genes that translate into protein levels within the affected tissue that differ from the gene expression and consequent protein levels found in healthy corneas. Expression studies have always been a valuable source of information regarding the functional genes and pathways important for KC pathogenesis, and recent research has demonstrated a link between gene expression and the biomechanical properties of the KC cornea [9]. These studies indicate an altered expression of genes involved primarily in collagen metabolism pathways, genes that translate to structural proteins such as *COL5A1, COL6A1, COL7A1, COL11A1*, genes within the extracellular matrix (ECM) like *FN1, TGFBI, MMP9*, and regulatory genes such as *TIMP1* and *TIMP2* [60].

For the phenotypes associated with CH and CRF, Simcoe et al. found a significant association in the expression of 86 genes with CH, and 107 with CRF. The strongest gene association for both CH and CRF was an increased expression of *ZNF469* and a noncoding RNA, *PRPF31* which lies upstream of *ZNF469* on chromosome 16 [12]. These results imply an association between the gene expression of the *ZNF469* gene and the genomic variants within *ZNF469* indicated by SNP-based GWASs as well variants uncovered in DNA sequencing studies [50, 51, 53].

A large transcriptome profiling experiment utilizing the RNA-seq platform uncovered an extensive disruption of collagen synthesis and maturation pathways along with the downregulation of the TGF-β, Hippo,and Wnt signaling pathways in human KC corneas [61]. This study conducted through the Department of Genetics and Pharmaceutical Microbiology at Poznan University in Poland, initially found as many as 5235 differentially expressed transcripts (1578 upregulated and 3657 downregulated). Earlier studies employing techniques such as microarray hybridization [62] or expressed sequence tag (EST) analysis coupled to traditional Sanger sequencing [63, 64] had uncovered differentially expressed genes that in some cases, did not agree with the results reported by the group at Poznan University. Specifically, genes such as *ACTN1, SERPINB1, LOX, SLPI, DSG3, FHL2, ANXA1, LGALS1, RPL23, S100A2,* and *GPNMB* that were expressed as upregulated with microarrays were found to be downregulated in the patients examined in the RNA-Seq study [61]. Often, genes that were shown to be important in earlier study designs with a specific patient group did not replicate in subsequent studies that used such state-of-the-art technologies as RNA-Seq. For example, the EST analysis mentioned above indicated an absence of transcripts for the *AQP5* gene in KC corneas, but this gene was not identified as being downregulated in other reports. This study did, however, indicate important links in gene expression associated with apoptosis, or programmed cell death. Genes associated with apoptosis appeared to be elevated in KC compared with normal donor corneas, and a regulatory long non-coding (lnc)-RNA, labeled *KC6* was also found to be abundantly expressed in KC corneas [63]. The diverse results from the large number of published work investigating gene expression within KC corneas illustrate that, like the research conducted into the genomic underpinnings of the disease, KC is a heterogenic disease of significant complexity.

5   Inflammatory Genes and Immunological Biomarkers Associated with KC

Historically, KC has been considered a noninflammatory corneal ectasia [3, 65]. However, current research has confirmed that tissue degradation in thinning disorders such as KC involves the expression of proinflammatory cytokines, cell adhesion molecules and matrix metalloproteinases [66]. The genes involved in these pathways are considered inflammatory mediator genes, and levels of pro-inflammatory cytokines, such as *IL-6* and *TNF-α*, and matrix metalloproteinase-9 (*MMP-9*) were found to be significantly increased in tears of patients with KC [67, 68]. The group conducting these studies at the University of Santiago de Compostela in Spain uncovered biomarkers for KC in the immune toll-like receptors 2 (TLR2) and 4 (TLR4) [66].

TLRs are a family of highly conserved innate immunity receptors that recognize damage-associated molecular patterns [69]. They are released as a consequence of tissue damage, and in individuals who have not been diagnosed with KC, but who have relatives that suffer from the disease, it was determined that *TLR2* and *TLR4* are overexpressed in corneal and conjunctival epithelial cells [70]. Additionally, it was found that *TLR2/TLR4* were over expressed in corneal and conjunctival epithelial cells in patients who suffer from PMD, a clinical variation of KC [71]. These biomarkers could therefore be used to monitor for early ocular changes in the corneal epithelial tissue in relatives of KC patients who do not show any abnormal clinical topographic or tomographic aberrations.

Allergies and eye rubbing, often termed environmental factors are widely accepted as agents in the progression of non-familial or non-genetic KC [3, 72]. It was noted in the studies reviewed above, that in the relatives of KC patients, allergic disease, eye itching or rubbing did not accompany the upregulated expression of *TLR2/TLR4* [70]. Previously, it was believed most KC cases were sporadic, brought on by environmental conditions and that only 5 to 23% of all cases possessed a genetic link [8]. The upregulated expression of inflammatory or immunological genes in the absence of itching or eye rubbing caused by allergies is further evidence for a genetic link to the etiology of KC. These findings warrant further study into the possibility that KC, caused by environmental factors has a genetic underpinning, and such research would provide additional insight into the complex molecular mechanism that leads to KC and to other corneal ectasias.

6   Current and Future Devices to Evaluate the Structural Properties of the Cornea and Its Biomechanics

The ability to specifically diagnose KC at an early-stage, prior to topographic involvement, remains a significant clinical challenge. Early diagnosis of KC has become increasingly important over the last two decades for two main reasons:

1. The availability and popularity of invasive refractive surgery procedures: More than 4 million procedures are carried out per year worldwide. Patients with undiagnosed KC are at significantly increased risk of complications, leading to post-surgical ectasias. This currently occurs in 0.04–0.6% [73] of the treatment population and is completely avoidable with access to screening tools capable of identifying early stage-disease.

2. The availability of minimally-invasive treatments such as CXL: These treatments are most effective if used at the earliest stages of the disease prior to the progression of topographic abnormalities. CXL increases the stiffness of the cornea counteracting the biomechanical weakening that occurs with KC, preventing the gradual changes to topography that would otherwise occur and lead to deterioration of vision. With timely CXL treatment severe visual abnormality can be avoided and long-term follow-up treatments such as hard contact lenses or IOLs would not be required.

7 Clinical Identification of Keratoconus

Corneal abnormalities in KC are initially topographically localized to small foci, but these initial slight structural abnormalities result in alterations of the biomechanical properties of the cornea at the defined locations. Progression of the disease then occurs as a result of biomechanical decompensation under exposure to various forces including IOP and forces from the eyelids during blinking and eye-rubbing [74]. As a result, the structural integrity and overall biomechanics of the system as a whole continue to degrade, and the abnormal region becomes exponentially larger. Since these subtle and localised biomechanical abnormalities significantly precede any topographic involvement, their detection is widely considered to be the key to identifying the disease at the earliest stage. However, mapping corneal biomechanics and identifying corneal biomechanical abnormality in the clinic remains a challenge yet to be adequately addressed. Current clinical assessment of keratoconus relies on a combination of information gained from the following three approaches:

1. A detailed patient clinical and family history, to determine genetic predisposition and risk factors associated with the development and acceleration of disease such as repetitive eye-rubbing or rapid changes to topography.
2. Topographic, pachymetic and tomographic evaluation, commonly via the Pentacam (OCULUS Optikgeräte GmbH, Wetzlar, DE) and/or Sirius (SCHWIND eye-tech-solutions, Kleinostheim, DE). Although other devices based around alternative technologies including optical coherence tomography (OCT) and high-frequency ultrasound (HFU) are also available and capable of providing similar data.
3. Evaluation of 'biomechanics' via the ORA (Reichert Ophthalmic Instruments, Inc., NY, USA) and/or CorVis ST (OCULUS Optikgeräte GmbH, Wetzlar, Germany).

Understanding a patient's family history can be useful for identifying individuals who may have a predisposition to the development of keratoconus. As discussed in detail in the preceding sections, several genes have been implicated in the development of keratoconus, recently leading to the development of genetic swab tests to screen individuals who may be at an increased risk (Avagen, Avellino Labs USA Inc., CA, USA). Once identified these patients can be monitored more closely for early signs of the disease and deterred from undertaking elective invasive refractive procedures even in cases of apparent normal topography, pachymetry and biomechanics. Clinical history is also important, tracking changes to topographic, pachymetric and tomographic measures over time is currently the gold-standard for identifying keratoconus.

7.1 Static Evaluation—Topographic, Tomographic and Pachymetric Assessment

Several topographic and tomographic measures have been shown to have good sensitivity and specificity for the diagnosis of keratoconus even in cases where visual acuity is normal, and the corneas have a normal appearance on slit-lamp examinations [75]. Two main devices are commonly used to obtain such measures, the Pentacam and the Sirius. Both devices employ a rotating Scheimpflug camera that obtains a 100 slit-lamp images of corneal cross-sections over a two-second measurement time, however the Sirius also incorporates placido disk topography to provide a more detailed assessment of anterior surface topography. Both devices provide whole corneal anterior and posterior surface elevation maps giving a 3-D view of the cornea.

Through viewing both the anterior and posterior surfaces of the cornea a large variety of different features can be analysed such as anterior/posterior radius of curvature, maximum thickness, minimum thickness, surface variance, symmetry and many more. Several of these factors have been confirmed to show changes with KC; however, there is generally a large cross-over between values for normal and keratoconic corneas [75]. Because of the large inter-patient variability in the measured properties, combined with the fact abnormalities are relatively subtle, especially in the early stages of disease, each one of these factors when evaluated in isolation has overall poor sensitivity for the disease and cannot be relied upon for diagnosis. This has led to the development of several integrated indices demonstrated to have higher predictive power, such as the Belin/Ambrosio enhanced ectasia total deviation value (BAD-D) [76] or the Pentacam Random Forest Index (PRFI) [77]. The BAD-D provides a comprehensive colour-coded overview to the clinician, detailing several tomographic and pachymetric parameters, highlighting in yellow and red values that are suspicious and abnormal respectively. Regression analysis is used to calculate an overall 'D' score where parameters are weighted based on their power with regards to identifying. The PRFI, uses artificial intelligence (AI) to evaluate data obtained from the Pentacam. The performance of these integrated indices for the detection of KC and subclinical KC across different studies is summarised in Table 2.

Table 2 Sensitivity and specificity of different topographic, tomographic and 'biomechanical' indices used in the assessment of keratoconus

Parameter	Data type	KC sensitivity (%)	KC specificity (%)	Subclinical-KC sensitivity (%)	Subclinical-KC specificity (%)	Comments
BAD-D	Pentacam tomographic	97–100 [78, 79]	61.4–94 [78, 79]	52–84 [78–80]	73–86 [78, 79]	
PRFI		94–99 [75, 77]	98–100 [75, 77]	71–86 [75]	84–88 [75]	
CH	ORA 'biomechanics'	77–87 [81–84]	63–98 [81–84]	76–91 [83, 85, 86]	62–76 [83, 86]	Both CH and CRF are generally lower in KC patients, but due to large overlaps in values with normal corneas they have poor sensitivity and specificity
CRF		68–90 [81–84]	66–96 [81, 83, 84]	74–96 [83, 85]	52–88 [83, 86]	
Waveform Analysis		74–78 [87]	84–91 [87]	66–76 [88]	66–76 [88]	It is possible to analyse 41 features of the waveform however further work is required to optimise the algorithms to gain maximum diagnostic potential
CBI	CorVis ST 'biomechanics'	90–99 [89–91]	93–99 [89–91]	63 [80]	80 [80]	Can detect outright keratoconus with good reliability however currently shows poor efficacy for true subclinical cases
TBI	CorVis ST 'biomechanics' and Pentacam tomographic	94–100 [91–93]	95–100 [91–93]	67–84 [75, 94, 95]	82–86 [75, 94, 95]	Similar to CBI the TBI can reliably detect outright keratoconus but cannot currently reliably detect subclinical cases

The current issue in many studies demonstrating the effectiveness of these parameters for diagnosing sub-clinical KC, is that what constitutes sub-clinical KC varies significantly between studies. In most instances the corneas classified as 'sub-clinical', or 'suspect' KC already present with some topographic or tomographic abnormality indicative of keratoconus that has progressed significantly enough to be identified. Therefore, we still do not truly understand the effectiveness of these methods for identifying the condition at its earliest stage. Furthermore, both indices have shown poor efficacy for KC staging, and hence currently cannot be used effectively to inform optimised and customised treatment.

7.2   Dynamic Evaluation—'Biomechanical' Assessment

In addition to the static measures performed, the dynamic response of a cornea to an air-puff is also routinely evaluated. This assessment is the current gold-standard in what clinicians and the ophthalmic community term to be 'biomechanical evaluation'. Two devices are commonly used, these are; the Ocular Response Analyser (ORA, Reichert Ophthalmic Instruments, Inc., NY, USA); and the CorVis Scheimpflug Tonometer (CorVis ST, OCULUS Optikgeräte GmbH, Wetzlar, Germany). The ORA is a point-based measurement method, evaluating the movement of the central cornea only. It focusses on determining corneal hysteresis (CH) [96], which is defined as the difference in the inward and outward applanation pressures and is suggested to relate to the viscoelastic properties of the cornea, hence its ability to store and dissipate energy. However, CH is affected by IOP and corneal thickness and therefore is a poor informant, in isolation, for identifying the presence of biomechanical abnormality. Attempts have been made to increase its power as a tool to identify abnormal biomechanics through concurrent analysis of factors that influence the deformation of the cornea.

Corneal Resistance Factor (CRF) was introduced to try to account for the influence of IOP in CH measurements; however, both factors so far have shown relatively low sensitivity for diagnosing KC with neither being able to reliably identify KC suspect cases (Table 2). Recently whole waveform analysis of the ORA signal has been trialled [87]; however, due to the large overlap between normal and keratoconic corneas across all of the indices evaluated, the ORA is not a reliable way of diagnosing KC especially at an early stage. This is not particularly surprising given the localised nature of early-stage disease and the fact the ORA only evaluates the movement of the cornea at a single point on the anterior surface.

Improving on the ORA, the CorVis ST evaluates the deformation of the cornea over an entire cross-section, hence many more indices can be quantified, it is not only possible to evaluate the magnitude of deformation at the central cornea but also factors such as the shape and symmetry of deformation. Once again however, there is a large overlap between normal and keratoconic corneas for many of the indices evaluated and factors such as IOP can influence the response. As a result, integrated indices have also been developed here, including the Corvis

Biomechanical Index (CBI) [89] and the tomographic/biomechanical Index (TBI) [97], which combines information from the Pentacam and the CorVis ST.

Both the CBI and TBI have demonstrated good efficacy for identifying KC and some ability to detect sub-clinical cases (Table 2), which is important when screening for refractive surgery procedures. However, the technique still has several important limitations when it comes to diagnosing KC. Firstly, as previously stated, we still have a poor understanding of its efficacy with regards to the detection of truly early-stage KC due to its variable definition between studies, it is likely the location of any biomechanical abnormality on the cornea and its proximity to the measured cross-section will have an impact here. Also, since the air puff force is directed at the centre, abnormalities closer to the central region, are likely to have a larger influence on the response and hence be easier to identify. The loading method itself is not ideal, if the load is not focussed on the central cornea it could influence the deformation of the cornea and as a result, conclusions drawn from the data. The load also pushes the cornea inwards resulting in compression of the anterior surface, the biomechanics of which have evolved to predominantly deal with tensile forces, meaning biomechanical abnormality with respect to this may go unnoticed. Above all, even if we can get to the point where we can use the CorVis ST to reliably identify sub-clinical cases of KC it does not provide enough information to make a specific diagnosis or inform targeted and customised treatments.

8 New Technologies Under Development for Clinical Assessment of Biomechanical Abnormality

It is evident that there is still some way to go when it comes to delivering timely, optimised and individualised patient care and a better understanding of corneal biomechanics, the biomechanics of KC and the effects of treatments. Laboratory-based studies alongside development of better clinical screening tools have a large role to play in this, and there is currently a significant amount of research being undertaken. To deliver customised and optimised treatment we need to not only be able to diagnose the presence of early-stage biomechanical abnor-mality with high sensitivity and specificity, but we need to be able to classify the abnormality in terms of severity and location. We then need to understand the long-term biomechanical and refractive effects of treatments such as CXL so that they can be delivered in a targeted way that optimises long-term refractive out-comes. This is summarised in Fig. 2 [98] which compares the current standard of care to that which would be possible with access to more information and advanced biomechanical screening.

Significant research is going into the development of devices capable of spatially mapping corneal biomechanical properties. To-date the term 'biomechanics' has been used very loosely within the ophthalmological industry especially when it comes to clinical assessment of 'corneal biomechanics'. Although the movement of

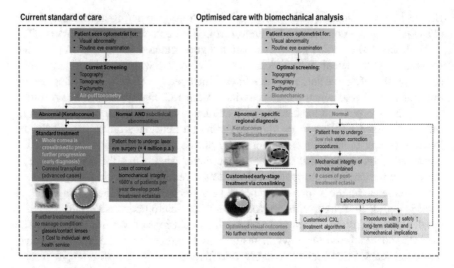

Fig. 2 A comparison of the current standard of care with that which would be possible with clinical tools capable of detailed biomechanical analysis and a better understanding of keratoconus as a disease and the biomechanical and refractive effects of CXL treatment protocols (adapted from [98])

the cornea in response to an air-puff has some relationship to its mechanical properties, we cannot derive specific mechanical properties such as stiffness from these tests, we also cannot use the data obtained from these tests to understand how the cornea behaves under normal forces such as IOP and how its mechanical properties contribute to this, as the loading used is not a normal physiological load.

Due to the relationship between the mechanical properties of the cornea, IOP and corneal shape, hence refractive properties, most research is now directed towards understanding and quantifying the mechanical properties of the cornea in response to fluctuations in IOP. Examining the response of the cornea in this way has several advantages. Firstly, IOP varies naturally diurnally and over the cardiac cycle, hence no external force is required to excite the cornea. Secondly, IOP fluctuations are simple to simulate during ex vivo experiments and can be directly related to in vivo behaviour. Thirdly, since the mechanical properties of the cornea under IOP are intrinsically linked to its shape, observing changes to the distribution of the response of the cornea to IOP fluctuations after treatments such as CXL can provide useful information regarding the likely topographic changes that will occur over the recovery period as the cornea returns to a steady-state in terms of biomechanics. And lastly the cornea is viscoelastic; hence, its mechanical properties are load and time dependent, therefore to gain useful and relevant information regarding its in vivo behaviour, its properties must be evaluated in response to physiologically representative loads.

Several methods are currently being used in ex vivo experiments to probe corneal biomechanics in response to IOP fluctuations with a number showing potential for in vivo application with further development. An important feature of any biomechanical measurement technique is the ability to spatially analyse the response of the cornea. The cornea has a complex and heterogeneous structure resulting in significant spatial and directional variability in mechanical properties. Recent studies [99–101] have demonstrated regional variability in mechanical properties of the cornea, especially highlighting differences in the properties of the limbus and peripheral cornea versus the central cornea [101]. These differences are extremely important, and their quantification will be key to the development of customised and targeted treatments for KC. Spatial analysis is also particularly important when considering early diagnosis of KC. As we have already described, KC is initially localised in nature, and it is the ability to spot these localised changes which will be the key to identifying the disease at the earliest stage. In addition, spatial analysis and whole-field imaging of the response of the cornea to IOP changes has a further advantage as it enables, not only, the overall magnitude of the response to be assessed but also the distribution. This is highly important in the case of the cornea, because as identified earlier there is large inter-patient variability in the response with factors such as age, hydration and ethnicity all playing a role, and as a result there is a large crossover between normal and pathological cases when relying on interpreting values for given properties. Analysis of the distribution of the response is helpful especially when trying to identify localised abnormalities, as the relative deformation in one region can be evaluated relative to the overall deformation of the cornea, removing the reliance on accurate quantification of specific mechanical properties. In fact, it has already been possible to identify similarities in the distribution of the anterior surface displacement of corneas to IOP variations and from this identify corneas that show abnormalities [101, 102].

8.1 Techniques Used to Spatially Map the Response of the Cornea to Fluctuations in IOP

Several techniques have been used to spatially map the response of the cornea to fluctuations in IOP, these are; Optical coherence tomography (OCT), High Frequency Ultrasound (HFU), Speckle interferometry (SI), Digital Image correlation (DIC) and Dynamic Videokeratoscopy (DV). OCT and HFU, are capable of through-thickness data acquisition so have been used to map the 3-D response of the cornea to IOP changes, whereas SI, DIC and DV look at the response of the anterior surface only. With both OCT and HFU, data is acquired through a single cross-section at a given time so they both require scanning to acquire data across the full cornea, meaning there is an inherent trade-off between resolution and measurement time. The newer systems are capable of fast measurement times [103, 104], acquiring data across full cross-sections in several milliseconds, but it still requires several seconds to minutes to generate 3-D data, and therefore, both systems struggle to cope with motion artefacts that occur during in vivo measurement when attempting whole corneal analysis. An additional drawback of both HFU and OCT currently is that they have only demonstrated the ability to collect data from the central 6 mm area of the cornea [103–105]. The curvature of the cornea presents issues with signal to noise and data interpretation approaching the periphery. A further disadvantage of HFU is it requires direct contact with the cornea, which is disadvantageous in a clinical setting, and involves some degree of discomfort for the patient. So far neither OCT or HFU have demonstrated efficacy for detecting biomechanical differences between normal or keratoconic corneas. This is because it is hard to undertake ex vivo experiments on keratoconic tissue due to a shortage of samples available for analysis, and neither have yet reached the stage where they can acquire reliable 3D in vivo data. However, both OCT and HFU have demonstrated efficacy for measuring changes to corneal biomechanics that occur after CXL, with HFU being used to evaluate a standard full-corneal CXL treatment [104] and OCT showing spatial changes to biomechanics that occur after patterned CXL in rats corneas [103].

Unlike OCT and HFU, with SI and DIC full-surface data is acquired in a snapshot, requiring only milliseconds. Data can also be obtained across the entire cornea and surrounding sclera providing a larger field of view and allowing the response at the limbus to be taken into account. Displacement speckle pattern interferometry, as has been used in previous studies [101, 102], has a displacement sensitivity of several nanometres and can therefore capture very high resolution displacement data over very small variations in IOP from 0.05 to 1 mmHg [101]. In contrast, OCT and HFU have slightly lower sensitivity requiring pressure variations of between 1 and 3 mmHg. The dynamic range of OCT and HFU based techniques is better, although the measurement range of SI techniques can be easily extended via regularly updating the reference image. However, the high sensitivity of SI does pose issues when considering in vivo translation. Unwanted eye movement can result in loss of data, and currently the methods are limited by inability to gain an adequate signal from the surface of the naked cornea due to its smoothness and transparency.

So far, SI has successfully demonstrated efficacy for mapping the displacement of the anterior surface of the cornea in response to IOP perturbations on the scale of those that occur during the cardiac cycle [101, 102, 106]. Recent investigations have shown similar displacement distributions of the anterior surface across different corneas, and due to this, it has been possible to identify corneas with superficial damage through identifying changes in the distribution of the displacement response from that of undamaged corneas [101]. The fact that information is acquired at the anterior surface only, does not seem to prevent damage from elsewhere in the structure from being identified, this is likely due to the fact the cornea is thin and has a highly integrated structure; hence, damage throughout its depth manifests as irregularities in the surface response. Using interferometry it has been possible to produce high resolution maps showing changes to the surface responses to pressure variations after patterned CXL (Fig. 3) [102, 107]. Use of SI based techniques combined with OCT/HFU will be key to understanding the

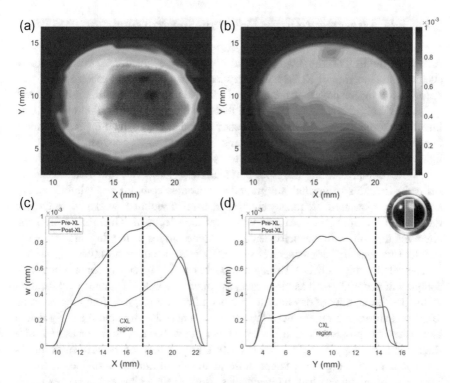

Fig. 3 Demonstration of the changes to the surface displacement of a human cornea in response to a pressure increase from 16.5 to 17.0 mmHg after CXL treatment along the central superior-inferior axis. **a** anterior surface displacement prior to CXL; **b** anterior surface displacement after CXL; **c** comparison of displacement before (blue) and after (red) CXL along the central nasal-temporal axis; **d** comparison of displacement before (blue) and after (red) CXL along the central superior-inferior axis (reproduced from [102])

biomechanical implications of CXL treatments and developing the treatment algorithms required to realise customised application.

In Dynamic videokeraoscopy a standard Placido topographer is used to capture data from the surface of the cornea at 2 different pressures to evaluate changes to surface curvature over a pressure change [108]. The measurement range of a standard topographer was extended by taking 5 measurements as the patient moved their eye to a different position so the limbal areas could be evaluated and the IOP was doubled via applying pressure to the eyelids with an ophthalmodynamometer. Ideally, it would be possible to identify biomechanical abnormality through identifying subtle changes to the curvature response across different regions. If this could be achieved, it would be a convenient method of analysis as most clinics already have access to a Placido disk topographer; however, due to the low sensitivity of the technique, it is unlikely that it will be capable of spotting truly early-stage disease. On the other hand, other variations on fringe reflection-based methods may have application here and remain to be investigated.

8.2   3-D Assessment Using Brillouin Spectroscopy

A final method that has shown potential for clinical evaluation of corneal biomechanics and detection of KC is Brillouin spectroscopy. Brillouin spectroscopy does
not measure the response of the cornea to IOP fluctuations, but instead measures
inelastic light scattered from the cornea that arises due to illumination of the tissue
initiating thermally excited hyper frequency sound waves, which leads to periodic
fluctuations in density [109]. The specific frequency shifts between the scattered
light and the incident light is referred to as the Brillouin modulus, which can be
related to compressibility in isotropic materials. However, the relationship of
Brillouin modulus to mechanical properties becomes complex in hydrated materials, as the measured frequency shift represents a volume weighted aggregate
modulus of the fluid and solid components of the specimen. Therefore, there is no
direct relationship with elasticity, leading to some groups cautioning against its use
as a tool to quantify biomechanical properties such as stiffness [110].

The relationship between Brillouin modulus and elasticity becomes especially
complex in materials such as the cornea, as corneal hydration changes with location
within the tissue, time of day and environmental conditions; therefore, it is essential
to get concurrent measurement of the water content if the aim is to precisely define
biomechanical properties. The water content could be accurately measured with
Ramen spectroscopy, but this presents a further problem, as the Ramen scatter is
dependent upon the precise temperature at the point and time of measurement.
Thus, measurements of true biomechanics using these techniques becomes extremely problematic and probably unsuitable for clinical applications.

However, despite the challenges associated with accurate quantification of
specific measures of elasticity, Brillouin spectroscopy may still prove to be a useful
tool for the early diagnosis of KC and has already been demonstrated to be capable
of in vivo measurement [111] and capable of distinguishing between normal corneas and those with outright KC [112]. Although, it has yet to show efficacy for
spotting suspect cases. Its ability to differentiate between corneas may be due to the
fact the presence of KC leads to density and hydration changes in the tissue and less
to do with its ability to measure biomechanics. The main challenge when considering the widespread application of Brillouin spectroscopy in a clinical setting to
detect KC is long-acquisition times. It currently requires several minutes to generate
a relatively low-resolution 40 point-scan; therefore, it would be time consuming to
incorporate into routine screening, and the low data resolution may mean cases are
missed. However, due to its ability to provide 3D data, if faster acquisition times
could be achieved it may prove to be a useful tool to inform more targeted
treatments.

Overall, it is likely a combination of the techniques discussed here will be used
to achieve optimal assessment of corneal biomechanics and the ability to identify
subtle and localised abnormalities in early-stage KC. Highly sensitive, whole surface evaluation techniques based around interferometric methods that are capable of
acquiring data in several milliseconds, combined with scanning-based techniques

that can provide 3-D data through the thickness of the cornea may provide the best approach through achieving an instant overview of the whole-corneal response, allowing more targeted assessment with the scanning-based 3-D measurement methods. In the meantime, continued ex vivo investigations using these techniques will provide the necessary data to optimise CXL procedures and pave the way for targeted and patient-individualised treatments with optimal refractive outcomes.

References

1. Loukovitis E, Sfakianakis K, Syrmakesi P, Tsotridou E, Orfanidou M, Bakaloudi DR, et al. Genetic aspects of keratoconus: a literature review exploring potential genetic contributions and possible genetic relationships with comorbidities. Ophthalmol Therapy. 2018;7:263–92. https://doi.org/10.1007/s40123-018-0144-8.
2. Kennedy RH, Bourne WM, Dyer JA. A 48-year clinical and epidemiologic study of keratoconus. Am J Ophthalmol. 1986;101:267–73. https://doi.org/10.1016/0002-9394(86)90817-2.
3. Rabinowitz YS. Keratoconus. Surv Ophthalmol. 1998;42:297–319. https://doi.org/10.1016/s0039-6257(97)00119-7.
4. Georgiou T, Funnell CL, Cassels-Brown A, O'Conor R. Influence of ethnic origin on the incidence of keratoconus and associated atopic disease in Asians and white patients. Eye. 2004;18:379–83. https://doi.org/10.1038/sj.eye.6700652.
5. Torres Netto EA, Al-Otaibi WM, Hafezi NL, Kling S, Al-Farhan HM, Randleman JB, et al. Prevalence of keratoconus in paediatric patients in Riyadh, Saudi Arabia. Br J Ophthalmol. 2018;102:1436–41. https://doi.org/10.1136/bjophthalmol-2017-311391.
6. Godefrooij DA, de Wit GA, Uiterwaal CS, Imhof SM, Wisse RPLL. Age-specific incidence and prevalence of keratoconus: a nationwide registration study. Am J Ophthalmol. 2017;175:169–72. https://doi.org/10.1016/j.ajo.2016.12.015.
7. Shetty R, D'Souza S, Khamar P, Ghosh A, Nuijts RMMA, Sethu S. Biochemical markers and alterations in keratoconus. Asia-Pacific J Ophthalmol. 2020;9:533–40. https://doi.org/10.1097/apo.0000000000000332.
8. Wheeler J, Hauser MA, Afshari NA, Allingham RR, Liu Y. The genetics of keratoconus: a review. Reprod Syst Sex Disord: Curr Res. 2012:1. https://doi.org/10.4172/2161-038X.S6-001.
9. Bykhovskaya Y, Rabinowitz YS. Update on the genetics of keratoconus. Exp Eye Res. 2021;202:108398. https://doi.org/10.1016/j.exer.2020.108398.
10. McComish BJ, Sahebjada S, Bykhovskaya Y, Willoughby CE, Richardson AJ, Tenen A, et al. Association of genetic variation with keratoconus. JAMA Ophthalmol. 2020;138:174–81. https://doi.org/10.1001/jamaophthalmol.2019.5293.
11. Lucas SEM, Zhou T, Blackburn NB, Mills RA, Ellis J, Leo P, et al. Rare, potentially pathogenic variants in 21 keratoconus candidate genes are not enriched in cases in a large Australian cohort of European descent. PLoS ONE. 2018;13:e0199178–e0199178. https://doi.org/10.1371/journal.pone.0199178.
12. Simcoe MJ, Khawaja AP, Hysi PG, Hammond CJ, Consortium UKBE and V. Genome-wide association study of corneal biomechanical properties identifies over 200 loci providing insight into the genetic etiology of ocular diseases. Human Mol Genet. 2020;29:3154–64. https://doi.org/10.1093/hmg/ddaa155.
13. Khawaja AP, Rojas Lopez KE, Hardcastle AJ, Hammond CJ, Liskova P, Davidson AE, et al. Genetic variants associated with corneal biomechanical properties and potentially conferring

susceptibility to keratoconus in a genome-wide association study. JAMA Ophthalmol. 2019;137:1005–12. https://doi.org/10.1001/jamaophthalmol.2019.2058.

14. Pearson AR, Soneji B, Sarvananthan N, Sandford-Smith JH. Does ethnic origin influence the incidence or severity of keratoconus? Eye (Lond). 2000;14(Pt 4):625–8. https://doi.org/10.1038/eye.2000.154.

15. Gokhale NS. Epidemiology of keratoconus. Indian J Ophthalmol. 2013;61:382–3. https://doi.org/10.4103/0301-4738.116054.

16. Millodot M, Shneor E, Albou S, Atlani E, Gordon-Shaag A. Prevalence and associated factors of keratoconus in Jerusalem: a cross-sectional study. Ophthalmic Epidemiol. 2011;18:91–7. https://doi.org/10.3109/09286586.2011.560747.

17. Hardcastle AJ, Liskova P, Bykhovskaya Y, McComish BJ, Davidson AE, Inglehearn CF, et al. A multi-ethnic genome-wide association study implicates collagen matrix integrity and cell differentiation pathways in keratoconus. Commun Biol. 2021;4:266. https://doi.org/10.1038/s42003-021-01784-0.

18. Naderan M, Shoar S, Rezagholizadeh F, Zolfaghari M, Naderan M. Characteristics and associations of keratoconus patients. Cont Lens Anterior Eye. 2015;38:199–205. https://doi.org/10.1016/j.clae.2015.01.008.

19. Sadoughi MM, Einollahi B, Einollahi N, Rezaei J, Roshandel D, Feizi S. Measurement of central corneal thickness using ultrasound pachymetry and orbscan ii in normal eyes. J Ophthalmic Vis Res. 2015;10:4–9. https://doi.org/10.4103/2008-322X.156084.

20. Lu Y, Vitart V, Burdon KP, Khor CC, Bykhovskaya Y, Mirshahi A, et al. Genome-wide association analyses identify multiple loci associated with central corneal thickness and keratoconus. Nat Genet. 2013;45:155–63. https://doi.org/10.1038/ng.2506.

21. Choquet H, Melles RB, Yin J, Hoffmann TJ, Thai KK, Kvale MN, et al. A multiethnic genome-wide analysis of 44,039 individuals identifies 41 new loci associated with central corneal thickness. Commun Biol. 2020;3:301. https://doi.org/10.1038/s42003-020-1037-7.

22. Dimasi DP, Burdon KP, Craig JE. The genetics of central corneal thickness. Br J Ophthalmol. 2009;94:971–6. https://doi.org/10.1136/bjo.2009.162735.

23. Bisceglia L, De Bonis P, Pizzicoli C, Fischetti L, Laborante A, Di Perna M, et al. Linkage analysis in keratoconus: replication of locus 5q21.2 and identification of other suggestive Loci. Invest Ophthalmol Vis Sci. 2009;50:1081–6. https://doi.org/10.1167/iovs.08-2382.

24. Hughes AE, Bradley DT, Campbell M, Lechner J, Dash DP, Simpson DA, et al. Mutation altering the miR-184 seed region causes familial keratoconus with cataract. Am J Hum Genet. 2011;89:628–33. https://doi.org/10.1016/j.ajhg.2011.09.014.

25. Bykhovskaya Y, Caiado Canedo AL, Wright KW, Rabinowitz YS. C.57 C > T mutation in MIR 184 is responsible for congenital cataracts and corneal abnormalities in a five-generation family from Galicia, Spain. Ophthalmic Genet. 2015;36:244–7. https://doi.org/10.3109/13816810.2013.848908.

26. Czugala M, Karolak JA, Nowak DM, Polakowski P, Pitarque J, Molinari A, et al. Novel mutation and three other sequence variants segregating with phenotype at keratoconus 13q32 susceptibility locus. Eur J Human Genet: EJHG. 2012;20:389–97. https://doi.org/10.1038/ejhg.2011.203.

27. Gajecka M, Radhakrishna U, Winters D, Nath SK, Rydzanicz M, Ratnamala U, et al. Localization of a gene for keratoconus to a 5.6-Mb interval on 13q32. Invest Ophthalmol Vis Sci. 2009;50:1531–9. https://doi.org/10.1167/iovs.08-2173.

28. Karolak JA, Kulinska K, Nowak DM, Pitarque JA, Molinari A, Rydzanicz M, et al. Sequence variants in COL4A1 and COL4A2 genes in Ecuadorian families with keratoconus. Mol Vis. 2011;17:827–43.

29. Karolak JA, Rydzanicz M, Ginter-Matuszewska B, Pitarque JA, Molinari A, Bejjani BA, et al. Variant c.2262A>C in DOCK9 leads to exon skipping in keratoconus family. Invest Opthalmol Vis Sci. 2015;56:7687. https://doi.org/10.1167/iovs.15-17538.

30. Lin Q, Zheng L, Shen Z, Jie L. A novel splice-site variation in COL5A1 causes keratoconus in an Indian family. J Ophthalmol. 2019;2019:2851380. https://doi.org/10.1155/2019/2851380.

31. Tyynismaa H, Sistonen P, Tuupanen S, Tervo T, Dammert A, Latvala T, et al. A locus for autosomal dominant keratoconus: linkage to 16q22.3-q23.1 in Finnish families. Invest Ophthalmol Vis Sci. 2002;43:3160–4.

32. Brancati F, Valente EM, Sarkozy A, Fehèr J, Castori M, Del Duca P, et al. A locus for autosomal dominant keratoconus maps to human chromosome 3p14-q13. J Med Genet. 2004;41:188–92. https://doi.org/10.1136/jmg.2003.012872.

33. Tang YG, Rabinowitz YS, Taylor KD, Li X, Hu M, Picornell Y, et al. Genomewide linkage scan in a multigeneration Caucasian pedigree identifies a novel locus for keratoconus on chromosome 5q14.3-q21.1. Genet Med. 2005;7:397–405. https://doi.org/10.1097/01.gim.0000170772.41860.54.

34. Bykhovskaya Y, Li X, Taylor KD, Haritunians T, Rotter JI, Rabinowitz YS. Linkage analysis of high-density SNPS confirms keratoconus locus at 5q chromosomal region. Ophthalmic Genet. 2016;37:109–10. https://doi.org/10.3109/13816810.2014.889172.

35. Khaled ML, Bykhovskaya Y, Gu C, Liu A, Drewry MD, Chen Z, et al. PPIP5K2 and PCSK1 are candidate genetic contributors to familial keratoconus. Sci Rep. 2019;9:19406. https://doi.org/10.1038/s41598-019-55866-5.

36. Bykhovskaya Y, Li X, Epifantseva I, Haritunians T, Siscovick D, Aldave A, et al. Variation in the Lysyl oxidase (LOX) gene is associated with keratoconus in family-based and case-control studies. Invest Ophthalmol Vis Sci. 2012;53:4152–7. https://doi.org/10.1167/iovs.11-9268.

37. Burdon KP, Coster DJ, Charlesworth JC, Mills RA, Laurie KJ, Giunta C, et al. Apparent autosomal dominant keratoconus in a large Australian pedigree accounted for by digenic inheritance of two novel loci. Hum Genet. 2008;124:379–86. https://doi.org/10.1007/s00439-008-0555-z.

38. Liskova P, Hysi PG, Waseem N, Ebenezer ND, Bhattacharya SS, Tuft SJ. Errors in end matter in: evidence for keratoconus susceptibility locus on chromosome 14: a genome-wide linkage screen using single-nucleotide polymorphism markers. Arch Ophthalmol. 2010;128:1431. https://doi.org/10.1001/archophthalmol.2010.247.

39. Li X, Rabinowitz YS, Tang YG, Picornell Y, Taylor KD, Hu M, et al. Two-stage genome-wide linkage scan in keratoconus sib pair families. Invest Opthalmol Vis Sci. 2006;47:3791. https://doi.org/10.1167/iovs.06-0214.

40. Davidson AE, Borasio E, Liskova P, Khan AO, Hassan H, Cheetham ME, et al. Brittle cornea syndrome ZNF469 mutation carrier phenotype and segregation analysis of rare ZNF469 variants in familial keratoconus. Invest Ophthalmol Vis Sci. 2015;56:578–86. https://doi.org/10.1167/iovs.14-15792.

41. Stabuc-Silih M, Ravnik-Glavac M, Glavac D, Hawlina M, Strazisar M. Polymorphisms in COL4A3 and COL4A4 genes associated with keratoconus. Mol Vis. 2009;15:2848–60.

42. Li X, Bykhovskaya Y, Canedo ALC, Haritunians T, Siscovick D, Aldave AJ, et al. Genetic association of COL5A1 variants in keratoconus patients suggests a complex connection between corneal thinning and keratoconus. Invest Ophthalmol Vis Sci. 2013;54:2696–704. https://doi.org/10.1167/iovs.13-11601.

43. Segev F, He´on E, Cole WG, Wenstrup RJ, Young F, Slomovic AR, et al. Structural abnormalities of the cornea and lid resulting from collagen V mutations. Invest Opthalmol Vis Sci. 2006;47:565. https://doi.org/10.1167/iovs.05-0771.

44. Lu Y, Dimasi DP, Hysi PG, Hewitt AW, Burdon KP, Toh T, et al. Common genetic variants near the brittle cornea syndrome locus ZNF469 influence the blinding disease risk factor central corneal thickness. PLoS Genet. 2010;6:e1000947–e1000947. https://doi.org/10.1371/journal.pgen.1000947.

45. Cornes BK, Khor CC, Nongpiur ME, Xu L, Tay W-T, Zheng Y, et al. Identification of four novel variants that influence central corneal thickness in multi-ethnic Asian populations. Hum Mol Genet. 2011;21:437–45. https://doi.org/10.1093/hmg/ddr463.

46. Hoehn R, Zeller T, Verhoeven VJM, Grus F, Adler M, Wolfs RC, et al. Population-based meta-analysis in Caucasians confirms association with COL5A1 and ZNF469 but not

COL8A2 with central corneal thickness. Hum Genet. 2012;131:1783–93. https://doi.org/10. 1007/s00439-012-1201-3.

47. Gao X, Gauderman WJ, Liu Y, Marjoram P, Torres M, Haritunians T, et al. A genome-wide association study of central corneal thickness in Latinos. Invest Ophthalmol Vis Sci. 2013;54:2435–43. https://doi.org/10.1167/iovs.13-11692.

48. Vitart V, Benčić G, Hayward C, Škunca Herman J, Huffman J, Campbell S, et al. New loci associated with central cornea thickness include COL5A1, AKAP13 and AVGR8. Hum Mol Genet. 2010;19:4304–11. https://doi.org/10.1093/hmg/ddq349.

49. Burkitt Wright EMM, Spencer HL, Daly SB, Manson FDC, Zeef LAH, Urquhart J, et al. Mutations in PRDM5 in brittle cornea syndrome identify a pathway regulating extracellular matrix development and maintenance. The Am J Hum Genet. 2011;89:346. https://doi.org/ 10.1016/j.ajhg.2011.07.013.

50. Vincent AL, Jordan CA, Cadzow MJ, Merriman TR, McGhee CN. Mutations in the Zinc finger Protein gene, ZNF469, contribute to the pathogenesis of keratoconus. Invest Opthalmol Vis Sci. 2014;55:5629. https://doi.org/10.1167/iovs.14-14532.

51. Zhang W, Margines J Ben, Jacobs DS, Rabinowitz YS, Hanser EM, Chauhan T, et al. Corneal perforation after corneal cross-linking in keratoconus associated with potentially pathogenic ZNF469 mutations. Cornea 2019;38:1033–9. https://doi.org/10.1097/ICO. 0000000000002002.

52. Sahebjada S, Schache M, Richardson AJ, Snibson G, MacGregor S, Daniell M, et al. Evaluating the association between keratoconus and the corneal thickness genes in an independent Australian population. Invest Opthalmol Vis Sci. 2013;54:8224. https://doi.org/ 10.1167/iovs.13-12982.

53. Yu X, Chen B, Zhang X, Shentu X. Identification of seven novel ZNF469 mutations in keratoconus patients in a Han Chinese population. Mol Vis. 2017;23:296–305.

54. Rong SS, Ma STU, Yu XT, Ma L, Chu WK, Chan TCY, et al. Genetic associations for keratoconus: a systematic review and meta-analysis. Sci Rep. 2017;7:4620. https://doi.org/ 10.1038/s41598-017-04393-2.

55. Gordon-Shaag A, Millodot M, Shneor E, Liu Y. The genetic and environmental factors for keratoconus. BioMed Res Int. 2015;2015:795738. https://doi.org/10.1155/2015/795738.

56. Cooke Bailey JN, Hoffman JD, Sardell RJ, Scott WK, Pericak-Vance MA, Haines JL. The application of genetic risk scores in age-related macular degeneration: a review. J Clin Med. 2016;5:31. https://doi.org/10.3390/jcm5030031.

57. Shijo T, Sakurada Y, Yoneyama S, Kikushima W, Sugiyama A, Matsubara M, et al. Association between polygenic risk score and one-year outcomes following as-needed aflibercept therapy for exudative age-related macular degeneration. Pharmaceuticals (Basel, Switzerland). 2020;13:257. https://doi.org/10.3390/ph13090257.

58. Qassim A, Souzeau E, Siggs OM, Hassall MM, Han X, Griffiths HL, et al. An intraocular pressure polygenic risk score stratifies multiple primary open-angle glaucoma parameters including treatment intensity. Ophthalmology. 2020;127:901–7. https://doi.org/10.1016/j. ophtha.2019.12.025.

59. De Stefano VS, Dupps WJ Jr. Biomechanical diagnostics of the cornea. Int Ophthalmol Clin. 2017;57:75–86. https://doi.org/10.1097/IIO.0000000000000172.

60. Bykhovskaya Y, Gromova A, Makarenkova HP, Rabinowitz YS. Abnormal regulation of extracellular matrix and adhesion molecules in corneas of patients with keratoconus. Int J Keratoconus and Ectatic Corneal Dis. 2016;5:63–70. https://doi.org/10.5005/jp-journals-10025-1123.

61. Kabza M, Karolak JA, Rydzanicz M, Szcześniak MW, Nowak DM, Ginter-Matuszewska B, et al. Collagen synthesis disruption and downregulation of core elements of TGF-β, Hippo, and Wnt pathways in keratoconus corneas. Eur J Hum Genet: EJHG. 2017;25:582–90. https://doi.org/10.1038/ejhg.2017.4.

62. Nielsen K, Birkenkamp-Demtro¨der K, Ehlers N, Orntoft TF. Identification of differentially expressed genes in keratoconus epithelium analyzed on microarrays. Invest Opthalmol Vis Sci. 2003;44:2466. https://doi.org/10.1167/iovs.02-0671.

63. Rabinowitz YS, Dong L, Wistow G. Gene expression profile studies of human keratoconus cornea for NEIBank: a novel cornea-expressed gene and the absence of transcripts for aquaporin 5. Invest Opthalmol Vis Sci. 2005;46:1239. https://doi.org/10.1167/iovs.04-1148.
64. Wistow G, Bernstein SL, Wyatt MK, Behal A, Touchman JW, Bouffard G, et al. Expressed sequence tag analysis of adult human lens for the NEIBank project: over 2000 non-redundant transcripts, novel genes and splice variants. Mol Vis. 2002;8:171–84.
65. Krachmer JH, Feder RS, Belin MW. Keratoconus and related noninflammatory corneal thinning disorders. Surv Ophthalmol. 1984;28:293–322. https://doi.org/10.1016/0039-6257 (84)90094-8.
66. Sobrino T, Regueiro U, Malfeito M, Vieites-Prado A, Pérez-Mato M, Campos F, et al. Higher expression of toll-like receptors 2 and 4 in blood cells of keratoconus patiens. Sci Rep. 2017;7:12975. https://doi.org/10.1038/s41598-017-13525-7.
67. Lema I, Duran J. Inflammatory molecules in the tears of patients with keratoconus. Ophthalmology. 2005;112:654–9. https://doi.org/10.1016/j.ophtha.2004.11.050.
68. Lema I, Sobrino T, Duran JA, Brea D, Diez-Feijoo E. Subclinical keratoconus and inflammatory molecules from tears. Br J Ophthalmol. 2009;93:820–4. https://doi.org/10. 1136/bjo.2008.144253.
69. Ueta M, Kinoshita S. Ocular surface inflammation is regulated by innate immunity. Prog Retin Eye Res. 2012;31:551–75. https://doi.org/10.1016/j.preteyeres.2012.05.003.
70. Regueiro U, López-López M, Hervella P, Sobrino T, Lema I. Corneal and conjunctival alteration of innate immune expression in first-degree relatives of keratoconus patients. Graefe's Arch Clin Exp Ophthalmol. 2020;259:459–67. https://doi.org/10.1007/s00417-020-04929-9.
71. Regueiro U, Pérez-Mato M, Hervella P, Campos F, Sobrino T, Lema I. Toll-like receptors as diagnostic targets in pellucid marginal degeneration. Exp Eye Res. 2020;200:108211. https:// doi.org/10.1016/j.exer.2020.108211.
72. Davidson AE, Hayes S, Hardcastle AJ, Tuft SJ. The pathogenesis of keratoconus. Eye (Lond). 2014;28:189–95. https://doi.org/10.1038/eye.2013.278.
73. Wolle MA, Randleman JB, Woodward MA. Complications of refractive surgery: Ectasia after refractive surgery. Int Ophthalmol Clin. 2016;56:127–39. https://doi.org/10.1097/IIO. 0000000000000102.
74. Roberts CJ, Dupps WJ. Biomechanics of corneal ectasia and biomechanical treatments. J Cataract Refract Surg. 2014;40:991–8. https://doi.org/10.1016/j.jcrs.2014.04.013.
75. Heidari Z, Hashemi H, Mohammadpour M, Amanzadeh K, Fotouhi A. Evaluation of corneal topographic, tomographic and biomechanical indices for detecting clinical and subclinical keratoconus: A comprehensive three-device study. Int J Ophthalmol. 2021;14:228–39. https://doi.org/10.18240/IJO.2021.02.08.
76. Belin MW, Ambrósio RJ. Scheimpflug imaging for keratoconus and ectatic disease. Indian J Ophthalmol. 2013;61.
77. Lopes BT, Ramos IC, Salomão MQ, Guerra FP, Schallhorn SC, Schallhorn JM, et al. Enhanced tomographic assessment to detect corneal ectasia based on artificial intelligence. Am J Ophthalmol. 2018;195:223–32. https://doi.org/10.1016/j.ajo.2018.08.005.
78. Shetty R, Rao H, Khamar P, Sainani K, Vunnava K, Jayadev C, et al. Keratoconus screening indices and their diagnostic ability to distinguish normal from Ectatic corneas. Am J Ophthalmol. 2017;181:140–8. https://doi.org/10.1016/j.ajo.2017.06.031.
79. Hashemi H, Beiranvand A, Yekta A, Maleki A, Yazdani N, Khabazkhoob M. Pentacam top indices for diagnosing subclinical and definite keratoconus. J Curr Ophthalmol. 2016;28:21–6. https://doi.org/10.1016/j.joco.2016.01.009.
80. Wang YM, Chan TCY, Yu M, Jhanji V. Comparison of corneal dynamic and tomographic analysis in normal, forme fruste keratoconic, and keratoconic eyes. J Refract Surg (Thorofare, NJ: 1995) 2017;33:632–8. https://doi.org/10.3928/1081597X-20170621-09.
81. Galletti JG, Pförtner T, Bonthoux FF. Improved keratoconus detection by ocular response analyzer testing after consideration of corneal thickness as a confounding factor. J Refract

Surg (Thorofare, NJ: 1995) 2012;28:202–8. https://doi.org/10.3928/1081597X-20120103-03.

82. Fontes BM, Ambrósio RJ, Velarde GC, Nosé W. Ocular response analyzer measurements in keratoconus with normal central corneal thickness compared with matched normal control eyes. J Refract Surg (Thorofare, NJ: 1995) 2011;27:209–15. https://doi.org/10.3928/1081597X-20100415-02.

83. Zhang H, Tian L, Guo L, Qin X, Zhang D, Li L, et al. Comprehensive evaluation of corneas from normal, forme fruste keratoconus and clinical keratoconus patients using morphological and biomechanical properties. Int Ophthalmol. 2021;9. https://doi.org/10.1007/s10792-020-01679-9.

84. Fontes BM, Ambrósio R, Jardim D, Velarde GC, Nosé W. Corneal biomechanical metrics and anterior segment parameters in mild keratoconus. Ophthalmology 2010;117:673–9. https://doi.org/10.1016/j.ophtha.2009.09.023.

85. Schweitzer C, Roberts CJ, Mahmoud AM, Colin J, Maurice-Tison S, Kerautret J. Screening of forme fruste keratoconus with the ocular response analyzer. Invest Ophthalmol Vis Sci. 2010;51:2403–10. https://doi.org/10.1167/iovs.09-3689.

86. Kirgiz A, Erdur SK, Atalay K, Gurez C. The role of ocular response analyzer in differentiation of forme fruste keratoconus from corneal astigmatism. Eye Contact Lens. 2019;45:83–7. https://doi.org/10.1097/ICL.0000000000000541.

87. Galletti JD, Ruiseñor Vázquez PR, Fuentes Bonthoux F, Pförtner T, Galletti JG. Multivariate analysis of the ocular response Analyzer's corneal deformation response curve for early keratoconus detection. J Ophthalmol. 2015;2015. https://doi.org/10.1155/2015/496382.

88. Luz A, Lopes B, Hallahan KM, Valbon B, Fontes B, Schor P, et al. Discriminant value of custom ocular response analyzer waveform derivatives in forme fruste keratoconus. Am J Ophthalmol. 2016;164:14–21. https://doi.org/10.1016/j.ajo.2015.12.020.

89. Vinciguerra R, Ambrósio R, Elsheikh A, Roberts CJ, Lopes B, Morenghi E, et al. Detection of keratoconus with a new biomechanical index. J Refract Surg. 2016;32:803–10. https://doi.org/10.3928/1081597X-20160629-01.

90. Steinberg J, Amirabadi NE, Frings A, Mehlan J, Katz T, Linke SJ. Keratoconus screening with dynamic biomechanical in vivo Scheimpflug analyses: a proof-of-concept study. J Refract Surg (Thorofare, NJ: 1995) 2017;33:773–8. https://doi.org/10.3928/1081597X-20170807-02.

91. Sedaghat M-R, Momeni-Moghaddam H, Ambrósio RJ, Heidari H-R, Maddah N, Danesh Z, et al. Diagnostic ability of corneal shape and biomechanical parameters for detecting frank keratoconus. Cornea 2018;37.

92. Kataria P, Padmanabhan P, Gopalakrishnan A, Padmanaban V, Mahadik S, Ambrósio R. Accuracy of Scheimpflug-derived corneal biomechanical and tomographic indices for detecting subclinical and mild keratectasia in a South Asian population. J Cataract Refract Surg. 2019;45:328–36. https://doi.org/10.1016/j.jcrs.2018.10.030.

93. Ferreira-Mendes J, Lopes BT, Faria-Correia F, Salomão MQ, Rodrigues-Barros S, Ambrósio RJ. Enhanced ectasia detection using corneal tomography and biomechanics. Am J Ophthalmol. 2019;197:7–16. https://doi.org/10.1016/j.ajo.2018.08.054.

94. Koc M, Aydemir E, Tekin K, Inanc M, Kosekahya P, Kiziltoprak H. Biomechanical analysis of subclinical keratoconus with normal topographic, topometric, and tomographic findings. J Refract Surg (Thorofare, NJ: 1995) 2019;35:247–52. https://doi.org/10.3928/1081597X-20190226-01.

95. Chan TCY, Wang YM, Yu M, Jhanji V. Comparison of corneal tomography and a new combined tomographic biomechanical index in subclinical keratoconus. J Refract Surg (Thorofare, NJ: 1995) 2018;34:616–21. https://doi.org/10.3928/1081597X-20180705-02.

96. Luce D. Determining in vivo biomechanical properties of the cornea with an ocular response analyzer. J Cataract Refract Surg. 2005;31:156–62. https://doi.org/10.1016/j.jcrs.2004.10.044.

97. Fernández J, Rodríguez-Vallejo M, Piñero DP. Tomographic and biomechanical index (TBI) for screening in laser refractive surgery. J Refract Surg (Thorofare, NJ: 1995) 2019;35:398. https://doi.org/10.3928/1081597X-20190520-01.

98. Wilson A, Marshall J. A review of corneal biomechanics: mechanisms for measurement and the implications for refractive surgery. Indian J Ophthalmol. 2020;68:2679–90. https://doi.org/10.4103/ijo.IJO_2146_20.

99. Boyce BL, Grazier JM, Jones RE, Nguyen TD. Full-field deformation of bovine cornea under constrained inflation conditions. Biomaterials. 2008;29:3896–904. https://doi.org/10.1016/j.biomaterials.2008.06.011.

100. Whitford C, Joda A, Jones S, Bao F, Rama P, Elsheikh A. Ex vivo testing of intact eye globes under inflation conditions to determine regional variation of mechanical stiffness. Eye and Vision. 2016;3:21. https://doi.org/10.1186/s40662-016-0052-8.

101. Wilson A, Jones J, Tyrer JR, Marshall J. An interferometric ex vivo study of corneal biomechanics under physiologically representative loading, highlighting the role of the limbus in pressure compensation. Eye Vis. 2020;7:43. https://doi.org/10.1186/s40662-020-00207-1.

102. Wilson A, Jones J, Marshall J. Interferometric ex vivo evaluation of the spatial changes to corneal biomechanics introduced by topographic CXL: a pilot study. J Refract Surg. 2021;37:263–73.

103. Kling S. Optical coherence elastography by ambient pressure modulation for high-resolution strain mapping applied to patterned cross-linking. J Royal Soc Interface 2020;17. https://doi.org/10.1098/rsif.2019.0786.

104. Clayson K, Pavlatos E, Pan X, Sandwisch T, Ma Y, Liu J. Ocular pulse elastography: imaging corneal biomechanical responses to simulated ocular pulse using ultrasound. Transl Vis Sci Technol. 2020;9:5. https://doi.org/10.1167/tvst.9.1.5.

105. Fu J, Haghighi-Abayneh M, Pierron F, Ruiz PD. Depth-resolved full-field measurement of corneal deformation by optical coherence tomography and digital volume correlation. Exp Mech. 2016;56:7. https://doi.org/10.1007/s11340-016-0165-y.

106. Wilson A, Marshall J, Tyrer JR. The role of light in measuring ocular biomechanics. Eye. 2016;30:234–40. https://doi.org/10.1038/eye.2015.263.

107. Wilson A, Marshall J. A speckle interferometric technique for the evaluation of corneal biomechanics under physiological pressure variations (Conference Presentation). In: Proceedings of SPIE, vol. 10880 Opti;2019. https://doi.org/10.1117/12.2507660.

108. Elsheikh A, McMonnies CW, Whitford C, Boneham GC. In vivo study of corneal responses to increased intraocular pressure loading. Eye Vis. 2015;2:1–22. https://doi.org/10.1186/s40662-015-0029-z.

109. Scarcelli G, Pineda R, Yun SH. Brillouin optical microscopy for corneal biomechanics. Invest Ophthalmol Vis Sci. 2012;53:185–90. https://doi.org/10.1167/iovs.11-8281.

110. Wu P-J, Kabakova IV, Ruberti JW, Sherwood JM, Dunlop IE, Paterson C, et al. Water content, not stiffness, dominates Brillouin spectroscopy measurements in hydrated materials. Nat Methods. 2018;15:561–2. https://doi.org/10.1038/s41592-018-0076-1.

111. Scarcelli G, Yun SH. In vivo Brillouin optical microscopy of the human eye. Opt Express. 2012;20:9197–202.

112. Seiler TG, Shao P, Eltony A, Seiler T, Yun SH. Brillouin spectroscopy of normal and keratoconus corneas. Am J Ophthalmol. 2019;202:118–25. https://doi.org/10.1016/j.ajo.2019.02.010.

Crosslinking in Children and Down Syndrome Patients

Robert Wisse and Daniel A. Godefrooij

1 Epidemiology of Keratoconus in Children

1.1 Incidence and Prevalence of Keratoconus

Keratoconus usually occurs during the second to fourth decade of life, although cases in children have been describes as young as 4 years old [1]. The incidence in the general population is approximately 13 new case per 100.000 people per year, although this number can vary strongly depending on the patient group and ethnicity; e.g. Asian people and people from Mediterranean descent tend to have more chance of getting Keratoconus than Caucasian people who are living in the same country [2]. The prevalence of keratoconus is 1 case per 375 people in the general population. Because keratoconus can stabilize but never completely resolves, the prevalence increases with age and therefore the prevalence is lowest in children [3].

1.2 Impact of Keratoconus on Quality of Life in Children

However, keratoconus in children can have an enormous impact because an inverse relationship has been found between patient age and disease severity; on average, pediatric cases are more severe and are more likely to develop progressive keratoconus. In children, the progression of keratoconus can be both rapid and devastating. As a result, younger patients have a higher likelihood of requiring corneal grafting surgery [4]. The main goal of keratoconus treatment is to maintain good visual acuity and good quality of life. In the early stages visual acuity can be

R. Wisse (✉) · D. A. Godefrooij
Department of Ophthalmology, University Medical Center Utrecht, Utrecht, the Netherlands
e-mail: r.p.l.wisse@umcutrecht.nl

corrected with spectacles and in cases with irregular astigmatism rigid gas permeable contact lenses can restore visual acuity. However, halting the disease in an early stage to prevent dependency on visual aids is beneficial, especially in children for whom it's harder to use those visual aids. Furthermore, halting disease progression can prevent the need for a corneal transplantation [5]. When a child gets to a stage of keratoconus where a corneal transplantation is necessary the quality of life of this child is impaired for the rest of its life. This further declines when both eyes require corneal transplantation, especially when the visual results of the corneal transplantation fall into the lower end of the possible outcomes [6].

And even in milder cases the progression of keratoconus can have a significant impact on the quality of life of a child. One study demonstrated that children with progressive keratoconus scored worse on mental health related quality of life, role difficulties, peripheral vision and vision related dependency [7]. Therefore, prompt management to halt the progression of the disease is crucial in order to not only retain vison, but also quality of life.

2 Diagnostic Challenges in Children and Patients with Down Syndrome

Often, the first symptoms of keratoconus are a deterioration of vison and/or an increase in refractive error; both myopisation and an increase in cylindrical power of the contact lens or spectacles can occur. Those symptoms will often not be experienced in an early stage by children or patients with Down syndrome, especially not when the keratoconus is unilateral or strongly asymmetrical and thus gives very limited binocular symptoms. In some cases of keratoconus in patients with Down syndrome the first time that any symptoms are experienced is when an acute hydrops occurs. When patients do seek professional help from an optometrist or ophthalmologist in an early stage the first clinical signs on slit lamp investigation are relatively subtle (corneal steepening, apical thinning, Vogt's striae and a Fleischer ring) and can be overlooked—especially when a child or patient with Down syndrome is not fully cooperative.

One of earliest classification systems for keratoconus was the Amsler-Krumeich classification which is divided into 4 stages according to the severity of the disease, incorporating myopia, astigmatism, keratometry readings, corneal thickness, and the transparency of the cornea. This classification system was the standard before more advanced corneal topography devices were adopted in clinical practice. Currently, Scheimpflug imaging is widely used because it can measure the corneal curvature of both the front and the back of the corneal as well as corneal thickness on several places of the cornea and local protrusions such as the maximum keratometry which often occurs inferior of the center of the cornea in keratoconus. Automated algorithms such as the Belin/Ambrosio Enhanced Ectasia Display program assesses the likelihood that a cornea is ectatic. It uses the above mentioned measurements and compares those to a reference standard and an abnormal corneal

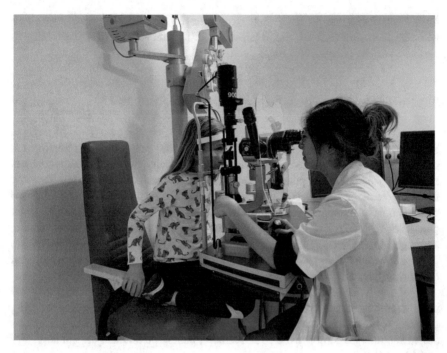

Fig. 1 A very cooperative girl behind a slit lamp who can be monitored with good precision and reliability

protrusion will automatically be highlighted as pathological [8]. However, for this type of investigation a patient is required to hold a steady focus while keeping the eye wide open for several seconds while the device projects moving lights on the cornea. When a patient is not fully cooperative the reliability drops rapidly, if any measurement can be taken at all. However, some young keratoconus patients are fully cooperative and can be monitored with the same precision and reliability as adults (see Fig. 1 of girl behind slitlamp).

In many cases of keratoconus in patients with Down syndrome it is not possible to monitor keratoconus based on corneal topography. Also, subjective complains are often not indicated clearly and subjective refraction is often not possible. In such cases the chance of progression of keratoconus should be based on the observations of caregivers indicating a deterioration in visual functioning, the amount of eye-rubbing, the age of the patient, and signs of hydrops.

It should be noted that follow-up based on auto-refraction is unreliable and should be avoided in keratoconus patients, especially when keratoconus is more advanced [9].

Because keratoconus progression in children can be more rapid than in adults, progression analysis intervals should be shorter to start with (e.g. 3 months) than analysis intervals in adults (e.g. yearly). Some authors have suggested that progression of keratoconus in children should not be awaited because the chances of (fast) progression are so large that treating at the time of diagnoses is justified without documentation of progression [10]. The indication of crosslinking in children will be discussed in more detail in the next section.

3   Indication for Crosslinking in Children

Since long, global consensus dictates that the main indication for CXL treatment is progression of keratoconus, regardless of visual acuity or age. Keratometry has traditionally been the key parameter to determine disease progression. For instance, the three seminal randomized clinical trials on CXL effectiveness based keratoconus progression on changes in keratometry readings. Keratometry is an important parameter with adequate repeatability. Keratoconus grading systems are available, although the Amsler-Krumeich classification is poorly suited for assessing disease progression, and the new ABCD grading is increasingly dependent on corneal tomography readings.

Importantly, none of the above-mentioned trials, guidelines, or grading systems incorporates extraocular factors such as eye rubbing, age, hormonal changes during pregnancy, contact lens tolerability, ethnic origin, or pericorneal diseases such as atopia and allergic conjunctivitis. Furthermore, patient preferences are not explicitly considered.

3.1   Prevent a Loss of Visual Acuity

Notwithstanding it is important to treat your patient and not a keratometry reading. The ultimate goal if crosslinking is to retain one's visual acuity and as such Quality of Vision and subsequently Quality of Life. These four concepts are inter-related, ranging from raw medical imaging data to measures of societal impact of keratoconus. Research by our group has indicated the cost-effectiveness of crosslinking for progressive keratoconus, most notably by preventing scenario's that lead to a reduced QoL later in life. The retainment of visual acuity is associated for the stabilization of many other aspects of vision, such as higher-order aberrations, contrast vision, straylight, halo's, glare and poor vision at night.

3.2   Prevent Dependencies of Visual Aids

In most keratoconus cases, visual acuity (VA) can be restored without surgery through the use of glasses; in advanced stages, specialized contact lenses may be indicated. A wide variety of CL types are currently available, including conventional soft lenses, silicone hydrogel lenses, rigidgas-permeable (RGP) corneal lenses, scleral lenses, hybrid lenses, occlusive lenses, iris print lenses, filter lenses, piggyback systems, and scleral prosthetics. Contact lenses can be a life-change aid for advanced keratoconus patients, though they come at a price: tailoring a lens to adequately fit the patient's needs requires a trained eye-care practitioner, particularly scleral lenses are costly and require yearly replacement, and poor tolerability in atopic can drastically reduce wearing times. Ample experience with various modalities in soft-, piggyback-, and scleral contact lenses in children is available and the age of the patient should not withhold a practitioner from offering these advanced lenses a priori.

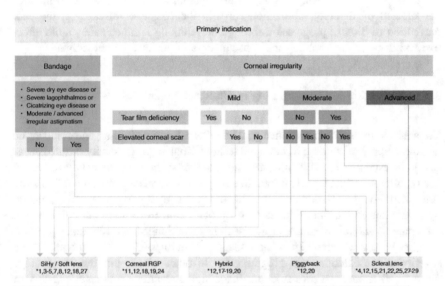

Contact lens selection algorithm. Description: A selection algorithm for selecting contact lenses for two principal medical uses: irregular astigmatism and bandage. SiHy=silicone hydrogel; RGP=rigidgas-permeable. Adapted from Visser ES et al. Cont Lens Anterior Eye. 2016, with a reference to the original publication: Visser ES, Wisse RP, Soeters N, Imhof SM, Van der Lelij A. Objective and subjective evaluation of the performance of medical contact lenses fitted using a contact lens selection algorithm. Cont Lens Anterior Eye. 2016 Aug;39(4):298-306. https://doi.org/ 10.1016/j.clae.2016.02.006. Epub 2016 Feb 23. PMID: 26917334. Mild corneal irregularity=acceptable subjective visual quality with SiHy; Moderate corneal irregularity=unacceptable subjective visual quality with SiHy, acceptable lens fit with RGP corneal; Advanced corneal irregularity=unacceptable subjective visual quality with SiHy, no acceptable lens fit with RGP corneal. Note: The grading of severe dry eye included grade IV and V based on the Oxford Index for staining and tear film break-uptime. SiHy or RGP corneal trial lenses were used to determine the grade of "mild", "moderate", or "advanced" corneal irregularity.

3.3   Prevent Surgery

Prior to the crosslinking era, more than 20% of patients ultimately may require corneal transplantation to restore VA. Both decreased visual performance and the need for corneal transplantation are associated with a significant decrease in the patient's quality of life (QoL), and its prevention proved to be the major driver of cost-effectiveness in our studies. Good news for our patients is that transplantation rates dropped considerably after the introduction of crosslinking.

Other modalities of corneal surgery, ranging from wavefront or topoguided PRK, to Intra Corneal Ring Segment implantation, to lenticular corneal implants, are affected by disease stabilization early in the course of disease. In the end, prevention of disease progression through crosslinking is much safer, more effective and cheaper than treating the consequences of advanced keratoconus.

3.3.1   Indication for Crosslinking in Children Versus Adults

Commensurate to abovementioned general criteria for crosslinking, one could argue that these apply to children in the same fashion. That is, progressivity of the disease should be established and treatment is indicated irrespective of subject age or visual acuity, after extra-ocular conditions like atopy or a vernal keratoconjunctivitis are controlled. Shetty et al. demonstrated that the treatment of peri-oculair inflammation by itself reduced the rate of keratoconus progression. In addition, all children and their parents should be educated on the risks of prolonged eye-rubbing.

It has become common knowledge that age is an important factor in both disease severity at presentation, and progressivity. In other words, children on average present with more severe keratoconus, have higher chances of disease progression, and this progression is more pronounced.

This does not imply that every pediatric patient with keratoconus should be treated, let aside bilaterally. Any surgical treatment incurs costs and risks, and there is no evidence that treatment of non-progressive keratoconus is ultimately cost-effective. Patient education on eye-rubbing is essential for disease control and treatment success. A solid identification of the patients most likely to show future disease progression is therefore helpful in deciding which patient to treat and which patient to follow-up conservatively.

3.3.2   The Factors That Determine Disease Progression

The following factors influence the rate of keratoconus progression: disease severity, age, peri-corneal inflammation such as atopia and allergic conjunctivits, eye-rubbing, hormonal changes, and potentially ethnic origin.

Assessing the need for crosslinking thus entails more than comparing topograms, even with elaborate progression analyses. Corneal topography is a reliable and reproducible anatomical imaging technique, though topograms can be variable, particularly in keratoconus, after contact lens wear, and after eye-rubbing. Your typical keratoconus patient will experience all this, making a clinical decision on one imaging parameter less reliable. Furthermore, the readings are device specific, hindering inter-device comparisons in clinical practice. From a patient perspective a topogram is merely an intermediate endpoint: patients experience changes in quality of vision, where visual acuity is the most common denominator. High-contrast visual acuity testing has limitations, but it is embedded in clinical practice and therefore the most practical proxy of visual functioning. Age is considered (and proven) as a surrogate of corneal biome- chanics owingto lower rates of disease progression at increasing age. Inversely, younger cases are in general more severe, and higher rates of disease progression are reported.

3.3.3 The DUtch Crosslinking for Keratoconus (DUCK) Score

Efforts to improve patient selection for any health intervention should focus on reducing overtreatment while preventing undertreatment. The ultimate aim is to reduce exposure to potential health risks associated with unnecessary treatments and to improve overall cost effectiveness. Analogous to existing algorithms that aid in clinical decision making such as the Glasgow Coma Scale score or Apgar score, the DUtch Crosslinking for Keratoconus (DUCK) score was conceptualized as an easy-to-use compound score to assess disease progression in keratoconus. The DUCK score is an assessment tool that provides quick insight in disease activity. It incorporates age, patient- reported quality of vision, objective visual acuity, manifest refraction, and keratometry [11].

Cutoff points for age were therefore chosen at younger than 18 years, 18 to 35 years, and older than 35 years. Quality of vision is arguably the most relevant ophthalmic parameter from a patient perspective. However, its quantification is cumbersome, and the association between patient-reported outcomes and refractive state is subject of debate. Uncorrected distance visual acuity (UDVA) was con- sidered the most sensitive parameter for changes in visual functioning for several reasons. First and foremost, early keratoconus can be corrected with glasses. Cases of progressive keratoconus amenable to a phoropter/spectacle correction would lead to a stable corrected distance visual acuity assessment and thus yield no viable data on keratoconus disease progression. A confounding effect of developing axial myopia on UDVA was considered negligible, based on the relatively short interval in measurements (12 months) and the age of typical keratoconus patients (older than 13 years; the Sorsby criterion).

Likewise, maximum keratometry was considered the most relevant reading for changes in keratometry because of its intrinsic volatility in progressive keratoconus with adequate repeatability and its widespread use in clinical trials and treatment guidelines. Alternative tomographic parameters either change less pronounced (corneal pachymetry, mean keratometry) or are less embedded in clinical practice (posterior curvature).

Changes in manifest refractive error were converted to spherical equivalents because both spherical and cylindrical power can increase with disease progression [6]. Patient-reported subjective quality of vision was scored as 0 (no complaints), 1 (complaints mildly affecting quality of life), or 2 (complaints severely affecting quality of life). All other domains were also scored 0, 1, or 2 points based on predefined cutoffs motivated by clinical experience and existing literature (Table 1). This leads to a DUCK score range of 0–10 points, with 10 indicating the highest rate of disease progression. According to current practice, differences were calculated by subtracting follow-up measurements from baseline measurements. This of course after controlling peri-ocular inflammation and educating on eye-rubbing risks.

In a multicenter clinical validation study, a total of 504 eyes of 388 patients were available for analysis on disease progression in the course of 12 and 24 months. Adhering to the DUCK score, rather than maximum keratometry, was associated with a reduction in overall treatment rate by 23% (95% CI, 18–30%), without increasing the risk of disease progression (ie, the rate of progression for both groups was equal; 0%). The DUCK score appears to better identify eyes that were duly

Table 1 The DUCK score[a]

Variable	Score 0	Score 1	Score 2
Age, y	>35	18–35	<18
Quality of vision	No impact on daily life	Mild impact on daily life	Severe impact on daily life
UDVA difference, Snellen line	<1	1–2	>2
Refraction difference (EE), D	<0.5	0.5–1.0	51.0
Maximum keratometry differs nee, D	<1	1–2	>2

Abbreviations D—diopter; DUCK—Dutch Crosslinking tor Keratoconus; SE—spherical equivalent; UDVA—uncorrected distance visual acuity.

[a]To assess differences, parameters should be documented at 2 separate moments. Always control extraocular inflammation and advise not to rub the eyes prior to treatment. A Duck score more than b indicates a crosslinking treatment tor progressive Keratoconus

withheld treatment by 35% (95% CI, 22–49%). Albeit this study was performed in adults, the outcomes relate to children equally. The DUCK methodology does not specifically state the interval between two measurements, as one might review a pediatric cases of the course over several months.

4   Indication for Crosslinking in Down Syndrome

The management of keratoconus in Down has overlap with pediatric keratoconus cases, particularly regarding diagnostic and therapeutic challenges. We therefore felt this specific group deserves mention in this book chapter.

4.1   Impact of Visual Acuity on QoL in Down Population

Keratoconus has long since been linked with Down syndrome. Reports show a 0.5–15% incidence of keratoconus in patients with Down syndrome, which is much higher than in the general population. The role of trisomy 21 in developing keratoconus remains somewhat unclear. A nonparametric linkage analysis suggested that a gene on chromosome 21 could be related to keratoconus, but this finding was never confirmed. Genetic studies have not yet deciphered the complex genetic architecture of keratoconus. This is perhaps in part due to differential distribution of the risk loci among ethnic populations or the relatively low contribution of genetic variants in developing keratoconus.

4.2   Late Referrals

Patients with Down syndrome often do not complain about their vision. Instead, the ailment is typically noticed by others in their environment due to changed behavior, resulting in a diagnosis in a more advanced disease state. Not seldom is a corneal hydrops the presenting sign of a keratoconus. The management of keratoconus in patients with Down syndrome varies, depending on the severity of keratoconus and the degree of Down syndrome characteristics.

As with all keratoconus cases, the overarching goal of crosslinking is to retain visual acuity and as such quality of vision. Therefore, when visual acuity already is severely compromised, the added benefit of a crosslinking treatment is reduced. This applies in particular for Down patients who present with a corneal hydrops, where not only visual acuity is compromised, but the scarred cornea is a contra-indication for crosslinking by itself. Importantly, the contralateral eye could be a very suitable candidate for crosslinking! The patients visual functioning now potentially depends on the non-hydrops eye. Loss of this vision has detrimental effects on self-reliance, independence, and quality of life.

4.3   Lack of Alternatives for Optimal Functioning

Another argument for a low threshold to offer crosslinking treatment in non-hydrops Down cases is that their alternatives for the amelioration of visual acuity are less accessible than for the regular patient. Naturally, this depends on the intellectual and behavioural capacities of the individual, but the adoption rate of scleral contact lenses is considered rather low. Virtual no literature or reports can be found on contact lens fitting in Down patients, a harbinger of poor suitability.

Performing a corneal transplantation in patients with Down syndrome entails considerable risks, and this surgery has a worse prognosis than other patients with keratoconus.

4.4   Diagnostic Challenges

Poor compliance and suboptimal adherence to instructions will lead to less then optimal data collection in Down patients. Particularly the corneal topography can prove a significant challenge. Therefore the clinician should check for clinical signs of keratoconus to establish the diagnosis (Munson sign, Fleischer ring, Stria, signs of previous corneal hydrops, floppy or lax eyelids, scissoring on retinoscopy). Signs of an active or previous hydrops can point toward a good indication for treatment in the contralateral eye. Observe the patient in behavior: is there eye-rubbing, does your patient understand verbal instructions, can you make eye-contact, and are topical eyedrops tolerated? In addition the clinician should judge the social environment and care-givers of the patient. Will these be able to deliver the required care after crosslinking, in particularly administer eyedrops, and duly make contact in case of emergency.

General (preop) assessment			
Spectacle tolerance		Yes	No
Eye contact		Yes	No
Verbal communication		Yes	No
Adequate Pentacam measurement		Yes	No
Treatment assessment			
Abrupt movements	With head	No	Yes
	With legs	No	Yes
	With arms	No	Yes
Passes 5-min supine position and fixation test		Yes	No
Can tolerate anaesthetic eye drop		Yes	No
Can tolerate eyelid touch		Yes	No
After-care assessment			
Eye rubbing		No	Yes
Follows instructions adequately		Yes	No
Cooperative parents/care givers		Yes	No
General impression		Good	Bad

Standardized clinical decision tool to judge the subject suitability of Down syndrome patients for a corneal crosslinking treatment under local anaesthesia

4.5 Therapeutic Challenges

Patients with Down syndrome show higher risks during general anaesthesia (bradycardia, natural air- way obstruction, difficult intubation, post-intubation croup, and bronchospasm); therefore, it is advisable to consider CXL under local anaesthesia. The abovementioned semi-structured scoring form on patient compliance and behavior is a helpful tool to assess whether Down patients are suitable for a treatment under local anaesthesia. A sedative administered 30 minutes prior to the treatment will relieve anxiety and abrupt movements. Naturally, many Down patients are not suitable for treatment under local anaesthesia. When performing crosslinking under general anaesthesia, we prefer to treat both eyes in one treatment to reduce the risks and costs of (repeated) anaesthesia.

It is desirable to halt keratoconus progression in an earlier stage and greatly minimize the need for future corneal surgery. To this end, corneal crosslinking is a minimally invasive procedure with an excellent safety profile: it has a low rate of vision threatening complications such as keratitis or corneal haze formation. A large retrospective series (N = 2550) identified significant higher risks for haze formation and sterile infiltrates in Down patients after CXL. In the early beginnings of crosslinking, devastating infectious complications after crosslinking in Down patients have been reported, and Down patients are prone to intractable eye-rubbing. A powerful method to prevent eye-rubbing and subsequent inoculation of the abraded cornea are *bilateral elbow plaster casts*. The surgeons plasterer can fit removable casts (with Velcro) prior to surgery, potentially when doing the pre-operative screening by ophthalmologist and anaesthesiologist. The casts are fixed after crosslinking, and removed after the corneal epithelium is completely healed.

Another clinical suggestion is to administer a subtenonal long-acting block (e.g. with levobupivacaine 5 mg/ml or lidocaine 10 mg/ml, ∼4 cc) after the laser treatment is finished. This approximately gives 3–6 hours of excellent pain control. Cave: a block will lead to mydriasis and should not be administered prior to the crosslinking treatment.

The specific effectiveness of both accelerated and conventional crosslinking has been prospectively investigated, and clinical outcomes do not deviate materially from other patient groups. Interestingly, here also accelerated crosslinking proved somewhat less powerful than conventional crosslinking regarding corneal flattening.

5 Therapeutic Challenges in Children and Patients with Down Syndrome

5.1 In-Office Preparations for Crosslinking in Children

Crosslinking is considered a standardized procedure which can be delegated to allied healthcare personnel such as nurse practitioners, optometrists or any other comparable functionary, if local regulation allows such. As in any ophthalmic procedure under local anesthesia, the cooperation of the patient is an important factor for a successful and safe procedure. In children, this requires attention and dedication by all the staff involved in the procedure. Both children and parents need to be at ease, with any pressing issues resolved: appointments in order, medication already stand by, basic knowledge of what to expect etc. etc. When properly addressed, pediatric crosslinking can be as predictable as a routine treatment in adults. Most children receiving crosslinking are old enough to understand the procedure and to be cooperative throughout the procedure. Poor compliance during the pre-operative exams, or a profound anxiety, can be indicative of poor compliance during the treatment.

Pearls for a smooth crosslinking procedure in children:

- Involve the child in clinical decision making. Talk to them, not over them, and ask on their opinion. You are legally required to do so (see below)
- Address particular questions and anxiety. Make them acquainted with the procedure, for instance by letting them touch and feel the speculum in office;
- A failed treatment due to lack of cooperation is a disappointment for all, but not the end of the world. A positive framing is that together you tried to prevent much more invasive general anaesthesia;
- The mental state of the parent reflects on the child. Address pressing issues, be it technicalities on appointment planning or particular anxieties on what to expect. Needless to say, 90% of this should have been done in the pre-operative consultations.

Informed consent for the treatment of children (and incapacitated patients):

The following abstract by De Lourdes Levy et al. is a practical synopsis, and applies to treatment decision in incapacitated patients (e.g. Down syndrome) as well. "Informed consent means approval of the legal representative of the child and/ or of the competent child for medical interventions following appropriate information. National legal regulations differ in regard to the question when a child has the full right to give his or her autonomous consent. Informed assent means a child's agreement to medical procedures in circumstances where he or she is not legally authorized or lacks sufficient understanding for giving consent competently. Doctors should carefully listen to the opinion and wishes of children who are not able to give full consent and should strive to obtain their assent. Doctors have the responsibility to determine the ability and competence of the child for giving his or her consent or assent. All children, even those not judged as competent, have a right to receive information given in a way that they can understand and give their assent or dissent."

Please consult your local legal advisor on the applicability of below mentioned statements. Based on our (Dutch) experience please consider the following.

- A child younger than 12 years of age has the right of information, but the legal representatives give consent to a treatment
- A child older than 16 years of age has the right of in consent, and the child may effectively refuse treatments that will not necessarily save their lives or prevent serious harm. If serious harm is expected by refusing treatment, the doctor has the duty to act in the best interest of the child.
- For children between 12 and 16 years of age consent should be acquired from both parents/representatives and the child.
- Normally, the child will be accompanied by its parents. Still, ascertain that the accompanying adult is actually the legal representative of the child, and in case only one parent is present, actively ask for the consent of the other parent. Particularly Down syndrome patients are frequently accompanied by

professional caregivers (e.g. a homecare nurse), who not necessarily are the legal representative, nor have the right to give informed consent. A follow-up telephonic conversation with the duly legal representative to obtain informed consent often from a family member, is considered the responsibility of the doctor.

5.2 Crosslinking Under Local Anesthesia: Choice of Treatment Modality

The clinician should always weigh the expected results and risks of a treatment. In our institution, we performed a head-to-head clinical trial in adults on trans-epithelial crosslinking and epi-off crosslinking, and found TE-CXL much less powerful in halting disease progression. Other studies reported the contrary, and we agree that the post-operative pain and infectious risks are the major downsides of crosslinking. Notwithstanding, current biological and clinical evidence indicate underperforming of TE-CXL, and therefore we advise to also treat children with conventional epithelium-off CXL.

5.3 Pain Management in Children

A prospective 3-armed study (n = 60) on post-operative pain management demonstrated clinical equivalence of the regimes in combating postoperative pain after routine CXL. Here, the effectiveness of bandage contact lenses, occlusive patching, and antibiotic ointment only was compared, in terms of post-operative pain and wound healing. Wound healing appeared quicker in the occlusive patch group (non-significant effect) and therefore might be the best standard of care after CXL. The clinical tradition of using bandage contact lenses should at least be questioned: we never put in contact lenses. This makes the post-operative visit slightly easier, particularly in anxious children or incapacitated Down patients [12].

Postoperative pain is managed conservatively with paracetamol max 60 mg/kg/day divided over 4 doses, with a minimum time in between of 6 hours. Effectively, we routinely prescribe paracetamol 500 mg 4 times daily. In addition, we prescribe oral NSAIDs: diclofenac 1–3 mg/kg/day divided over 3 doses, with a maximum dosing of 150 mg/day. Effectively, we routinely prescribe diclofenac 50 mg 2 times daily, with a dosage reduction to 25 mg 2 times daily when the child is <40 kg. When this resulted in insufficient reduction of pain, oxycodone (10 mg, 1–3 per day) is prescribed as rescue medication.

To some shock, our study also highlighted that the actual dosing of pain medication was far from the proposed *pain ladder.*In particular, paracetamol was under-used, and oxycodone over-used. Careful and repeated instructions of your patients will reduce the amount of post-operative pain due to inadvertent non-compliance, and increase overall medication safety.

5.4 Therapeutic Challenges in Down Syndrome

Patients with Down syndrome show higher risks during general anaesthesia (bradycardia, natural air- way obstruction, difficult intubation, post-intubation croup, and bronchospasm); therefore, it is advisable to consider CXL under local anaesthesia. The abovementioned semi-structured scoring form on patient compliance and behavior is a helpful tool to assess whether Down patients are suitable for a treatment under local anaesthesia. A sedative administered 30 minutes prior to the treatment will relieve anxiety and abrupt movements. Naturally, many Down patients are not suitable for treatment under local anaesthesia. When performing crosslinking under general anaesthesia, we prefer to treat both eyes in one treatment to reduce the risks and costs of (repeated) anaesthesia.

It is desirable to halt keratoconus progression in an earlier stage and greatly minimize the need for future corneal surgery. To this end, corneal crosslinking is a minimally invasive procedure with an excellent safety profile: it has a low rate of vision threatening complications such as keratitis or corneal haze formation. A large retrospective series (N = 2550) identified significant higher risks for haze formation and sterile infiltrates in Down patients after CXL. In the early beginnings of crosslinking, devastating infectious complications after crosslinking in Down patients have been reported, and Down patients are prone to intractable eye-rubbing. A powerful method to prevent eye-rubbing and subsequent inoculation of the abraded cornea are *bilateral elbow plaster casts*. The surgeons plasterer can fit removable casts (with Velcro) prior to surgery, potentially when doing the pre-operative screening by ophthalmologist and anaesthesiologist. The casts are fixed after crosslinking, and removed after the corneal epithelium is completely healed. See Fig. 2.

As mentioned before, we do not use bandage contact lenses in our routine crosslinking cases, nor for patients with Down Syndrome. This eliminates the need to remove those after crosslinking, which can be quite burdensome in an uncooperative individual.

Another clinical suggestion is to administer a subtenonal long-acting block (e.g. with levobupivacaine 5 mg/ml or lidocaine 10 mg/ml, ~4 cc) after the laser treatment is finished. This approximately gives 3–6 hours of excellent pain control. Cave: a block will lead to mydriasis and should not be administered prior to the crosslinking treatment.

The specific effectiveness of both accelerated and conventional crosslinking has been prospectively investigated, and clinical outcomes do not deviate materially from other patient groups. Interestingly, here also accelerated crosslinking proved

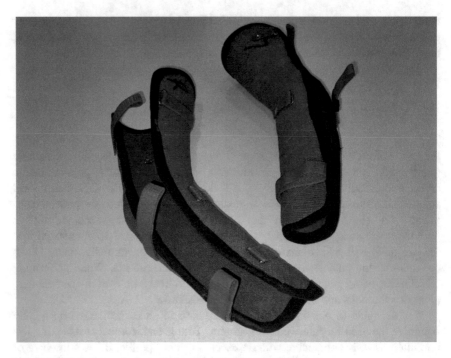

Fig. 2 Bilateral elbow plaster casts for the right (R) and left (L) arm

somewhat less powerful than conventional crosslinking regarding corneal flattening.

6   Treatment Efficacy and Long-Term Follow-Up of Pediatric Crosslinking

6.1   Various CXL Treatment Protocols

6.1.1   Conventional Versus Modified CXL

The original crosslinking protocol included the removal of the central corneal epithelium, application of riboflavin 0.1% as a photosensitizer and an irradiation time of 30 minutes using 370 nm ultraviolet-A (UVA) light with an irradiance of 3 mW/cm^2. This protocol is commonly referred to as the Dresden protocol. Adaptations of this protocol aimed at avoiding the need for epithelium removal (transepithelial CXL) and shortening the treatment time (accelerated CXL). This was attempted in order to prevent postoperative pain and the risk of infection due to epithelium removal and to circumvent the need for the patient to lie still for an extended period of time. This is especially relevant for children because the tolerance of pain and the ability to lie still are usually less at this age. However, so far the efficacy of transepithelial CXL in halting the progression of keratoconus is inferior to CXL with epithelial removal when comparing keratometry values. This is mostly due to the fact that the inability of riboflavin to pass through the intact epithelium. A method that aims to circumvent the removal of the epithelium while enabling the riboflavin to penetrate the cornea stroma is iontophoresis-assisted transepithelial CXL. However, interest in this treatment has diminished since it has been demonstrated to be less effective than standard CXL with epithelium removal in a head-to-head comparison.

Over the years many smaller and larger adaptations from the Dresden protocol have been used and investigated including the abovementioned transepithelial treatment and accelerated treatment. Also, different riboflavin solutions have been used of which not all the treatment effects were comparable. Figure 3 displays the treatment effect of a combination of different ribovlavin solutions, accelerated crosslining and transepithelial crosslinking in adult keratoconus patients. Note the much larger spread of the crosslinking treatment effect on maximum keratometry compared to mean keratometry.

Another modification of the conventional crosslinking protocol is pulsed CXL. During photosensitization, oxygen in the corneal stroma is an important component of the chemical reactions. In accelerated CXL protocols where the irradiation time is markedly reduced, it is thought that there may be insufficient time for replenishment of oxygen levels in the stroma, leading to decreased treatment efficacy. Therefore, by pulsing the UVA irradiation during the exposure time allows oxygen to diffuse deeper into the corneal stroma during pauses in the UVA, which may increase the treatment depth and the resultant corneal stiffening. Although the depth of treatment might be deeper in rabbit corneas, the clinical results in terms of refractive and tomographic results appear to be inferior.

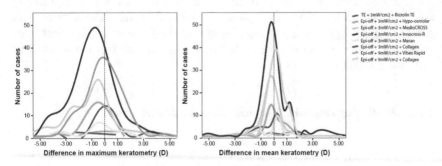

Fig. 3 Distribution of maximum keratometry (Kmax) and mean keratometry (Kmean) measured in in keratoconus patients one year after treatment with the indicated treatment modalities. The difference in Kmax (**a**) and Kmean (**b**) indicates the relative change in values between baseline) and 12 months after treatment. The diagram legend displays the composition of the eight different treatment modalities. TE = transepithelial; Epi-off = epithelium-off

6.2   Topography-Guided CXL

A treatment protocol that has the potential to replace the standard CXL protocol is topography-guided CXL. The rationale of this treatment is that CXL can be altered based on each individual's cone shape; the ultraviolet light intensity is augmented based on the corneal topography which can result in more flattening of the ectatic area of the cornea. Topography-guided CXL has led to superior results in corneal flattening, spherical equivalent and visual acuity after 12 months compared to standard CXL in a randomized controlled trial. However, those studies were executed in adults and it is plausible but not certain that those results can be applied to pediatric keratoconus.

6.2.1   Long Term Results and Treatment Failure

Cohort studies up to 7.5 years have been reported on epithelium off crosslinking for pediatric keratoconus. In one study on 20 pediatric eyes keratometry values stabilized and corrected distance visual acuity improved while no eyes lost any lines of corrected distance visual acuity while no complications were observed. In another study on 54 pediatric eyes average keratometry, uncorrected distance visual acuity and corrected distance visual acuity on average improved. However, one eye with pre-operative corrected distance visual acuity of 1.2 (Snellen) deteriorated to 0.9 and 0.8 at the one-year and two-year follow-up visits, respectively; this decline in corrected distance visual acuity was due to persistent haze. Furthermore, 12 eyes (22%) showed progression by the time of the last follow-up visit leading to the suggestion that progression after crosslinking might be more common in a pediatric population. Interestingly, none of these patients suffered a decline of one or more Snellen lines. The authors concluded that the underlying cause of progression was a more decentralized cone those pediatric patients due to less UV light exposure of the peripheral cornea with a UV light source centered on the center of the cornea. Most novel UV light sources designed after this study spread the UV light more uniformly over the cornea, potentially preventing the under-treatment of more decentralized cones.

6.2.2   Strategies Towards Repeated CXL Treatment

Retreatment with CXL in case of persistent progression of keratoconus after initial CXL is controversial and the evidence of this procedure is limited. The evidence consists mostly on case reports and small case series.

6.3   Pseudo-Progression Versus Real Progression

The classical definition of progression of keratoconus was an increase of maximum keratometry of >1.0 D in 2 consecutive measurements—using the same imaging method—during a time interval of 12 months. However, it should be noted that the repeatability of keratometry readings vastly inreases when keratoconus is more advanced. In keratoconic cornea's with maximum keratometry readings below 50.0 D the measurement error is approximately 0.4 D, but in keratoconic cornea's with maximum keratometry readings above 55.0 D the measurement error would increase to 1.7 D. When taking this into account the criterion for (repeated) CXL treatment in case of a maximum keratometry increase of >1.0 D in 2 consecutive measurements is clearly irrational. The authors of a perspective on retreatment article make a useful distinction between pseudo-progression and real progression. Pseudo-progression is a situation in which keratometry values deteriorate without actual keratoconus progression. Apart from measurement errors in keratometry values the authors name superficial punctate keratopathy, corneal stromal scarring, use of contact lenses and even vernal or atopic keratoconjunctivitis as possible causes of pseudo-progression. Therefore, indicating repeated CXL at times of superficial punctate keratopathy or vernal or atopic keratoconjunctivitis is not advisable. One of the strategies to prevent diagnosing real progression in cases of pseudo-progression would be to make multiple cornea topographic measurements separated in time to reduce the measurement error. Although this strategy might be useful in patients using spectacle correction or no refractive correction at all, this strategy is less attractive in patients who are dependent on (rigid) contact lens correction for their visual rehabilitation. Patients who wear (rigid) contact lenses are advised not to wear their lenses one or a several weeks before corneal topography measurements, making multiple measurements separated in time unattractive. The effect of contact lens wear on corneal curvature and pachemetry can be significant; directly after scleral lens removal, the average maximum keratometry was 1.1 D lower compared to ≥ 1 week after scleral lens removal in 20 keratoconus eyes of 14 patients. Furthermore, the average keratometry value was 0.7 D lower. As stated earlier in this chapter assessing the need for crosslinking thus entails more than comparing topograms, even with elaborate progression analyses.

Since the evidence for the efficacy of repeated CXL in cases of progression after CXL treatment is limited, the ideal strategy for progression after CXL treatment is simply unknown. We advise to incorporate more factors than keratometry only in this clinical decision, such as the age of the patient, the patient- reported quality of vision, the objective visual acuity and the manifest refraction—which were already discussed in the section on indication for (initial) crosslinking above. Repeated-CXL seems to be a safe procedure based on the relatively small case series that have been published.

Acknowledgements We would kindly like to thank Julia Wisse and Hannah Hardjosantoso for their participation in the beautiful slit lamp photograph.

References

1. Gunes A, Tok L, Tok Ö, Seyrek L. The youngest patient with bilateral keratoconus secondary to chronic persistent eye rubbing. Semin Ophthalmol. 2015;30(5–6):454–6.https://doi.org/10.3109/08820538.2013.874480.Epub 2014 Feb 7 PMID: 24506444.
2. Pearson AR, Soneji B, Sarvananthan N, Sandford-Smith JH. Does ethnic origin influence the incidence or severity of keratoconus? Eye (Lond). 000;14(4):625–8.
3. Godefrooij DA, de Wit GA, Uiterwaal CS, Imhof SM, Wisse RP. Age-specific incidence and prevalence of keratoconus: a nationwide registration study. Am J Ophthalmol. 2017; 175:169–172. https://doi.org/10.1016/j.ajo.2016.12.015.Epub 2016 Dec 28 PMID: 28039037.
4. Al Suhaibani AH, Al-Rajhi AA, Al-Motowa S, et al. Inverse relationship between age and severity and sequelae of acute corneal hydrops associated with keratoconus. Br J Ophthalmol. 2007;91:984–5.
5. Godefrooij DA, Mangen MJ, Chan E, O'Brart DPS, Imhof SM, de Wit GA, Wisse RPL. Cost-effectiveness analysis of corneal collagen crosslinking for progressive keratoconus. Ophthalmology. 2017;124(10):1485–95. https://doi.org/10.1016/j.ophtha.2017.04.011. Epub 2017 May 19 PMID: 28532974.
6. Godefrooij DA, de Wit GA, Mangen MJ, Wisse RP. Comment on 'Cost effectiveness of collagen crosslinking for progressive keratoconus in the UK NHS'. Eye (Lond). 2016;30 (8):1150–2. https://doi.org/10.1038/eye.2016.82. Epub 2016 Apr 22. PMID: 27101748; PMCID: PMC4985680.
7. Steinberg J, Bußmann N, Frings A, Katz T, Druchkiv V, Linke SJ. Quality of life in stable and progressive 'early-stage' keratoconus patients. Acta Ophthalmol. 2020. https://doi.org/10.1111/aos.14564. Epub ahead of print. PMID: 32914586.
8. Olivo-Payne A, Abdala-Figuerola A, Hernandez-Bogantes E, Pedro-Aguilar L, Chan E, Godefrooij D. Optimal management of pediatric keratoconus: challenges and solutions. Clin Ophthalmol. 2019;13:1183–91.https://doi.org/10.2147/OPTH.S183347.PMID:31371915; PMCID:PMC6628904.
9. N Soeters MB Muijzer J Molenaar DA Godefrooij RPL Wisse 2018 Autorefraction versus manifest refraction in patients with keratoconus J Refract Surg 34 1 30 34 https://doi.org/10.3928/1081597X-20171130-01 PMID: 29315439
10. N Chatzis F Hafezi 2012 Progression of keratoconus and efficacy of pediatric [corrected] corneal collagen cross-linking in children and adolescents J Refract Surg 28 11 753 758 https://doi.org/10.3928/1081597X-20121011-01.Erratum.In:JRefractSurg.2013Jan;29(1):72 PMID: 23347367
11. Wisse RPL, Simons RWP, van der Vossen MJB, Muijzer MB, Soeters N, NuijtsRMMA, Godefrooij DA. Clinical evaluation and validation of the dutch crosslinking for keratoconus score. JAMAOphthalmol. 2019 Jun 1;137(6):610–616. https://doi.org/10.1001/jamaophthalmol.2019.0415. PMID: 30920597; PMCID:PMC6567860.
12. Soeters N, Hendriks I,Godefrooij DA, Mensink MO, Wisse RPL. Prospective 3-arm study on pain and epithelial healing after cornealcrosslinking. J Cataract Refract Surg. 2020 Jan;46 (1):72–77. https://doi.org/10.1016/j.jcrs.2019.08.036. PMID: 32050235.

Accelerated Crosslinking: The New Epithelium-Off

Frederik Raiskup and Robert Herber

One major disadvantage of the standard corneal crosslinking (S-CXL) procedure so far is the long total treatment time of 1 hour in case of considering only "pure incision-suture" time. Taking into account the time of patient´s preparation before the procedure and follow-up of patient immediately after the crosslinking, is the duration of the actual personnel engagement in only one case even longer than one hour. Therefore, in order to increase patient's comfort and the surgeon's workflow in a clinical practice, a shorter CXL procedure would be desirable.

1 Theoretical Approach and in Vitro Evidence of Efficacy of Accelerated CXL

According to the photochemical law of reciprocity (Bunsen-Roscoe law), the same photochemical effect can be achieved with reduced illumination time and correspondingly increased irradiation intensity, meaning that 10-minute irradiation at 9.0 mW/cm^2 (A-CXL(9*10)), 5-minute irradiation at 18.0 mW/cm^2 (A-CXL (18*5)) and 3-minute irradiation at 30 mW/cm^2 (A-CXL(30*3)), should provide the same effect obtained with a 30-minute irradiation at 3.0 mW/cm^2 (S-CXL (3*30)), all delivering 5.4 J/cm^2 of energy [1].

In 2011, Schumacher et al. published an experimental study that used higher intensity and a shorter treatment time and showed an equivalent result in the biomechanical stability of the corneal stroma with S-CXL (3*30) and A-CXL (9*10). Using stress–strain measurements in porcine corneas, they found a similar increase in stiffness in both groups [1]. In an in vitro study using different irradi-

F. Raiskup (✉) · R. Herber
Department of Ophthalmology, C.G. Carus University Hospital, TU Dresden, Fetscherstr. 74, 01307 Dresden, Germany
e-mail: frederik.raiskup@uniklinikum-dresden.de

119

ances (2, 3, 9, 15 mW/cm^2 continuously and 15 mW/cm^2 fractionated with alternate cycles of 30 s "on" and 30 s "off"), Krueger et al. found comparable efficacy in stiffening corneal collagen with the standard method and methods that achieved equivalent exposure of 5.4 J/cm^2. They used extensiometry to determine the stiffness and strength of treated porcine corneas [2].

A large ex vivo study investigated the efficacy of CXL at higher intensities and corneal stiffness changes to irradiances between 3 mW/cm^2 and 90 mW/cm^2 with illumination times between 30 minutes and 1 minute, respectively. Their results showed that the Bunsen-Roscoe reciprocity law is valid only for illumination intensities up to 40–50 mW/cm^2 with illumination longer than 2 minutes. At higher intensities and shorter duration, the stiffness could rapidly decrease [3].

Hafezi et al. observed even more pronounced decreased stiffening effect with increasing UV-A intensity. Young's modulus at 10% strain showed significant differences between 3 mW/cm^2 and used higher UV-A intensities (9 and 18 mW/cm^2). The biomechanical effect of CXL decreased significantly when using high irradiance and short irradiation time settings. These results confirmed authors' hypothesis that intrastromal oxygen diffusion capacity and increased oxygen consumption associated with higher irradiances may be a limiting factor leading to reduced treatment efficiency [4].

In addition, Bao et al. investigated different CXL protocols using inflation tests. They found that the shorter the treatment time, the lower is the stiffening effect at 4% strain (lower strain than the one used in Young's modulus). This strain level corresponds with the physiological strain of the cornea at regular IOP conditions [5, 6]. In extensiometry (stress–strain measurements) at the same strain level (4%), S-CXL was significantly more effective in stiffening than A-CXL (18*5). However, A-CXL (9*10) increased corneal stiffness significantly compared to controls. Similar findings could obtained using air-puff tonometry (Corvis ST, Oculus, Wetzlar, Germany) ex vivo, where S-CXL changed corneal biomechanical related parameters (DCR parameters) more effective than A-CXL protocols, however, no significance was achieved. Significant alteration were observed in all used protocols for specific DCR parameters before and after CXL indicating corneal stiffening [7].

1.1 Surgical Procedure

Considering the results of experimental studies, we decided to use for our clinical setting in patients with progressive keratoconus an accelerated protocol UV-intensity of 9 mW/cm^2 for 10 minutes. As a riboflavin solution we use 0.1% riboflavin in 1.1% hydroxypropylmethylcellulose (HPMC). The recent ex vivo animal experiments with porcine corneas measuring riboflavin concentration gradient in the anterior corneal stroma showed, that riboflavin concentration decreased with increasing depth and increased with longer application times. In the deep layers of corneal stroma yielded HPMC-assisted riboflavin imbibition high concentrations [8].

The HPMC-assisted imbibition of corneal stroma leads to a mild tissue swelling and that's why it is suitable as a first choice riboflavin solution option also for a treatment of corneas with thickness after epithelial removal is slightly under 400 μm (up to 380 μm). If the corneal thickness is after epithelial removal under 380 μm, we use hypoosmolar riboflavin solution [9].

The crosslinking procedure is performed in an outpatient service. Thirty minutes before the procedure, pain medication is administered and if necessary also tranquilizers. The procedure is conducted under sterile conditions in operating room. After topical anesthesia of proxymetacaine hydrochloride 0.5% (Proparakain-POS, URSAPHARM, Saarbrücken, Germany) eyedrops is administered, lid speculum is applied, corneal thickness measured and the corneal epithelium is removed in a central 8-mm–diameter area with a hockey-knife or an Epi-Bowman Keratectomy knife (EBK). The EBK aims to alter the Bowman layer less than a conventional hockey knife. A study by Shetty et al. found a smoother Bowman layer after debridement and therefore a significant faster recovery of the epithelium and less pain after CXL compared to a hockey knife [10]. We could support these findings by our own clinical experience over a cohort of around 100 patients. After measuring the corneal thickness again, is 0.1% riboflavin solution in HPMC instilled every minute for 15 minutes. After this period of time is the riboflavin solution layer removed from the corneal surface with a lancet sponge (Pro-ophta, Lohmann&Rauscher International GmbH & Co.KG, Rengsdorf, Germany) and the corneal thickness is measured again to prove, that corneal thickness before irradiation is above 400 μm. When required, a hypoosmolar riboflavin solution is instilled to promote corneal swelling. A calibrated ultraviolet A meter (LaserMate-Q; Laser 2000, Wessling, Germany) is used before treatment to check the irradiance at a 1.0-cm distance. A 7.5-mm (diameter 1, "S") or 9.5 mm (diameter 2, "M") diameter of the central cornea then is irradiated with an irradiance of 9 mW/cm^2 (UV-X 2000, former IROC Innocross AG, Zug, Switzerland) for 10 minutes. During irradiation time, the riboflavin solution is not applied on the ocular surface anymore. Topical anesthesia is added as needed during the procedure.

A soft therapeutic contact lens (Pure Vision, Dr. Gerhard Mann Chem.-Pharm. Fabrik GmbH, Bausch & Lomb Inc., Berlin, Germany) is applied until re-epithelialization of cornea is complete. After surgery, analgesics systemically are prescribed and antibiotic ofloxacin eye drops (Floxal® EDO, Dr. Mann Pharma Berlin, Germany) 3 times a day and artificial tears at least 6 times a day are applied. Postoperative follow-up examinations are performed daily until complete reepithelialization. After the corneal reepithelialization (3–4 days) is the contact lens removed and antibiotic eye drops discontinued. The application of dexamethasone steroid eye drops (Dexa® EDO, Dr. Mann Pharma Berlin, Germany) 3 times a day for 3 weeks is initiated together with further continuation of artificial tears application.

Further follow-up examinations are regularly scheduled at 1, 3 (optional), 6, and 12 month and then annually. At each examination, refraction, best corrected visual acuity with glasses or with contact lenses, corneal topography, tomography, ocular response analyzer and intraocular pressure are recorded. At 6-month follow-up is a fitting of a new contact lens or glasses recommended.

1.2 Clinical Outcomes

A study analyzing the 12-month results of 3 protocols of ACXL—9, 30 mW/cm^2 with continuous-light, and 30 mW/cm^2 with pulsed-light compared these results with those achieved with conventional (3 mW/cm^2) procedure [11]. Although 30 mW accelerated CXL treatment modalities appeared to be effective in stabilizing keratoconus progression, they seemed less effective in achieving topographic improvement.

In another study were data from ninety-three eyes of 67 patients collected retrospectively from 3 separate study groups. The aim of this study was to compare functional outcomes using standard protocol (3 mW/cm^2 for 30 min, 5.4 J/cm^2) and accelerated protocol with equivalent total irradiance (9 mW/cm^2 for 10 min, 5,4 J/cm^2) and accelerated with increased total irradiance (30 mW/cm^2 for 4 min, 7.2 J/cm^2). All 3 protocols showed improvements in Kmax, CDVA, and other variables, with similar functional outcomes for each despite greater change in keratoconus indices after standard protocol [12].

Several recent meta-analyses observing trials comparing efficacy of standard with accelerated procedure tend to have similar conclusions. Wen et al. included in their meta-analysis eleven trials. These trials showed, that standard CXL had a greater effect in terms of reduction in Kmax than accelerated procedure, while A-CXL induced less reduction in central corneal thickness (CCT) and endothelial cell density (ECD) than S-CXL [13].

Meta-analysis of German authors investigated results of 22 studies with 1158 eyes. In their observations, consideration of less corneal thinning, similarly as in previous meta-analysis, favours A-CXL, whereas the deeper demarcation line and greater changes in minimum keratometric values in S-CXL may indicate a higher treatment efficacy. The authors claim, that altogether, S-CXL, as well as A-CXL, provide successful results in the strengthening of corneal tissue [14].

Two independent Japanese authors performed a comprehensive search using the Cochrane methodology to evaluate the clinical outcomes of S-CXL and A-CXL for treating progressive keratoconus. They identified 6 randomized controlled trials that met the eligibility criteria. Their observations showed that A-CXL showed a comparable efficacy and safety profile at the 1-year follow-up, but it had less impact on improving best spectacle-corrected visual acuity when compared with the Dresden protocol. Overall, both methods similarly stopped the disease progression [15].

1.3 Complications and Side Effects of A-CXL

Complications and side effects after CXL procedure are in general very rare. The corneal wound healing process postoperatively is accompanied by an apoptosis of keratocytes and a simultaneous appearance of corneal haze. The repopulation of keratocytes last for around 3 months [16] whereas the corneal clearance recovers to baseline after 6 up to 12 months [17]. In the early postoperative period (2–4 weeks), a demarcation line is visible in the mid-stroma by slit-lamp [18] or anterior optical coherence tomography [19]. The demarcation line represents the transition zone between cross-linked and untreated stromal tissue [18]. It is known, that demarcation line depth of A-CXL is shallower than S-CXL [14, 20]. The appearance of the demarcation line is more a qualitative sign than a predictive value of treatment success (if detected by topography and tomography) [21].

Other complications described after A-CXL are delayed epithelial healing, sterile infiltrates, infectious keratitis, scarring or the loss of visual acuity [14, 22].

1.4 Clinical Evaluation of Treatment Success

Important criterion of evaluating the effectiveness of a procedure is the failure rate. In case the keratoconus continues to progress despite the initial treatment, we perform usually a re-treatment at the earliest after 12 months concerning the consensus of a change of 1 D increase in Kmax-values within six or 12 months. We also indicate a re-treatment procedure in the case of a new progression of corneal ectasia after a long period of stable findings.

We have analyzed a cohort of patients who have undergone different modes of primary CXL procedure. We were interested in if the re-treatment rate / failure rate of A-CXL (9*10) is higher than compared to S-CXL. All patients in our cohort underwent at least a three-year (36 months) follow up at our Department of Ophthalmology at University Hospital Carl Gustav Carus, Technical University Dresden. CXL was performed between 2006 and 2015. The study was approved by the ethics committee of our Institution (NCT04251143, Dresden Corneal Disease and Treatment Study). In case of a progressive KC, corneas were cross-linked using S-CXL [23] or A-CXL (9*10) [24] protocol. Each patient received a complete eye examination (medical history, topography, tomography, visual acuity and slit lamp examination). 230 eyes of 155 patients were enrolled with a minimal follow up of 36 months. The demographic data are presented in Table 1. Those patients whose corneas received S-CXL were significantly younger and slight more advanced concerning KC stage (higher Kmax value, higher LogMar BCVA). Table 2 summarizes the CXL settings used in our patients.

The mean follow-up time at last visit were 99.8 ± 29.2 months and 51.3 ± 12.7 for S-CXL and A-CXL after CXL, respectively, which was statistically significant ($P < 0.001$, linear mixed model, LMM [25]). This could be explained by the longer period that the S-CXL procedure is performed in our keratoconus clinic. However, all patients received a minimum follow-up of 36 months as described before. Concerning the complete follow-up, best-corrected visual acuity (BCVA in LogMar) improved statistically significant after S-CXL and A-CXL (both $P < 0.001$, LMM, Table 3), while the improvement of BCVA was more pronounced in S-CXL although they have shown worse preoperative BCVA. Statistically significant flattening of maximum keratometry (Kmax) was also found

Table 1 Demographic data of S-CXL and A-CXL group

	S-CXL (n = 120)	A-CXL (n = 110)	
Parameter	Mean ± SD	Mean ± SD	P value
Age (years)	24.7 ± 7.8	27.3 ± 9.9	**0.025***
Kmax preop (D)	63.6 ± 12.3	58.3 ± 8.5	**<0.001***
MCT preop (µm)	456.6 ± 54.5	455.5 ± 45.4	0.862*
BCVA (logMAR)	0.50 ± 0.33	0.35 ± 0.27	**< 0.001***

BCVA, best-corrected visual acuity; Kmax, maximum keratometry; MCT, minimal corneal thickness. *P values were obtained using the linear mixed model to consider inter-eye correlations [25]. P < 0.05 was considered as significance

Table 2 CXL settings used in this study

Parameter	S-CXL	A-CXL
Treatment target	Progressive keratoconus	Progressive keratoconus
Fluence (total) (mJ/cm^2)	5.4	5.4
Soak Time (interval)	20 min (q2)	20 min (q2)
Intensity (mW/cm^2)	3	9
Treatment time (min)	30	10
Light source	UV-X 1000	UV-X 2000
Irradiation mode	Continuous	Continuous
Epithelium status	Off	Off
Chromophore (centration)	Riboflavin (0.1%)	Riboflavin (0.1%)

in both groups (P < 0.001, LMM, Table 3), with a stronger, more pronounced improvement for S-CXL. Minimal corneal thickness (MCT) decreased significantly after S-CXL (P < 0.001, LMM, Table 3), while no change was found after A-CXL (P = 0.229, LMM, Table 3). In summary, these findings are in accordance to previously described studies and meta-analysis [11–15].

1.5 Failure Rates of S-CXL and A-CXL

Re-treatments were necessary in 26 (22%) cases treated with S-CXL and 19 (17%) cases treated with A-CXL (P = 0.412, Fisher exact test). The mean time between initial CXL and re-treatment were 62.6 ± 41.9 months and 29.2 ± 19.2 months for S-CXL and A-CXL (P = 0.020, LMM). Kaplan–Meier-Analysis revealed a survival rate (cumulative prediction rate) after CXL of 75.2% and 69.5% for S-CXL and A-CXL, respectively (Fig. 1). These values were not statistically significant (P = 0.103, Log-rank test). To compare the failure rates between both protocols without the impact of different follow-up periods we should focus especially at the time frame of 36 months. In Fig. 1 (right plot), Kaplan–Meier-Analysis revealed a

Table 3 Pre- and postoperative data of visual acuity, maximum keratometry and minimal corneal thickness for S-CXL and A-CXL group with a minimum of 36 months follow-up

	S-CXL Mean ± SD			A-CXL Mean ± SD		
	Pre-CXL	Last visit	P value	Pre-CXL	Last visit	P value
BCVA (LogMar)	0.46 ± 0.30	0.32 ± 0.27	<0.001*	0.33 ± 0.28	0.26 ± 0.27	<0.001*
Kmax (D)	61.7 ± 11.1	56.5 ± 7.8	<0.001*	57.3 ± 8.3	55.3 ± 8.0	<0.001*
MCT (μm)	460.9 ± 51.4	434.9 ± 63.0	<0.001*	459.1 ± 47.4	454.4 ± 48.8	0.229*
Mean Follow-up (months)		99.8 ± 29.2	-		51.3 ± 12.7	< 0.001*
Re-treatments over complete follow-up		26 (22%)	-		19 (17%)	0.412+
Time to re-treatment [months]		62.6 ± 41.9	-		29.2 ± 19.2	0.020*

BCVA, best-corrected visual acuity; Kmax, maximum keratometry, MCT, minimal corneal thickness. * P values were obtained using the linear mixed model to consider inter-eye correlations [25]. + P values were obtained using Fisher exact test. P < 0.05 was considered as significance.

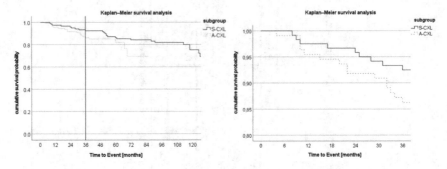

Fig. 1 Kaplan–Meier-Analysis for the S-CXL and A-CXL concerning complete follow-up (left) and 36 months (right)

cumulative prediction rate after CXL of 92.5% and 86.4% for S-CXL and A-CXL, respectively (P = 0.130, Log-rank test).

We have analyzed the risk factors for re-treatment for all included patients (n = 230). We have focused on age, preoperative MCT, preoperative Kmax, gender and atopic diseases (neurodermitis, asthma, food allergy, and allergic rhinitis) of treated patients and CXL protocol (S-CXL or A-CXL). To determine the odds ratio (OR) of risk factors, generalized estimating equations (GEE) were used to consider the inter-eye correlation. First, each of the previously mentioned factors were separately analyzed. It has been shown, that a thinner preoperative MCT (OR = 0.991, P = 0.012, GEE), a higher preoperative Kmax (OR = 1.057, P < 0.001, GEE) and the presence of neurodermatis combined with other atopic diseases (OR = 4.29, P = 0.012, GEE) were statistically significant risk factors for a progressing KC after initial CXL (Table 4). The mode of used protocol (S-CXL or A-CXL) had no statistically significant impact on further KC progression. Second, three of the significant risk factors (preoperative MCT, preoperative Kmax, and neurodermitis combined with other atopic diseases) detected by univariate analysis were used for a multivariate model. It has been shown that higher preoperative Kmax and presence of neurodermitis combined with other atopic diseases remained statistically significant (Table 4).

In conclusion, A-CXL (in modus of 9 mW/cm^2 for 10 min) has been proved as an effective treatment modality to halt KC progression that allows shortening the overall duration of procedure in the long-term follow-up according to the *Siena Eye Cross Study 2* [26]. This is an important positive finding enabling the well-being of patients during procedure and bringing at the same comforting of clinical workflow in reducing the necessity of qualified personnel engagement. Based on our clinical experience and literature research, the improvement of keratometric values and visual acuity after A-CXL might be less pronounced as it was found in S-CXL. However, MCT did not change as much as in S-CXL. This fact is important regarding treatment of thin corneas. To be able to "individualize" the treatment for each patient—medical history (signs of atopy, especially neurodermitis or habits, e.g. eye rubbing) as well as the value of Kmax and MCT should be considered in

Table 4 Risk factors of re-treatment of CXL using a univariate and multivariate analysis

Parameter	Univariate analysis			Multivariate analysis			
	OR	95% CI		P value[a]	OR	95% CI		P value[a]
Age	0.962	0.918	1.01	0.116	–			
Preoperative MCT	0.991	0.983	0.998	**0.012**	0.998	0.989	1.007	0.654
Preoperative Kmax	1.057	1.029	1.086	**< 0.001**	1.052	1.02	1.086	**0.001**
Gender	1.11	0.458	2.691	0.817	–			
Neurodermitis	2.316	0.95	5.643	0.065	–			
Atopy except neurodermitis	1.05	0.448	2.463	0.91	–			
Neurodermitis combined with other atopic disease	4.291	1.378	13.359	**0.012**	3.886	1.277	11.823	**0.017**
CXL protocol (S-CXL or A-CXL)	0.695	0.382	1.264	0.233	–			

[a]Determined by generalized estimating equation (GEE), P < 0.05 was considered as sig

physician's decision about modality of CXL procedure planned in each specific case. S-CXL might be more favored as a primary procedure in patients presenting with risk factors for treatment failure (e.g. atopy, eye rubbing) or in re-treatment procedure where A-CXL modality as an initial procedure already failed.

References

1. Schumacher S, Oeftiger L, Mrochen M. Equivalence of biomechanical changes induced by rapid and standard corneal cross-linking, using riboflavin and ultraviolet radiation. Invest Ophthalmol Vis Sci. 2011;52:9048–52. https://doi.org/10.1167/iovs.11-7818.
2. Krueger RR, Herekar S, Spoerl E. First proposed efficacy study of high versus standard irradiance and fractionated riboflavin/ultraviolet a cross-linking with equivalent energy exposure. Eye Contact Lens. 2014;40:353–7. https://doi.org/10.1097/ICL.0000000000000095.
3. Wernli J, Schumacher S, Spoerl E, Mrochen M. The efficacy of corneal cross-linking shows a sudden decrease with very high intensity UV light and short treatment time. Invest Ophthalmol Vis Sci. 2013;54:1176–80. https://doi.org/10.1167/iovs.12-11409.
4. Hammer A, Richoz O, Arba Mosquera S, Tabibian D, Hoogewoud F, Hafezi F. Corneal biomechanical properties at different corneal cross-linking (CXL) irradiances. Invest Ophthalmol Vis Sci. 2014;55:2881–4. https://doi.org/10.1167/iovs.13-13748.
5. Bao F, Zheng Y, Liu C, Zheng X, Zhao Y, Wang Y, Li L, Wang Q, Chen S, Elsheikh A. Changes in corneal biomechanical properties with different corneal cross-linking irradiances. J Refract Surg. 2018;34:51–8. https://doi.org/10.3928/1081597X-20171025-01.
6. Xue C, Xiang Y, Shen M, Wu D, Wang Y. Preliminary investigation of the mechanical anisotropy of the normal human corneal stroma. J Ophthalmol. 2018;2018:5392041. https://doi.org/10.1155/2018/5392041.

7. Herber R, Francis M, Spoerl E, Pillunat LE, Raiskup F, Sinha Roy A. Comparison of waveform-derived corneal stiffness and stress-strain extensometry-derived corneal stiffness using different cross-linking irradiances: an experimental study with air-puff applanation of ex vivo porcine eyes. Graefes Arch Clin Exp Ophthalmol. 2020;258:2173–84. https://doi.org/10.1007/s00417-020-04792-8.

8. Ehmke T, Seiler TG, Fischinger I, Ripken T, Heisterkamp A, Frueh BE. Comparison of corneal riboflavin gradients using dextran and HPMC solutions. J Refract Surg. 2016;32:798–802. https://doi.org/10.3928/1081597X-20160920-03.

9. Raiskup F, Spoerl E. Corneal cross-linking with hypo-osmolar riboflavin solution in thin keratoconic corneas. Am J Ophthalmol. 2011;152:28-32 e21. https://doi.org/10.1016/j.ajo.2011.01.016.

10. Shetty R, Nagaraja H, Pahuja NK, Jayaram T, Vohra V, Jayadev C. Safety and efficacy of epi-bowman keratectomy in photorefractive keratectomy and corneal collagen cross-linking: a pilot study. Curr Eye Res. 2016;41:623–9. https://doi.org/10.3109/02713683.2015.1045082.

11. Toker E, Cerman E, Ozcan DO, Seferoglu OB. Efficacy of different accelerated corneal crosslinking protocols for progressive keratoconus. J Cataract Refract Surg. 2017;43:1089–99. https://doi.org/10.1016/j.jcrs.2017.05.036.

12. Lang PZ, Hafezi NL, Khandelwal SS, Torres-Netto EA, Hafezi F, Randleman JB. Comparative functional outcomes after corneal crosslinking using standard, accelerated, and accelerated with higher total fluence protocols. Cornea. 2019;38:433–41. https://doi.org/10.1097/ICO.0000000000001878.

13. Wen D, Li Q, Song B, Tu R, Wang Q, O'Brart DPS, McAlinden C, Huang J. Comparison of standard versus accelerated corneal collagen cross-linking for keratoconus: a meta-analysis. Invest Ophthalmol Vis Sci. 2018;59:3920–31. https://doi.org/10.1167/iovs.18-24656.

14. Shajari M, Kolb CM, Agha B, Steinwender G, Muller M, Herrmann E, Schmack I, Mayer WJ, Kohnen T. Comparison of standard and accelerated corneal cross-linking for the treatment of keratoconus: a meta-analysis. Acta Ophthalmol. 2019;97:e22–35. https://doi.org/10.1111/aos.13814.

15. Kobashi H, Tsubota K. Accelerated versus standard corneal cross-linking for progressive keratoconus: a meta-analysis of randomized controlled trials. Cornea. 2020;39:172–80. https://doi.org/10.1097/ICO.0000000000002092.

16. Mazzotta C, Balestrazzi A, Traversi C, Baiocchi S, Caporossi T, Tommasi C, Caporossi A. Treatment of progressive keratoconus by riboflavin-UVA-induced cross-linking of corneal collagen: ultrastructural analysis by Heidelberg Retinal Tomograph II in vivo confocal microscopy in humans. Cornea. 2007;26:390–7. https://doi.org/10.1097/ICO.0b013e318030df5a.

17. Ziaei M, Gokul A, Vellara H, Patel D, McGhee CNJ. Prospective two year study of changes in corneal density following transepithelial pulsed, epithelium-off continuous and epithelium-off pulsed, corneal crosslinking for keratoconus. Cont Lens Anterior Eye. 2020;43:458–64. https://doi.org/10.1016/j.clae.2020.03.004.

18. Seiler T, Hafezi F. Corneal cross-linking-induced stromal demarcation line. Cornea. 2006;25:1057–9. https://doi.org/10.1097/01.ico.0000225720.38748.58.

19. Doors M, Tahzib NG, Eggink FA, Berendschot TT, Webers CA, Nuijts RM. Use of anterior segment optical coherence tomography to study corneal changes after collagen cross-linking. Am J Ophthalmol. 2009;148:844-851 e842. https://doi.org/10.1016/j.ajo.2009.06.031.

20. Kymionis GD, Tsoulnaras KI, Grentzelos MA, Plaka AD, Mikropoulos DG, Liakopoulos DA, Tsakalis NG, Pallikaris IG. Corneal stroma demarcation line after standard and high-intensity collagen crosslinking determined with anterior segment optical coherence tomography. J Cataract Refract Surg. 2014;40:736–40. https://doi.org/10.1016/j.jcrs.2013.10.029.

21. Pircher N, Lammer J, Holzer S, Gschliesser A, Donner R, Pieh S, Schmidinger G. Correlation between central stromal demarcation line depth and changes in K values after corneal cross-linking (CXL). Graefes Arch Clin Exp Ophthalmol. 2018;256:759–64. https://doi.org/10.1007/s00417-018-3922-z.

22. Cakmak S, Sucu ME, Yildirim Y, Kepez Yildiz B, Kirgiz A, Bektasoglu DL, Demirok A. Complications of accelerated corneal collagen cross-linking: review of 2025 eyes. Int Ophthalmol. 2020;40:3269–77. https://doi.org/10.1007/s10792-020-01512-3.
23. Wollensak G, Spoerl E, Seiler T. Riboflavin/ultraviolet-a-induced collagen crosslinking for the treatment of keratoconus. Am J Ophthalmol. 2003;135:620–7. https://doi.org/10.1016/s0002-9394(02)02220-1.
24. Herber R, Kunert KS, Velika V, Spoerl E, Pillunat LE, Raiskup F. Influence of the beam profile crosslinking setting on changes in corneal topography and tomography in progressive keratoconus: Preliminary results. J Cataract Refract Surg. 2018;44:718–24. https://doi.org/10.1016/j.jcrs.2018.03.025.
25. Herber R, Kaiser A, Grahlert X, Range U, Raiskup F, Pillunat LE, Sporl E. Statistical analysis of correlated measurement data in ophthalmology: tutorial for the application of the linear mixed model in SPSS and R using corneal biomechanical parameters. Ophthalmology. 2020;117:27–35. https://doi.org/10.1007/s00347-019-0904-4.
Mazzotta C, Raiskup F, Hafezi F, Torres-Netto EA, Armia Balamoun A, Giannaccare G, Bagaglia SA. Long termresults of accelerated 9 mW corneal crosslinking for early progressive keratoconus: the Siena Eye-Cross Study 2. EyeVis (Lond). 2021 May 1;8(1):16. https://doi.org/10.1186/s40662-021-00240-8.

Enhanced Trans-Epithelial Accelerated Crosslinking Protocols: The Way Out of Future CXL

Cosimo Mazzotta, Adel Barbara, Alessandro Di Maggio, and Pierpaolo Pintore

1 Introduction

Riboflavin/Ultraviolet-A (UVA) corneal collagen cross-linking (CXL) has become the standard of conservative treatment for disease related or iatrogenic corneal ectasias [1, 2]. Although remarkable improvements have been made in the treatment protocols, most of the CXL procedures are actually efficaciously performed with removal of the central 7–9 mm of the corneal epithelium. Epithelium removal represents, for standard or accelerated CXL, a crucial step in order to enable riboflavin and oxygen diffusion in the corneal stroma, which are necessary to enable and optimize the photo-oxydative reaction leading to efficient collagen cross-linking [1, 3, 4]. Disruption of the epithelial barrier exposes the cornea to some risks such as infectious keratitis, wound heling stimulation (haze and thinning) and temporary glare disability making visual recovery longer and often associated to greater patient's discomfort [5–8]. In order to overcome these problems, the research for new therapeutic innovations is focusing on "*enhanced*" or "*compensated*" accelerated trans-epithelial CXL protocols with high energies or fluencies, Table 1.

C. Mazzotta (✉)
Departmental Ophthalmology Unit, USL Toscana Sud Est, Alta Val D'Elsa Hospital, Campostaggia, Siena, Italy

C. Mazzotta
Siena Crosslinking Center, Siena, Italy

A. Barbara
Vision Without Glasses Medical Center, Haifa, Israel

A. Di Maggio
Post Graduate Ophthalmology School, University of Siena, Siena, Italy

P. Pintore
Ophthalmology Operative Unit, Alghero Hospital, Alghero, Italy

© The Author(s), under exclusive license to Springer Nature Switzerland AG 2022   131
A. Armia and C. Mazzotta (eds.), *Keratoconus*,
https://doi.org/10.1007/978-3-030-84506-3_7

Table 1 Enhanced higher fluence trans-epithelial accelerated crosslinking protocols

Enhanced higher fluence trans-epithelial accelerated crosslinking protocols
Enhanced fluence pulsed light epi-on ACXL with Iontophoresis and without supplemental oxygen (EFPL I-CXL) [23, 24] Fluence 7 J/cm^2—Pulsed Light 1:1 s– UV-A Power 18mW/cm^2
Enhanced Fluence Pulsed Light Mazzotta—TECXL without Iontophoresis and without supplemental oxygen (EFPL-M-TECXL) Fluence 7 J/cm^2—Pulsed Light 1:1 s—UV-A Power 18 mW/cm^2
Customized epi-on ACXL with supplemental oxygen Fluences 7.2 J/cm^2—10 J/cm^2—Pulsed Light—30mW/cm^2 [30]

Original Epi-On procedures had unsatisfactory outcomes as showed by Koppen et al. in a cohort study evaluating the efficacy of Epi-on CXL by using proparacaine drops 0.5% plus preserved with BAC 0.005%, proving that despite no complications or haze occurred, the trans-epithelial CXL with 5.4 J/cm^2 fluence was not effective in stabilizing progressive keratoconus, documenting a statistically significant continuous maximum K increasing and thinnest point decreasing (i.e. KC progression) throughout the study in 100% of eyes [10].

On the same route, Caporossi et al. reported a 50% of retreatments 24-months after trans-epithelial CXL in paediatric patients that required an additional S-CXL with epithelium removal between the 15th and the 24th month after treatment [11]. Gatzioufas et al. in a prospective, interventional multicenter study assessing the efficacy of an enhanced Riboflavin solution containing 0.01% BAK for Epi On-CXL, confirmed the clinical inefficacy of the original treatment, documenting that K max, uncorrected and corrected distance visual acuity did not change significantly after 12-months follow-up and a progression of KC (defined by an increase in K max greater than 1.00 D) occurring in 46% of treated eyes [12].

There is no doubt that, an intact corneal epithelium represents a hindrance for riboflavin solutions, which are not capable to adequately penetrate the tight junctions and uniformly diffuse into the corneal stroma [5]. Indeed, being riboflavin a large hydrophilic molecule, with an approximate weight of 340 Da, its transportation through a lipophilic epithelium, relatively low permissive for molecules >80 Da, was an indubitable issue to overcome [5, 9, 13, 14].

The barrier effect of corneal epithelium has been widely described in literature and confirmed by a number of spectrophotometry experiments, demonstrating the low diffusion even with commercially available trans-epithelial riboflavin formulations [5, 9, 11, 13]. However, several strategies have been postulated to increase epithelial permeability to riboflavin, such as the mechanical focal disruption of the epithelium, the increased exposure time, multiple pre-operative administration of preservative-based anaesthetic drops, application of 20% alcohol solution, but all showed to achieve an inhomogeneous loading between the 20 and 50% compared with passive diffusion and gradient of concentration of riboflavin solutions after epithelium removal [5, 9, 13, 14]. Of course, this one parameter does not necessarily imply an undisputed ineffectiveness of the treatment as no one knows exactly the necessary concentration of riboflavin and the what we call the "*crosslinking alchemy*" is given by the combination of multiple interactions including UV-A rays impact and mode of exposure (continuous or pulsed), oxygen availability and intraoperative diffusion, collagen and proteoglycans molecules, as well as riboflavin gradient of concentration and no less to the difference between one KC and the other in clinical, biologic and genetic terms as well as concomitant environmental factors (hormones, allergy, comorbidities, eye-rubbing) influencing the specific response to treatment on a case-by-case basis. [15, 16].

Numerous trans-epithelial riboflavin formulations have been marketed, most of which are dextran-free because of the high molecular weight of dextran, which is believed to hinder riboflavin penetration across the epithelium. In such formulations riboflavin vehiculation is entrusted to 1% hydroxypropyl methycellulose (HPMC) while epithelial permeability is enhanced through addition of chemical agents, such as benzalkonium chloride (BAC), trometamol (TRIS) and ethylenediamine tetra-acetic acid (EDTA) [10, 13, 15]. Despite these chemical enhancers, clinical studies using trans-epithelial riboflavin formulations have shown contradictory results, most of which were inferior compared to Epi-off CXL in stabilizing corneal ectasia in the long-term follow-up, especially in younger patients [9–11].

Being riboflavin water-soluble and negatively charged at physiological pH, its transportation through the epithelium can be facilitated by the application of low intensity electrical gradient (1 m Ampere × 5 minutes). This procedure, already used in several fields of medicine to enhance drugs absorption, is called Iontophoresis [13–20]. Increased permeation of the riboflavin into the stroma, compared to the Epi-On procedures, has been confirmed by several laboratory studies, showing an average riboflavin concentration that was two folds higher throughout all corneal depth, with deeper and more homogeneous distribution into the corneal stroma, but, at the same time, its concentration was halved if compared to that of standard Epi-Off CXL [9, 13, 14]. This doesn't necessarily mean that riboflavin concentration with Iontophoresis is not sufficient to adequately link corneal collagen, although long term follow-ups indicated that the Iontophoresis-assisted CXL halted the progression of keratoconus less efficiently than did Epi-off CXL with a 23 to 25% retreatment rate [18–20].

Besides riboflavin issues, there are other important determinants for an efficient by a photochemical point of view and a clinically efficacious corneal cross-linking requiring compensation in relation to the principles of photochemistry: the total energy dose (fluence) delivered to the stroma through the epithelium in situ; epithelium oxygen metabolic consumption; intra-stromal oxygen availability, diffusion and reactive oxygen species availability enabling crosslinking reaction. The compensation levels adopted to increase the overall efficiency and clinical outcome of modern trans-epithelial higher energies ACXL treatments [23, 24, 31] are displayed in Table 2.

Table 2 Photochemistry compensations of "*enhanced*" Trans-epithelial ACXL Protocols

Photochemistry compensations of enhanced Trans-Epithelial CXL Protocols
Increased **Riboflavin Concentration** in the range between 0.14 and 0.25% up to 0.3%
Increased **UV-A Fluence** in the range between 7 and 10 J/cm^2 up to 15 J/cm^2 according to epithelial UV-A attenuation at 370 nm waveband
Use of **Pulsed UV-A Light Exposure** to increase intraoperative oxygen diffusion, demarcation line depth, inducing less microstructural damage
Use **Intraoperative Supplemental Oxygen** to boost-up oxygen diffusion
Use of developing **Chemically Boosted Riboflavin Solutions** for CXL capable to increase ROS intra-stromal release also in low oxygen concentration or anaerobic environment

Our goal in trying to improve the efficiency and feasibility of the Epi-On CXL protocols, considering them the best "*way out of CXL*" in the near future, is largely based on consideration of all the benefits of trans-epithelial procedures such as the elimination of the corneal infectious risk, the elimination of the risk of stromal scarring and thinning, the speeding up of functional patient recovery, the reduction of postoperative pain duration, the minimization of microstructural damage to the ocular surface, the prevention of dry eye, the possibility of quickly rehabilitating the patient to school and work activities in a few days, the possibility of carrying out the procedure comfortably in outpatient mode and reducing costs. Nevertheless, we are interested in the possibility, which must absolutely be combined with the early diagnosis of keratoconus in paediatric age, to reduce the risk profile of the CXL therapy, in order to propose also it in the preventive use, in the absence of ascertained clinical worsening or for the less affected eye in combination with Epi-off CXL in the worst eye and for simultaneous bilateral treatments. The potential

Table 3 Advantages of enhanced trans-epithelial CXL procedures

Advantages of Trans-Epithelial Enhanced CXL Protocols
Reduction/elimination of corneal infection risk
Reduction/elimination of corneal wound healing stimuli (haze, scarring, extreme thinning)
Faster patients recovery and visual rehabilitation
Minimization of microstructural damage to the ocular surface
Prevention of dry eye preserving the neve plexus structure
Simultaneous bilateral treatment
Quick rehabilitation of the patient to school and work activities
Full outpatient procedure
Preventive use of CXL without awaiting progression at any age
Reduced costs

benefits of transepithelial enhanced or "compensated" CXL procedures are listed in Table 3.

Recently new techniques and strategies have been proposed [23, 24, 31] that are reducing the gap of efficacy with the Epi-off treatments as showed in Table 1. Moreover, we have tested a new protocol named Enhanced Fluence Pulsed Light M (Mazzotta) trans-epithelial CXL without iontophoresis mediated riboflavin soaking and without supplemental oxygen (EFPL-M-TECXL), adopting a higher Fluence of 7 J/cm^2 for a UV-A exposure time of 12 minutes and 58 seconds—Pulsed Light (1 sec on 1 sec off cycle)—UV-A Power 18mW/cm^2, as in the same way as the new enhanced Fluence pulsed light iontophoresis (EFPL I-CXL) [23, 24] without using the iontophoresis and without adding intraoperative oxygen supplement, with the advantage of additional simplification of the procedure, improving patient comfort and reducing costs, thus requiring no adjunctive kits and being less invasive and completely feasible in outpatient modality. Moreover, the recent introduction in the CXL panorama of new "*chemically boosted*" riboflavin solutions for Epi-off CXL may further increase the efficiency of trans-epithelial CXL also in low oxygen environment or anaerobic condition increasing the release of reactive oxygen species (ROS), thus enhancing CXL efficiency as first reported in the literature [32].

The role of corneal epithelium in UV absorbing process has been largely described in literature [21, 22]. Ultraviolet rays stimulate reactive oxygen species production, which have been shown to induce cell death in cultured corneal cells and play a major role in several intraocular pathological conditions. In order to protect against these effects, high levels of anti-oxidant enzymes, ascorbate and tryptophan residues are stored in the corneal epithelium, significantly increasing absorption coefficient for UV rays in the 240- to 400-nm range [21]. The UV-A energy photo-attenuation provided by corneal epithelium and Bowman's lamina radical absorbers, in the waveband of 365 nm set in all the CXL therapy, is approximately the 30% of UV-A radiation. [21] This partially explain the inefficiency of first Iontophoresis assisted CXL (I-CXL) protocol, using standard 5.4 J/cm^2 Fluence [18–20]. Compensation of epithelial UV-A absorption is fundamental achieving a sufficient energy delivery throughout the entire treatment stromal volume thus increasing crosslinks formation and saturation, justifying Fluence increase from 5.4 to 7 J/cm^2 up. Safety and efficacy of higher irradiances exposure has been described in literature by Mazzotta et al. [23, 24]. Studies analysing corneal microstructure using in vivo scanning laser confocal microscopy (IVCM) showed that in topography-guided CXL protocols by means of energy doses higher than conven-tional 5.4 J/cm^2 (from 7 up to 15 J/cm^2), the depth of keratocytes apoptosis was directly proportional to the Fluence, and this was also evident with corneal OCT, where multiple demarcation lines were appreciable on month after the treatment, underlying the different energy doses and UV-A exposure times used [25]. According to the "equal-dose" physical principle set in the Bunsen-Roscoe's low of reciprocity, the same amount of energy dose can be delivered by modifying both UV-A power and exposure time accelerating the treatment, so that a total energy of 5.4 J/cm^2 can be administered either with 3 mW/cm^2 for 30 min or 9 mW/cm^2 for

10 min, 15 mW for 6 minutes or 18 mW/cm^2 for 5 min, 30 mW/cm^2 for 3 min or 45 mW/cm^2 for 2 min. Several laboratory and clinical studies investigated the possible application of pulsed UV-A light, describing deeper demarcation line compared to continuous light CXL maintaining the same irradiance and the same energy [26]. This could be explained by the overall longer irradiation time using pulsed light while the linking efficiency may be increased by facilitating diffusion of oxygen in corneal stroma during the light-off or dark phase [27].

The Bunsen-Roscoe's law doesn't apply in full to crosslinking because oxygen diffusion, consumption and replenishment plays a crucial role in corneal CXL since the photo-oxydative reaction can be carried out in either an aerobic or an anaerobic pathway, but the first one assures a higher concentration of oxygen radicals, making the linking process (stromal crosslinks formation) more efficacious [28]. Maintaining an adequate oxygen concentration throughout the entire treatment is an important issue to overcome in case of Epi-on CXL, as oxygen concentration rapidly cuts out during UV-A illumination (10–15 seconds) and slowly recovers when the light source is switched off [29].

Main factors impacting on oxygen availability in case of trans-epithelial procedures are the barrier effect on passive diffusion and the epithelial oxygen consumption, which has been estimated in about 40% [22]. Several trials demonstrated that a stable hyperoxic environment in the operating field can counteract these effects, with material benefits in high-irradiance (higher oxygen consumption) Epi-on (low oxygen diffusion) protocols [29, 30, 32–36].

2   Enhanced Fluence Pulsed Light Iontophoresis Protocol (EFPL I-CXL)

Riboflavin delivery throughout the whole corneal stromal thickness represents one of the major issues in case of epithelium on procedures, being the riboflavin a relatively large, water-soluble, negatively charged molecule. This last characteristic represents the mainstay of the iontophoresis assisted CXL protocols, in which a low electrical gradient (1 mA × 5 min) is applied in order to support riboflavin penetration into the stroma [18, 19]. The result is an almost doubled stromal concentration if compared to previous epi-on procedures and halved if compared to passive diffusion after standard CXL with epithelium removal, with a more homogeneous distribution throughout the corneal layers [9, 13, 14]. However, the original iontophoresis CXL protocols (I-CXL) showed less satisfactory results on both anatomical and/or functional side having photochemical limitations in adopting the same fluence of Epi-off CXL and limitation in oxygen diffusion [40]. The demarcation line after I-CXL was inconsistent and superficially visible only in 35–45% of treated corneas vs the 95% after standard epithelium-off CXL, with a mean depth of 212 ± 36.5 μm, shallower compared with 97% of the standard CXL at 345 ± 24.5 μm [20].

It was demonstrated that to achieve a long-term follow-up ectasia stabilization after a CXL procedure it is advisable to achieve a treatment depth of at least 250 μm epithelium included [37–39]. On the other hand, functional results were shown to be less reproducible and quite contrasting [18, 20]. While some study reported encouraging functional results, with statistically significant improvement of uncorrected and corrected visual acuity, reduction of maximum keratometry and coma aberration [19]. The incomplete success of above mentioned studies may be explained by the fact that despite the presence of epithelium in situ, the UV-A Fluence delivered to corneal stroma was identical to that used in the Epi-off CXL Dresden protocol with (5.4 J/cm^2) with a continuous UV-light irradiation [1]. As previously described and referenced in the chapter introduction, the linking effect of the procedure is not only related to stromal riboflavin concentration, since other factors play a crucial role, such as UV-light photo-attenuation and oxygen kinetics.

The photo-attenuation activity exerted by the corneal epithelium and Bowman's lamina has been largely described, thus highlighting the need for a compensation of the absorbed energy which has been estimated in around 25–30% of the total dose. Laboratory studies just reported how a 25% increase in UV-A radiance (from 5.4 J to 6.5 J/cm^2) significantly increased the corneal resistance against enzymatic degradation in case of Epi-On CXL, although inferior to Epi-off CXL [41]. Mazzotta et al. medium to long-term follow-up clinical studies, in line with the results of these laboratory tests, demonstrated an improved visibility of DL in over 80% of patients treated by enhancing the fluence of the original I-CXL of 30% (from 5.4 to 7 J/cm^2), with an average depth of 285 ± 20 μm, thus improving the photochemical kinetic of the original I-CXl and this new tans-epithelial protocol was named Enahanced Fluence Pulsed Light Iontophoresis (EFPL I-CXL) [23, 24].

2.1 EFPL I-CXL Surgical Procedure

The EFPL I-CXL technique is displayed in Table 4 and showed in Fig. 1. After topical anaesthesia (oxybuprocaine hydrochloride drops) instilled 10 minutes before treatment and a Barraquer's closed valve eye-lid speculum application, the ocular surface is dried with a micro-sponge, iontophoresis suction ring is placed and centred on the corneal surface. Stromal imbibitions is performed with the Ricrolin + ® riboflavin solution (Sooft, Montegiorgio, Italy) delivered by the electric generator I-ON CXL® (Fidia - Sooft, Montegiorgio, Italy), at 1 m Ampere × 5 min. After 5 minutes of imbibition, the exceeding solution is aspired by a syringe, suction interrupted, ocular surface rinsed abundantly with sterile saline Na-Cl solution for 15–20 seconds, eliminating all the residual riboflavin on the corneal surface and pulsed light UV-A exposure started. The UV-A source used was the KXL I system (Glaukos - Avedro, Waltam, MA, USA) setting a Fluence of 7 J/cm^2 delivered by an UV-A power of 18mW/cm^2 with pulsed light emission (1 sec on/ 1 sec off) in a total UV-A exposure time of 12.58 minutes in order to maintain the overall treatment time under 20 minutes. During the pulsed UV-A

Table 4 Enhanced fluence pulsed light iontophoresis (EFPL I-CXL) protocol

Mazzotta Enhanced Fluence Pulsed Light Iontophoresis Protocol (EFPL I-CXL) [23, 24]	
Parameter	Variable
Treatment target	KC stabilization
Fluence (total) (Joule/cm^2)	7 J/cm^2
Soak time and interval (minutes)	Ricrolin + (5 minutes + 5 for kit placement)
Intensity (mW)	18 mW/cm^2
Irradiation Time	12 minutes and 58 seconds
Epithelium status	On
Chromophore	Riboflavin 0.15%
Chromophore carriers	Trometamol (Tris), Na-EDTA, no Dextran
Chromophore osmolarity	hypotonic
Chromophore concentration	0.1%
Light source	KXL I (Glaukos-Avedro, Waltam MA, USA)
Irradiation mode (interval)	Pulsed (1 sec on—1 sec off)
Protocol modifications	I-CXL
Protocol abbreviation	EFPL I-CXL (Mazzotta New Iontophoresis) or Ionto PLUS

light emission the epithelial surface is washed with the Na-Cl solution every 1–2 minutes. At the end of the UV-A irradiation the corneal surface is medicated with antibiotics, hyaluronic acid and dressed with a therapeutic soft contact lens for 24 hours.

The higher fluence compensated the 28–30% UV-A energy photo-attenuation provided by the corneal epithelium in situ and Bowman's layer antioxidants systems. Moreover, Mazzotta and coll, added the Pulsed-light illumination facilitating the intraoperative oxygen kinetics and diffusion, thus increasing the treatment penetration as confirmed by the postoperative detection of the demarcation lines, Fig. 1.

Today, the 5-years statistically significant data showed that average UDVA decreased from 0.50 ± 0.10 to 0.35 ± 0.06 Log MAR, average K max decreased from 52.94 ± 1.34 D to 51.2 ± 1.50 D (Delta: −1.7 ± 0.5 D), average Coma improved from 0.24 ± 0.05 μm to 0.10 ± 0.02 μm (p = 0.001) and Symmetry Index (SI) decreased from 4.22 ± 1.01 D to 3.49 ± 0.90 D. Corneal OCT showed a demarcation line detection at 285.8 ± 20.2 μm average depth in over 80% at first month follow-up. The EF I-CXL pulsed-light protocol showed its capability in stabilizing progressive Keratoconus in absence of adverse events in the long-term over 3-years follow-up. The new iontophoresis, also knowed as Ionto Plus, reached clinical results closer to S-CXL and superior to the original epithelium-on I-CXL protocol with standard Fluence of 5.4 J/cm^2 in terms of average K max flattening, high order aberration reduction and functional outcomes. No additional intraoperative oxygen supplementation was used for this "*compensated*" technique [23, 24].

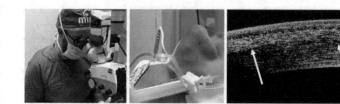

Fig. 1 Enhanced fluence pulsed light iontophoresis (EFPL I-CXL) or Ionto PLUS showing the demarcation line at one month (white arrows)

3 Enhanced Fluence Pulsed Light M—Trans-Epithelial Crosslinking Protocol (EFPL-M-TECXL)

More recently the 18 mW/7J/cm^2 Transepithelial Enhanced Fluence Pulsed Light Accelerated Crosslinking (ACXL) irradiation protocol developed by Mazzotta et al. [23, 24] for the new iontophoresis (Ionto PLUS), as described in the previous paragraph, has been successfully simplified and applied in the treatment of progressive keratoconus in young-adult patients over 21 years, without using the iontophoresis method for corneal soaking. The iontophoresis technique however, presents a certain invasiveness for young patients and the risk of damaging the epithelium during the positioning of the suction ring. Moreover, many cases of subconjunctival hemorrhages, chemosis and damage of the conjunctiva, which can be captured by error of decentralized positioning of the suction ring, are described often resulting in postoperative painful symptoms despite epithelium-on technique. Another disadvantage of iontophoresis is the possibility of loss of suction and the waste of riboflavin during treatment, forcing the use of a second kit which inevitably increase the costs of the procedure. Beyond the higher cost of the necessary kit it absolutely requires a reclining chair or an operating bed and good patient compliance due to suction ring correct positioning and maintaining a perpendicular position of the eye for at least 6–7 minutes to avoid suction loss and inducing a well-centred riboflavin loading. In order to reduce invasiveness, optimizing patient compliance and reducing the costs of adjunctive kits, transforming the procedure in a full outpatient technique without the necessity of operating beds or reclining chairs, also giving the possibility to use the technique at slit lamp, we used chemically enhanced 0.25 and 0.22% Riboflavin Solutions (ParaCel™ 1 and ParaCel™ 2, Avedro-Glaukos, Waltam MA, USA) for 10 minutes corneal soaking, performing the treatment at 21% air room oxygenation without supplemental oxygen. The new trans-epithelial protocol parameters developed by Mazzotta, are displayed in Table 5.

The prospective open non-randomized interventional study included 40 patients with early (Stage I and II) progressive KC undergoing the EFPL-M-TECXL 18 mW/7 J/cm^2, Table 4. The study cohort mean age was 25.2 years (22–36 y). The 12 minutes and 58 seconds pulsed 1on/1off seconds UV-A exposure treatments were performed after a 10 minutes corneal soaking with ParaCel I™ 0.25%

Table 5 Enhanced fluence pulsed light Mazzotta trans-epithelial crosslinking protocol (EFPL-M-TECXL)

Enhanced fluence pulsed light M trans-epithelial crosslinking protocol (EFPL-M-TECXL)	
Parameter	Variable
Treatment target	KC stabilization
Fluence (total) (Joule/cm^2)	7 J/cm^2
Soak time and interval (minutes)	ParaCel I (4 minutes) + ParaCel II (6 minutes)
Intensity (mW)	18 mW/cm^2
Irradiation Time	12 minutes and 58 seconds
Epithelium status	On
Chromophore	Riboflavin
Chromophore carriers	Trometamol, Na-EDTA, no Dextran
Chromophore osmolarity	Isotonic + hypotonic
Chromophore concentration	0.25% + 0.22%
Light source	KXL I (Glaukos-Avedro, Waltam MA, USA)
Irradiation mode (interval)	Pulsed (1 sec on—1 sec off)
Protocol modifications	EFPL I—CXL
Protocol abbreviation	EFPL M—TECXL

(administered each minute for 4 minutes) and ParaCel II 0.22% (administered every 30 seconds for 6 minutes) Riboflavin Solutions (Glaukos-Avedro, Waltham, USA) at air room 21% oxygenation and by using the New KXL I™ (Glaukos-Avedro, Waltham, USA). UDVA, CDVA, K MAX, AK, Coma HOA and Minimum Corneal Thickness (MCT) were measured and Corneal OCT performed to compare the demarcation line detection with new iontophoresis protocol as showed in Table 3. All patients examined completed the 24 follow-up. UDVA improved significantly (Δ + 1.2 lines), P < 0.05. Also K Max improved significantly (Δ—1.3 D) from the baseline value. Apical Curvature (AK) significantly flattened (Δ—1.6 D) and also COMA aberration value reduced (Δ—0.3 µm). No adverse events or complications were recorded during the follow-up. The postoperative spectral-domain corneal OCT performed on month after treatments revealed a mean demarcation line depth at 282.6 ± 43.6 µm, Fig. 2.

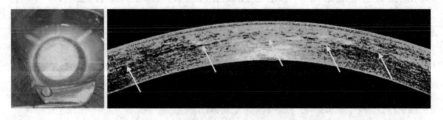

Fig. 2 Enhanced fluence pulsed light Mazzotta trans-epithelial crosslinking protocol (EFPL M TECXL)

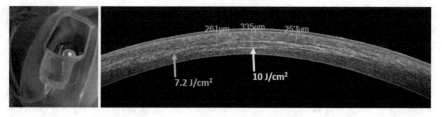

Fig. 3 Customized trans-epithelial CXL with supplemental oxygen via boost goggles (CuRV)®. Double demarcation line (green arrow 7.2 J/cm^2 and white arrow 10 J/cm^2) according to different treatment fluences

The EFPL M TECXL developed by Mazzotta showed that, by using chemically enhanced 0.25 and 0.22% riboflavin solutions, and increasing the Fluence to 7 J/cm^2 with the pulsed light illumination 1 second on and 1 second off for 12 minutes and 58 seconds, adequately washing the corneal surface with BSS for 15 seconds before starting the UV-A light, in order to eliminate the adjunctive riboflavin shielding effect over the epithelial surface, and at air room 21% oxygen, halted KC progression and improved functional outcomes without adverse events similarly to the EFPL I-CXL protocol being non-invasive and optimally tolerated. Differently from the EFPL I-CXL (iontophoresis soaking) method, this simplified approach was preferred by the patients being less invasive (avoiding suction ring required), cost-effective (no adjunctive iontophoresis or supplemental oxygen kit costs), offering the possibility of full outpatient treatments thus optimizing clinic workflow. Of course, it is actually indicated in young adult patients over 21 years, bilateral treatments (also in same-day procedures) and low-compliant patients with and without intellectual disability. Nobody knows the exact concentration of riboflavin to achieve optimal CXL, however the Dresden protocol, used as standard benchmark, is giving way to accelerated protocols [4]. A limitation could be the reduced amount and inhomogeneous stromal distribution of riboflavin that in the Iontophoresis-mediated soaking is superior, however the demarcation line and the clinical results after a 2-years follow-up are similar of those obtained with the new enhanced iontophoresis stromal soaking method. Comparative mid to long-term studies are under investigation at *Siena Crosslinking Center*, also increasing the Fluence up to 10J/cm.^{2}

4 Customized Trans-Epithelial Corneal Crosslinking with Supplemental Oxygen

While corneal cross-linking can occur both under anaerobic (photodynamic Type II pathway) and aerobic (Type I pathway) conditions, the aerobic pathway seems to be more efficient in generating reactive oxygen species x molecule of riboflavin, by re-oxidizing reduced riboflavin to its original state [28]. Reaching and maintaining an adequate oxygen concentration throughout the whole corneal volume is desirable in order to carry-out a more efficient oxygen of CXL [27, 29–31, 34]. That of oxygen concentration represents of course an important issue in case of epithelium-on procedures. Reduced passive oxygen diffusion, epithelial oxygen consumption, which has been estimated in about 40%) [22], higher consumption rate in case of higher Fluence accelerated CXL procedures [28], highlighted the necessity for oxygen compensation by increasing environmental oxygen concentration [30]. Seiler et al. recently described oxygen kinetics during corneal CXL using different UVA irradiance, with and without supplementary oxygen [34]. As already known, oxygen concentration quickly decreases when UV irradiation is started, rapidly stabilizing at an equilibrium. The highest oxygen availability at equilibrium was found in the $3mW/cm^2$ subgroup in 100 μm with $2.3 \pm 2.5\%$ in the normoxic and $50.2 \pm 6.2\%$ in the hyperoxic environment. In all subgroups, decreasing oxygen levels were observed when measured in deeper corneal layers or higher irradiances, while depletion rates increase with higher applied irradiances and decrease with depth [35]. This study does not take into account the "saturation threshold" of crosslinks x stromal volume, so a markedly hyperoxic environment would bring no advantage once the "*saturation value*" for the formation of cross-links in a given volume of stroma has been reached as demonstrated in the literature by Mazzotta et al. [39]. As reported in the biochemical studies by Weadock et al. [42] was clearly proved that collagen molecules possess many amino acid reactive residues, such as lysine and proline, constituting over the 80% of collagen amino acids, that are recruited in the strong chemical (aldehydes-mediated) CXL, while only a limited amount (less than 20%) of free reactive residues of aromatic amino-acids, such as tyrosine and phenylalanine, are involved in the short-wave UV-mediated CXL. Thus the "*cross-linking density*" can rise only up to an upper bound value, i.e., the saturation value. The cross-linking density in the superficial layers ends after reaching the saturation and cannot be increased indefinitely [43] so its overall efficiency attains a homogeneous distribution into the stroma both horizontally but also in a "*depth-dependent curve*". These concepts imply that oxygen kinetic could be sufficient to generate a "*saturating level of crosslinks amount*" also in a normoxic or even hypoxic environment.

The first international clinical experience of the accelerated customized trans-epithelial CXL technique in keratoconic patients was reported by Mazzotta et al. [30] with the aim to induce a customized remodeled vision while reinforcing the corneal stroma contemporary stabilizing corneal ectasia and providing a customized refractive empowerment to the technique based on computational corneal modeling simulations. The concept was first introduced and demonstrated in the 2011 by Roy et al. [44] and re-discussed in the 2014 review article by Roberts et al. [45]. The authors described the potential of customized CXL treatments to reduce asymmetry in ectatic corneas with resultant benefits in visual outcomes and According to computational modeling analysis it was calculated that smaller-diameter simulated CXL treatments centered on the cone area could theoretically provide greater reductions in corneal curvature and corneal higher-order aberrations (HOA) than the conventional broad-beam CXL pattern. An array of standard and alternative CXL patterns were simulated on central and eccentric cones, and the authors found that the greatest topographic flattening effect could be achieved by inducing greater differential stiffening of the apical area of the kera-toconus cone relative to the surrounding cornea [44–47]. This has become possible through the introduction of specially designed oxygen delivery goggles. Supplemental oxygen is delivered through the goggles to increase the rate of dif-fusion of oxygen to the corneal stroma to replenish oxygen consumed during the cross-linking reaction8. This technique has previously been applied in trans-epithelial, pulsed, high dose, photorefractive intra-stromal CXL in the treat-ment of low-grade myopia and hyperopia providing greater flattening than the earlier protocols, including the Epi-off approach [32–36].

Transposition in the field of progressive KC has shown promising results as documented in a recent prospective interventional case series conducted by Mazzotta et al. [30] who reported high-irradiance Epi-On customized CXL with supplemental oxygen to be effective in halting KC progression, with statistically significant reductions in corneal curvature and improvements in corneal HOA without significant adverse events. AS OCT revealed the good penetration-power of this technique, with a mean depth of the demarcation line of 218.23 ± 43.32 μm in the corneal area treated at 7.2 J/cm^2 fluence and 325.71 ± 39.70 μm in the steeper corneal area (apical region of the cone) treated with 10 J/cm^2 fluence, Fig. 3.

Customized Trans-Epithelial CXL with Supplemental Oxygen: Surgical technique

The surgical procedure, displayed in Table 6, was performed as follows: one drop of topical pilocarpine 2% was administered 30 minutes (min) before the surgery, topical anesthetic 0.4% Oxybuprocaine Hydrocloride drops were instilled (1 drop/min × 3 min) and a lid speculum applied. The corneal epithelial surface was gently cleared of surface mucin layer with a cellulose spear moistened with ParaCel Part 1 (0.25% riboflavin ophthalmic solution, Glaukos—Avedro, Waltham, MA, USA), swiping approximately 4 × each in both horizontal and vertical meridians. The cornea was coated with 2–4 drops of ParaCel Part 1 and the induction timer of the UV-A delivery device (Mosaic System, Avedro Inc., Waltham, MA, USA) was started. An additional 2–4 drops of ParaCel Part 1 were instilled every 60 seconds (sec) for 4 min. After 4 min, ParaCel Part 1 was rinsed away with ParaCel Part 2 (0.22% riboflavin ophthalmic solution, Glaukos - Avedro), starting the Part 2 induction timer. An additional 2–4 drops of ParaCel Part 2 were instilled every 30 seconds for 6 min. Residual ParaCel was rinsed from the epithelial surface with BSS for at least 15 seconds to remove any residual riboflavin biofilm shield. After rinsing the excess ParaCel Part 2 from the eye, oxygen goggles (Boost, Glaukos-Avedro Inc., Waltham, MA, USA) were applied and connected by tubing to a humidifier bottle and oxygen cylinder, checking that oxygen regulator is set to a flow rate of 2.5 LPM. Oxygen concentration in the goggles was confirmed using an oxygen analyzer (NTH-PSt7 sensor with OXY-4 meter, PreSens Precision Sensing GmbH, Germany). Thirty to sixty sec were necessary for measured oxygen concentration to stabilize at $\geq 90\%$. The epi-on, customized cross-linking protocol

Table 6 Customized Epi-on CXL with supplemental oxygen via boost goggles (CuRV)®

Customized trans-epithelial CXL with supplemental oxygen via boost goggles (CuRV)®	
Parameter	Variable
Treatment target	KC stabilization + refractive empowerment
Fluence (total) (Joule/cm^2)	10 J/cm^2 (range 7.2–10 J/cm^2)
Soak time and interval (minutes)	ParaCel I (4 minutes) + ParaCel II (6 minutes)
Intensity (mW)	30 mW/cm^2
Irradiation Time	11 minutes and 6 seconds
Epithelium status	On
Chromophore	Riboflavin
Chromophore carriers	HPMC 1%
Chromophore osmolarity	Isotonic
Chromophore concentration	0.25% + 0.22%
Light source	Mosaic® (Glaukos-Avedro, Waltam MA, USA)
Irradiation mode (interval)	Pulsed (1 sec on—1 sec off)
Supplemental Oxygen	On $\geq$ 90% via Boost Goggles—Flow rate 2.5 LPM
Protocol modifications	TE—CXL
Protocol abbreviation	CuRV®

with supplemental oxygen was carried out with the Mosaic System (Glaukos-Avedro, Waltam, MA, USA) using a 30 mW/cm^2 UV-A irradiance with pulsed-light emission (1 second on/1 second off) for 11 min and 6 seconds, with maximum UV-A dose of 10 J/cm^2. Drops of BSS were instilled at 1–2 min intervals, or more frequently as needed to maintain hydration during UV-A exposure. The UV-A treatment shape (round or oval) and diameter of the irradiation zones were customized according to the preoperative tomographic examination, with a total dose of 7.2 J/cm^2 applied to the flattest part of the cone area (4.5–5.5 mm spot diameter, applied for 8 min) and 10 J/cm^2 in the steepest part (2–2.5 mm spot diameter, applied for the remaining 2 min 54 sec).

The localization of the treatment on the corneal surface after alignment under the Mosaic System was predetermined using the x–y polar coordinates of the location of thinnest pachymetry obtained from the corneal tomographic examination. A drop of anesthetic was instilled prior to start UV-A irradiation. After UV-A irradiation, the goggles were removed and the corneal surface was rinsed with BSS, and medicated with preservative-free antibiotic-steroid drops, cyclopentolate, preservative-free hyaluronate-carbopol gel and dressed with a soft bandage contact lens for 48 hours. The preliminary results of this pilot study demonstrate the high potentiality of epithelium-on, customized corneal crosslinking with supplemental oxygen to reduce corneal higher-order aberrations (HOA) and flattening corneal curvature in patients with progressive keratoconus, Fig. 4.

Eyes treated with customized topography-guided Epi-on CXL in a high oxygen environment ($\geq$ 90% oxygen) showed a significantly larger improvement in visual

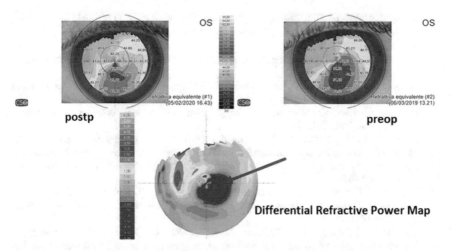

Fig. 4 Customized trans-epithelial CXL with supplemental oxygen differential refractive power map showed higher corneal flattening (red arrow)

outcomes than eyes treated in room-air environment ($\sim 20\%$ oxygen) in low-grade myopia, supporting the rationale to use intraoperative high oxygen concentration also in KC eyes to improve the overall oxygen kinetic of trans-epithelial accelerated CXL and to induce a higher flattening of corneal ectasia. Indeed, the degree of corneal flattening, HOA reduction and symmetry achieved after the customized epi-on treatments with topography-guided higher fluence and supplemental oxygen in this series, as documented for the first time at international level in KC by Mazzotta et al. [30], was comparable or even superior to Epi-off Dresden protocol outcomes as showed in Fig. 4, conferring a refractive power to trans-epithelial customized accelerated CXL beyond ectasia stabilization. More recently the efficacy of trans-epithelial customized crosslinking with intraoperative oxygen supplement was also conformed after 12-months follow-up as reported in the literature [48, 49].

References

1. Raiskup F, Spoerl E. Corneal crosslinking with riboflavin and ultraviolet A. I. Principles. Ocul Surf. 2013;11(2):65–74.
2. Lang PZ, Hafezi NL, Khandelwal SS, Torres-Netto EA, Hafezi F, Randleman JB. Comparative functional outcomes after corneal crosslinking using standard, accelerated, and accelerated with higher total fluence protocols. Cornea. 2019;38(4):433–41.
3. Kobashi H, Tsubota K. Accelerated versus standard corneal cross-linking for progressive keratoconus: a meta-analysis of randomized controlled trials. Cornea. 2020;39(2):172–80.
4. Mazzotta C, Raiskup F, Hafezi F, Torres-Netto EA, Armia Balamoun A, Giannaccare G, Bagaglia SA. Long term results of accelerated 9 mW corneal crosslinking for early progressive keratoconus: The Siena eye-cross study 2. Eye Vis (Lond). 2021;8(1):16.

5. Baiocchi S, Mazzotta C, Cerretani D, Caporossi T, Caporossi A. Corneal crosslinking: riboflavin concentration in corneal stroma exposed with and without epithelium. J Cataract Refract Surg. 2009;35(5):893.
6. Leccisotti A, Islam T. Transepithelial corneal collagen cross-linking in keratoconus. J Refract Surg. 2010;26(12):942–8.
7. Ghanem VC, Ghanem RC, de Oliveira R. Postoperative pain after corneal collagen cross-linking. Cornea. 2013;32(1):20–4.
8. Dhawan S, Rao K, Natrajan S. Complications of corneal collagen cross-linking. J Ophthalmol. 2011;2011:869015.
9. Franch A, Birattari F, Dal Mas G, Lužnik Z, Parekh M, Ferrari S, Ponzin D. Evaluation of intrastromal riboflavin concentration in human corneas after three corneal cross-linking imbibition procedures: a pilot study. J Ophthalmol. 2015;2015:794256. https://doi.org/10.1155/2015/794256.
10. Koppen C, Wouters K, Mathysen D, Rozema J, Tassignon MJ. Refractive and topographic results of benzalkonium chloride-assisted transepithelial crosslinking. J Cataract Refract Surg. 2012;38(6):1000–5.
11. Caporossi A, Mazzotta C, Paradiso AL, Baiocchi S, Marigliani D, Caporossi T. Transepithelial corneal collagen crosslinking for progressive keratoconus: 24-month clinical results. J Cataract Refract Surg. 2013;39(8):1157–63.
12. Gatzioufas Z, Raiskup F, O'Brart D, Spoerl E, Panos GD, Hafezi F. Transepithelial corneal cross-linking using an enhanced riboflavin solution. J Refract Surg. 2016;32(6):372–7.
13. Mastropasqua L, Nubile M, Calienno R, Mattei PA, Pedrotti E, Salgari N, Mastropasqua R, Lanzini M. Corneal cross-linking: intrastromal riboflavin concentration in iontophoresis-assisted imbibition versus traditional and transepithelial techniques. Am J Ophthalmol. 2014;157(3):623–30.
14. Laborante A, Longo C, Mazzilli E, Giardinelli K. Corneal iontophoresis and cross linking: a preliminary report of our experience. Clin Ter. 2015;166(4):e254–6. https://doi.org/10.7417/T.2015.1869 PMID: 26378758.
15. Mazzotta C, Traversi C, Mellace P, Bagaglia SA, Zuccarini S, Mencucci R, Jacob S. Keratoconus progression in patients with allergy and elevated surface matrix metalloproteinase 9 point-of-care test. Eye Contact Lens. 2018;44(Suppl 2):S48–53.
16. Claessens JLJ, Godefrooij DA, Vink G, Frank LE, Wisse RPL. Nationwide epidemiological approach to identify associations between keratoconus and immune-mediated diseases. Br J Ophthalmol. 2021;bjophthalmol-2021-318804. https://doi.org/10.1136/bjophthalmol-2021-318804. Epub ahead of print. PMID: 33879468.
17. Hayes S, Morgan SR, O'Brart DP, O'Brart N, Meek KM. A study of stromal riboflavin absorption in ex vivo porcine corneas using new and existing delivery protocols for corneal cross-linking. Acta Ophthalmol. 2016;94(2):e109–17.
18. Bikbova G, Bikbov M. Transepithelial corneal collagen cross-linking by iontophoresis of riboflavin. Acta Ophthalmol. 2014;92(1):e30–4.
19. Vinciguerra P, Romano V, Rosetta P, et al. Transepithelial iontophoresis versus standard corneal collagen cross-linking: 1-year results of a prospective clinical study. J Refract Surg. 2016;32(10):672–8.
20. Jouve L, Borderie V, Sandali O, et al. Conventional and iontophoresis corneal cross-linking for keratoconus: efficacy and assessment by optical coherence tomography and confocal microscopy. Cornea. 2017;36(2):153–62.
21. Kolozsvári L, Nógrádi A, Hopp B, Bor Z. UV absorbance of the human cornea in the 240- to 400-nm range. Invest Ophthalmol Vis Sci. 2002;43(7):2165–8.
22. Freeman RD. Oxygen consumption by the component layers of the cornea. J Physiol. 1972;225(1):15–32.
23. Mazzotta C, Bagaglia SA, Vinciguerra R, Ferrise M, Vinciguerra P. Enhanced-fluence pulsed-light iontophoresis corneal cross-linking: 1-year morphological and clinical results. J Refract Surg. 2018;34(7):438-44.

24. Mazzotta C, Bagaglia SA, Sgheri A, Di Maggio A, Fruschelli M, Romani A, Vinciguerra R, Vinciguerra P, Tosi GM. Iontophoresis corneal cross-linking with enhanced fluence and pulsed UV-A light: 3-year clinical results. J Refract Surg. 2020;36(5):286–92.
25. Mazzotta C, Moramarco A, Traversi C, Baiocchi S, Iovieno A, Fontana L. Accelerated corneal collagen cross-linking using topography-guided UV-A energy emission: preliminary clinical and morphological outcomes. J Ophthalmol. 2016;2016:2031031.
26. Mazzotta C, Traversi C, Caragiuli S, Rechichi M. Pulsed vs continuous light accelerated corneal collagen crosslinking: in vivo qualitative investigation by confocal microscopy and corneal OCT. Eye (Lond). 2014;28(10):1179–83.
27. Kamaev P, Friedman MD, Sherr E, Muller D. Photochemical kinetics of corneal cross-linking with riboflavin. Invest Ophthalmol Vis Sci. 2012;53(4):2360–7.
28. Richoz O, Hammer A, Tabibian D, Gatzioufas Z, Hafezi F. The biomechanical effect of corneal collagen cross-linking (cxl) with riboflavin and UV-A is oxygen dependent. Transl Vis Sci Technol. 2013;2(7):6.
29. Hill J, Liu C, Deardorff P, Tavakol B, Eddington W, Thompson V, Gore D, Raizman M, Adler DC. Optimization of oxygen dynamics, UV-A delivery, and drug formulation for accelerated epi-on corneal crosslinking. Curr Eye Res. 2020;45(4):450–8.
30. Mazzotta C, Sgheri A, Bagaglia SA, Rechichi M, Di Maggio A. Customized corneal crosslinking for treatment of progressive keratoconus: clinical and OCT outcomes using a transepithelial approach with supplemental oxygen. J Cataract Refract Surg. 2020;46 (12):1582–7.
31. Mazzotta C, Ferrise M, Gabriele G, Gennaro P, Meduri A. Chemically-boosted corneal cross-linking for the treatment of keratoconus through a riboflavin 0.25% optimized solution with high superoxide anion release. J Clin Med. 2021;10(6):1324.
32. Fredriksson A, Näslund S, Behndig A. A prospective evaluation of photorefractive intrastromal cross-linking for the treatment of low-grade myopia. Acta Ophthalmol. 2020;98(2):201–6.
33. Sachdev GS, Ramamurthy S, Dandapani R. Photorefractive intrastromal corneal crosslinking for treatment of low myopia: clinical outcomes using the transepithelial approach with supplemental oxygen. J Cataract Refract Surg. 2020;46(3):428–33.
34. Seiler TG, Komninou MA, Nambiar MH, Schuerch K, Frueh BE, Büchler P. Oxygen kinetics during corneal cross-linking with and without supplementary oxygen. Am J of Ophth. 2021;223:368–76.
35. Wang J, Wang L, Li Z, Wang YM, Zhu K, Mu G. Corneal biomechanical evaluation after conventional corneal crosslinking with oxygen enrichment. Eye Contact Lens. 2020;46 (5):306–9.
36. Stodulka P, Halasova Z, Slovak M, et al. Photorefractive intrastromal crosslinking for correction of hyperopia: 12-month results. J Cataract Refract Surg. 2020;46(3):434–40.
37. Kohlhaas M, Spoerl E, Schilde T, Unger G, Wittig C, Pillunat LE. Biomechanical evidence of the distribution of cross-links in corneas treated with riboflavin and ultraviolet A light. J Cataract Refract Surg. 2006;32(2):279–83.
38. Mazzotta C, Romani A, Burroni A. Pachymetry-based accelerated cross-linking: the "M Nomogram" for standardized treatment of all-thickness progressive ectatic corneas. Int J Keratoconus Ectatic Corneal Dis. 2019;7(2):137–44.
39. Mazzotta C, Wollensak G, Raiskup F, Pandolfi AM, Spoerl E. The meaning of the demarcation line after riboflavin-UVA corneal collagen crosslinking. Expert Rev Ophthalmol. 2019;115–31. https://doi.org/10.1080/17469899.2019.1611425.
40. Torres-Netto EA, Kling S, Hafezi N, Vinciguerra P, Randleman JB, Hafezi F. Oxygen diffusion may limit the biomechanical effectiveness of iontophoresis-assisted transepithelial corneal cross-linking. J Refract Surg. 2018;34(11):768–74.
41. Aldahlawi NH, Hayes S, O'Brart DP, et al. An investigation into corneal enzymatic resistance following epithelium-off and epithelium-on corneal cross-linking protocols. Exp Eye Res. 2016;153:141–51.

42. Weadock KS, Miller EJ, Bellincampi LD, Zawadsky JP, Dunn MG. Physical crosslinking of collagen fibers: comparison of ultraviolet irradiation and dehydrothermal treatment. J Biomed Mater Res. 1995;29(11):1373–9.
43. Lanchares E, del Buey MA, Cristóbal JA, Lavilla L, Calvo B. Biomechanical property analysis after corneal collagen cross-linking in relation to ultraviolet A irradiation time. Graefes Arch ClinExp Ophthalmol. 249(8):1223–7.
44. Roy AS, Dupps WJ Jr. Patient-specific computational modeling of keratoconus progression and differential responses to collagen cross-linking. Invest Ophthalmol Vis Sci. 2011;52 (12):9174–87.
45. Roberts CJ, Dupps WJ Jr Biomechanics of corneal ectasia and biomechanical treatments. J Cataract Refract Surg. 2014;40(6):991–8.
46. Sinha Roy A, Rocha KM, Randleman JB, Stulting RD, Dupps WJ Jr. Inverse computational analysis of in vivo corneal elastic modulus change after collagen crosslinking for keratoconus. Exp Eye Res. 2013;113:92–104.
47. Seven I, Sinha Roy A, Dupps WJ Jr. Patterned corneal collagen crosslinking for astigmatism: computational modeling study. J Cataract Refract Surg. 2014;40(6):943–53.
48. Kamiya K, Kanayama S, Takahashi M, Shoji N. Visual and topographic improvement with epithelium-on, oxygen-supplemented, customized corneal cross-linking for progressive keratoconus. J Clin Med. 2020;9(10):3222.
49. Aydın E, Aslan MG. The efficiency and safety of oxygen-supplemented accelerated transepithelial corneal cross-linking. Int Ophthalmol. 2021. https://doi.org/10.1007/s10792-021-01859-1. Epub ahead of print. PMID: 33876334.

Corneal Cross-Linking at the Slit Lamp

Emilio A. Torres-Netto, Mohamed Hosny, and Farhad Hafezi

Corneal cross-linking (CXL) is a well-established method for slowing or halting the treatment of corneal ectasias like keratoconus or post-refractive surgery ectasia [1, 2]. Like most procedures in ophthalmology, CXL has typically been performed in an operating room (OR), with the patient lying in a supine position throughout most of the procedure, including the riboflavin instillation, corneal pachymetry, and UV irradiation. In these situations, only the pre- or post-operative slit lamp exams are performed with the patient sitting upright.

E. A. Torres-Netto (✉) · F. Hafezi
ELZA Institute, Dietikon/Zurich, Switzerland
e-mail: emilio.torres@cabmm.uzh.ch

E. A. Torres-Netto · F. Hafezi
Laboratory of Ocular Cell Biology, Center for Applied Biotechnology and Molecular Medicine, University of Zurich, Zurich, Switzerland

E. A. Torres-Netto
Department of Ophthalmology, Paulista School of Medicine, Federal University of Sao Paulo, Sao Paulo, Brazil

E. A. Torres-Netto · F. Hafezi
Faculty of Medicine, University of Geneva, Geneva, Switzerland

E. A. Torres-Netto
Department of Ophthalmology, University Hospital Zurich, University of Zurich, Zurich, Switzerland

M. Hosny
Department of Ophthalmology, Cairo University, Cairo, Egypt

F. Hafezi
USC Roski Eye Institute, University of Southern California, Los Angeles, CA, USA

F. Hafezi
Department of Ophthalmology, University of Wenzhou, Wenzhou, China

© The Author(s), under exclusive license to Springer Nature Switzerland AG 2022   149
A. Armia and C. Mazzotta (eds.), *Keratoconus*,
https://doi.org/10.1007/978-3-030-84506-3_8

However, as our knowledge of CXL, the UV-riboflavin photochemical reaction, and its mechanisms of action has expanded, it has become increasingly clear that CXL can be performed outside of the OR—ideally at the slit lamp. This approach could bring numerous advantages, as it lowers costs by removing the administrative and cost burden of booking and operating an OR, and brings cross-linking technology away from ORs in hospitals that are predominantly concentrated in large population centers, to even the most rural clinic locations in low-to-middle-income countries (LMICs), where procedure cost is particularly sensitive.

This chapter discusses how crosslinking technology can be safely incorporated into the medical office (Fig. 1) in its various clinical indications, whether in remote areas where an operating room is not available or in large centers where the efficiency and costs can be optimized.

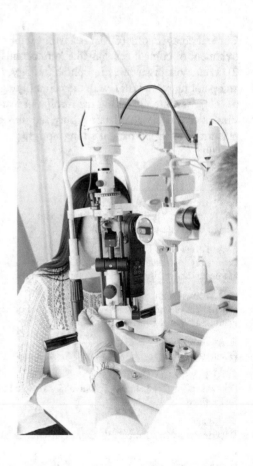

Fig. 1 Cross-linking with a portable slit lamp-mounted cross-linking device

1 Bringing Surgical Procedures Out of the OR

Across ophthalmology, and medicine in general, there is a trend to take procedures that were once performed in an OR, out into a minor procedure room, or even the doctor's office, as long as safety can be maintained. In these cases, the purpose is not only to optimize costs, but also to increase patient convenience and efficiency. In reality, this is not a novelty in ophthalmology: for many years now, a large proportion of intravitreal injections for retinal disorders have been performed in the office, not the OR [3]. In 2014, Tabandeh et al. performed a retrospective consecutive case series review of over 11,700 intravitreal injections of anti-VEGF agents or triamcinolone acetonide for the treatment of retinal disease, and found endophthalmitis rates to be both low and similar, irrespective of whether the procedure was performed in the office or in an OR [3].

A study that evaluated cataract surgery, performed as an in-office procedure, instead of an OR in more than 21,000 eyes, and with an average patient age of 72 years, has been shown that this approach can be as safe and effective as cataract surgery performed in an OR, in terms of not only visual outcomes, but also rates of adverse events and endophthalmitis [4]. The US Medicare Program has stated that cataract surgeries, particularly routine cases, that it is possible and advantageous to perform the procedure outside a traditional operating room, and in an "office-based surgical suite." [5].

On the other hand, ORs are comfortable places for the surgeon to operate. They are sterilized thoroughly before every procedure, and there is a familiarity for surgeons in that environment: everything is in the same place, every time. Despite this, OR use comes with administrative and financial costs. ORs need to be booked in advance (and surgeons often compete for OR time), and there is a cost attached to using them. The running, cleaning, and staff costs are not trivial, and performing a procedure in an OR certainly adds to the cost of the procedure to both doctor and patient. A "clean, but not sterile" environment, similar to the environment in which many retina specialists administer intravitreal anti-VEGF injections, is more than sufficient for a CXL procedure.

2 CXL 'sterilizes' the Cornea

CXL has one major advantage over the procedures mentioned above: it reduces the microbiological load of microorganisms on the irradiated surface of the cornea [6, 7].

When the UV light interacts with riboflavin molecules in the stroma, it produces photoactivated (reduced) riboflavin molecules and other reactive oxygen species (ROS) [1]. These react in multiple ways (Fig. 2). The first (and intended) effect of CXL in treating ectasia is that these molecules covalently bind and "cross-link" the molecules on the surface of the collagen fibrils or between the fibrils and the proteoglycan extrafibrillar matrix [8]. This results in a tougher, stronger, stiffer

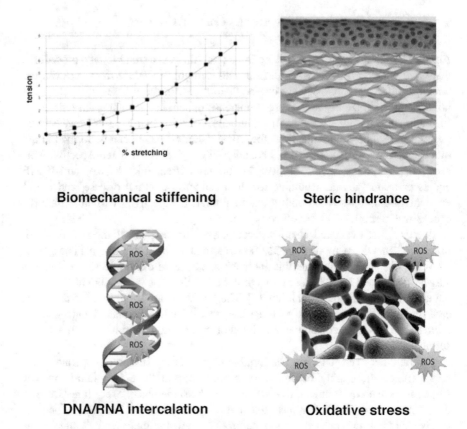

Biomechanical stiffening   **Steric hindrance**

DNA/RNA intercalation   **Oxidative stress**

Fig. 2 The four main effects corneal cross-linking has on the cornea

cornea that is more resistant to outward distortion by intraocular pressure and the physical damage to the stroma that can be caused by chronic eye rubbing. This cross-linking process also means that there are fewer binding sites for matrix metalloproteinases to bind (i.e. steric hindrance), making it harder for proteases generated as part of inflammatory processes to digest the stroma.

Photoactivated riboflavin and ROS also attack and damage cell membranes and intercalate and oxidatively damage nucleic acids [9–12]. The corneal stroma, where the effect is limited by careful direction of UV energy, consists of mostly collagen and proteoglycans, and is essentially an acellular zone, and the corneal epithelium is usually removed prior to riboflavin application (otherwise only a small amount of riboflavin will reach the stroma). Interestingly, this sterilizing effect has led to CXL being used to treat infectious keratitis of bacterial, fungal, and mixed bacterial/fungal origin, in a procedure called photoactivated chromophore for keratitis–corneal cross-linking (PACK-CXL) [13].

There is little point in 'sterilizing' a room to perform a procedure that 'sterilizes' the organ and tissue being operated on, especially when antimicrobial prophylaxis is administered immediately after the cross-linking procedure is completed. The greatest concern regarding infection after CXL (or any other corneal procedure) is how the open corneal surface is handled postoperatively. A second important point is related to the treatment of infectious keratitis with PACK-CXL. Here it makes even less sense to bring an active infection into an operating room, considering that the treatment could be performed at the slit lamp effectively elsewhere.

3 Adapting CXL for Keratoconus to the Slit Lamp

Cross-linking, performed according to the classic, gold-standard Dresden protocol [2], involves quite an extended period of irradiation—30 minutes—which might favor a patient lying supine to receive the UV irradiation, as patients may eventually feel uncomfortable if sat upright for that duration. However, after more than 20 years of CXL development, effective, accelerated protocols that cut the UV irradiation time by one-third and can be used in the vast majority of cases to halt ectasia progression are now available.

Initially, it was believed that the UV-riboflavin photochemical reaction adheres to a principle of photochemistry called the Bunsen-Roscoe law of reciprocity. In essence, this means that if the total light energy delivered into a photochemical reaction remains the same, it does not matter whether that energy (the total fluence) is delivered quickly or slowly: the same amount of reaction will occur. This means that irrespective of whether 3 mW/cm^2 of UV energy is delivered for 30 minutes, or 9 mW/cm^2 is delivered over a 10-minute period, the cross-linking effect should be essentially the same [14].

However, after we identified oxygen as a central element in the CXL photochemical reactions [15], several studies have shown this law of reciprocity starts to break down as the reaction is accelerated beyond a certain point [16, 17]. Oxygen availability in the riboflavin-saturated stroma is the rate-limiting step, and the UV-riboflavin photochemical reaction consumes oxygen and depleting the cornea of oxygen rapidly. The rate at which the reaction progresses is therefore dependent on how quickly oxygen can diffuse into the stroma. Attempts to accelerate the reaction by irradiating with high intensities and short duration times limit the total amount of oxygen that can diffuse into the stroma, and accordingly, reduces the overall biomechanical strengthening effect that the procedure achieves [18, 19]. As it turns out, trying to increase intensity beyond ∼9 mW/cm^2 starts to result in a diminished stiffening effect [14, 15, 19, 20]. Therefore, we believe that a good balance between efficiency of the procedure and irradiation time is when 9 mW/cm^2 is delivered over a 10-minute UV irradiation. This could be offered for a large fraction of the eyes while maintaining a satisfactorily stabilizing effect and patient convenience [14, 21, 22]. In summary, a 10 minutes treatment is an attractive proposition for patients to sit at the slit lamp, and should be well within most patients' comfort zones.

One question that has been raised about performing cross-linking in patients who are sat upright is that riboflavin might be redistributed in the cornea thanks to gravity, particularly if the patient is sat upright for extended periods, which could lead to an uneven crosslinking effect. We addressed this point through a laboratory study in 2017 and the experiments have shown no significant settling or shift in riboflavin concentration in the stroma, even after 1 hour of sitting upright after saturation [23].

PACK-CXL: Treating Infectious Keratitis

The World Health Organization has called infectious keratitis a "silent epidemic." [24, 25]. It is a leading cause of visual impairment worldwide, particularly in developing countries, where those who fall victim to it are usually agricultural workers in the most productive years of their lives. Infectious keratitis progresses rapidly, and therefore prompt diagnosis and emergent treatment are critical.

Infections in temperate and developed countries tend to be bacterial in origin, largely due to micro-abrasions from contact lens wear. In developing countries with warmer, more humid environments, many of these cases are fungal, or worse, mixed (i.e., bacterial and fungal) infections. Our phase III clinical trial (Hafezi et al., submitted) has shown that PACK-CXL has the potential to effectively treat early bacterial, fungal, and mixed infections, in a single sitting accelerated treatment, without antimicrobial drugs as effectively as current standard-of-care antimicrobial therapy, and crucially, in a manner that sidesteps the issue of antimicrobial resistance (AMR). Although more studies are needed to assess the optimal role of this treatment as a standalone therapy for infectious keratitis, several studies have already shown the positive impact of PACK-CXL as an adjuvant treatment [26–29].

PACK-CXL also cross-links the cornea, which increases the corneal resistance to digestion by pathogen-produced proteases, with the potential benefit of reducing the eventual scar size. Interestingly, the pathogen-killing component of PACK-CXL appears to be even less dependent on oxygen than CXL to stabilize keratoconus or iatrogenic ectasias. So, when it comes to treating infectious keratitis, higher intensities and shorter treatment times should be feasible in this context [27, 30].

A central point in the killing rate of microorganisms with PACK-CXL is the total energy used [31]. The Dresden protocol delivers a total fluence of 5.4 J/cm^2, and initial PACK-CXL protocols studied also delivered the same fluence. We have since learned that higher fluences are more effective at killing pathogens than the fluence delivered with the Dresden protocol and its derivatives, meaning that high-fluence PACK-CXL should be even more effective than it has been in earlier clinical studies [7, 32, 33].

Crucially, this potentially one-shot treatment performed outside of the OR should be considerably less expensive for patients in low-to-middle-income countries (LMICs). Repeated doctor visits and intensive, hourly topical antimicrobial drug administration is beyond the means of many in developing countries. PACK-CXL, with its ability in many cases, to treat in a single treatment, should mean that far more people receive effective and affordable infectious keratitis treatment, no matter where they live in the world.

4 Summary

Given that (1) CXL reduces the microbial load on the cornea so much it can be used to even treat bacterial and fungal corneal infections, (2) patients can sit at the slit lamp for 10 minutes to receive an accelerated CXL protocol, (3) riboflavin is not significantly redistributed in the cornea due to gravity, and (4) operating rooms are expensive to run and attract an administrative burden, there is little to argue against performing CXL, safely and effectively, at the slit lamp (Fig. 3). CXL at the slit lamp has the advantage of not only lowering costs, but also opening up the procedure to areas of the world where access to an OR is limited, but where tertiary eyecare centers are present—all of which all have the near-ubiquitous slit lamp available. This opens up not only CXL to more ophthalmologists and therefore more patients around the world, but potentially more importantly, PACK-CXL to a far larger global demographic: the chronically underserved in LMICs. In conclusion, CXL at the slit lamp has a number of advantages: it lowers costs for patients and doctors, it permits treatment to be brought to a far greater population in need of treatment, and PACK-CXL at the slit lamp may potentially save many thousands of people's vision, who in the past would have been blinded by infectious keratitis.

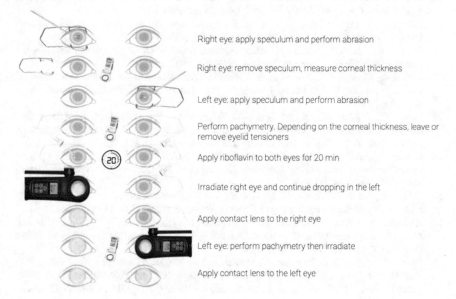

Fig. 3 The key steps involved in performing CXL at the slit lamp, exemplified here by a simultaneous bilateral treatment

References

1. Randleman JB, Khandelwal SS, Hafezi F. Corneal cross-linking. Surv Ophthalmol. 2015;60 (6):509–23.
2. Wollensak G, Spoerl E, Seiler T. Riboflavin/ultraviolet-a-induced collagen crosslinking for the treatment of keratoconus. Am J Ophthalmol. 2003;135(5):620–7.
3. Tabandeh H, Boscia F, Sborgia A, et al. Endophthalmitis associated with intravitreal injections: office-based setting and operating room setting. Retina. 2014;34(1):18–23.
4. Ianchulev T, Litoff D, Ellinger D, Stiverson K, Packer M. Office-based cataract surgery: population health outcomes study of more than 21 000 cases in the United States. Ophthalmology. 2016;123(4):723–8.
5. U.S. Department of Health and Human Services CfMaMS. Medicare program; Re- visions to payment policies under the physician fee schedule and other revisions to Part B for CY 2016; Proposed rule. Federal Register 2015. 2016;80:41700.
6. Hafezi F, Randleman JB. PACK-CXL: defining CXL for infectious keratitis. J Refract Surg. 2014;30(7):438–9.
7. Kling S, Hufschmid FS, Torres-Netto EA, et al. High fluence increases the antibacterial efficacy of PACK cross-linking. Cornea. 2020;39(8):1020–6.
8. Hayes S, Boote C, Kamma-Lorger CS, et al. Riboflavin/UVA collagen cross-linking-induced changes in normal and keratoconus corneal stroma. PLoS One. 2011;6(8):e22405.
9. Martins SA, Combs JC, Noguera G, et al. Antimicrobial efficacy of riboflavin/UVA combination (365 nm) in vitro for bacterial and fungal isolates: a potential new treatment for infectious keratitis. Invest Ophthalmol Vis Sci. 2008;49(8):3402–8.
10. Naseem I, Ahmad M, Hadi SM. Effect of alkylated and intercalated DNA on the generation of superoxide anion by riboflavin. Biosci Rep. 1988;8(5):485–92.
11. Pileggi G, Wataha JC, Girard M, et al. Blue light-mediated inactivation of Enterococcus faecalis in vitro. Photodiagnosis Photodyn Ther. 2013;10(2):134–40.
12. Tsugita A, Okada Y, Uehara K. Photosensitized inactivation of ribonucleic acids in the presence of riboflavin. Biochim Biophys Acta. 1965;103(2):360–3.
13. Richoz O, Kling S, Hoogewoud F, et al. Antibacterial efficacy of accelerated photoactivated chromophore for keratitis-corneal collagen cross-linking (PACK-CXL). J Refract Surg. 2014;30(12):850–4.
14. Lang PZ, Hafezi NL, Khandelwal SS, Torres-Netto EA, Hafezi F, Randleman JB. Comparative functional outcomes after corneal crosslinking using standard, accelerated, and accelerated with higher total fluence protocols. Cornea. 2019;38(4):433–41.
15. Richoz O, Hammer A, Tabibian D, Gatzioufas Z, Hafezi F. The Biomechanical effect of corneal collagen cross-linking (cxl) with riboflavin and UV-A is oxygen dependent. Transl Vis Sci Technol. 2013;2(7):6.
16. Webb JN, Su JP, Scarcelli G. Mechanical outcome of accelerated corneal crosslinking evaluated by Brillouin microscopy. J Cataract Refract Surg. 2017;43(11):1458–63.
17. Hammer A, Richoz O, Mosquera S, Tabibian D, Hoogewoud F, Hafezi F. Corneal biomechanical properties at different corneal collagen cross-linking (CXL) irradiances. Invest Ophthalmol Vis Sci. 2014;55(5):2881–4.
18. Hammer A, Richoz O, Tabibian D, Hafezi F. The increase in biomechanical stiffness in corneal collagen cross-linking (CXL) is oxygen dependent. In: Paper presented at 106th general assembly of the Swiss Ophthalmological Society; August 28–31, 2013, 2013; Locarno, Switzerland.
19. Torres-Netto EA, Kling S, Hafezi N, Vinciguerra P, Randleman JB, Hafezi F. Oxygen diffusion may limit the biomechanical effectiveness of iontophoresis-assisted transepithelial corneal cross-linking. J Refract Surg. 2018;34(11):768–74.
20. Hammer A, Richoz O, Arba Mosquera S, Tabibian D, Hoogewoud F, Hafezi F. Corneal biomechanical properties at different corneal cross-linking (CXL) irradiances. Invest Ophthalmol Vis Sci. 2014;55(5):2881–4.

21. Shajari M, Kolb CM, Agha B, et al. Comparison of standard and accelerated corneal cross-linking for the treatment of keratoconus: a meta-analysis. Acta Ophthalmol. 2019;97(1): e22–35.
22. Turhan SA, Yargi B, Toker E. Efficacy of conventional versus accelerated corneal cross-linking in pediatric keratoconus: two-year outcomes. J Refract Surg. 2020;36(4):265–9.
23. Salmon B, Richoz O, Tabibian D, Kling S, Wuarin R, Hafezi F. CXL at the slit lamp: no clinically relevant changes in corneal riboflavin distribution during upright UV irradiation. J Refract Surg. 2017;33(4):281.
24. Whitcher JP, Srinivasan M. Corneal ulceration in the developing world–a silent epidemic. Br J Ophthalmol. 1997;81(8):622–3.
25. World Health Organization. Antimicrobial resistance: global report on surveillance. http://www.who.int/drugresistance/documents/surveillancereport/en/ . Published 2014. Accessed 29 Oct 2020.
26. Wei A, Wang K, Wang Y, Gong L, Xu J, Shao T. Evaluation of corneal cross-linking as adjuvant therapy for the management of fungal keratitis. Graefes Arch Clin Exp Ophthalmol. 2019;257(7):1443–52.
27. Knyazer B, Krakauer Y, Tailakh MA, et al. Accelerated corneal cross-linking as an adjunct therapy in the management of presumed bacterial keratitis: a cohort study. J Refract Surg. 2020;36(4):258–64.
28. Bonzano C, Di Zazzo A, Barabino S, Coco G, Traverso CE. Collagen cross-linking in the management of microbial keratitis. Ocul Immunol Inflamm. 2019;27(3):507–12.
29. Price MO, Price FW Jr. Corneal cross-linking in the treatment of corneal ulcers. Curr Opin Ophthalmol. 2016;27(3):250–5.
30. Knyazer B, Krakauer Y, Baumfeld Y, Lifshitz T, Kling S, Hafezi F. Accelerated corneal cross-linking with photoactivated chromophore for moderate therapy-resistant infectious keratitis. Cornea. 2018;37(4):528–31.
31. Kling S, Hufschmid FS, Torres-Netto EA, et al. High fluence increases the antibacterial efficacy of PACK cross-linking. Cornea. 2020;39(8):1020-26.
32. Hafezi F, Torres-Netto EA, Hillen MJP. Re: Prajna et al.: Cross-Linking-Assisted Infection Reduction: a randomized clinical trial evaluating the effect of adjuvant cross-linking on outcomes in fungal keratitis (Ophthalmology. 2020;127:159–66). Ophthalmology. 2021;128 (1):e6.
33. Uysal BS, Yaman D, Sarac O, Akcay E, Cagil N. Sterile keratitis after uneventful corneal collagen cross-linking in a patient with Axenfeld-Rieger syndrome. Int Ophthalmol. 2019;39 (5):1169–73.

Corneal Cross-Linking in Ultrathin Corneas

Farhad Hafezi and Emilio A. Torres-Netto

Introduced into clinical practice in 2003, corneal cross-linking (CXL) is a treatment modality that biomechanically stiffens the cornea, and can arrest the progression of corneal ectatic disorders like keratoconus, post-operative ectasia, and pellucid marginal degeneration [1–3]. The original CXL ("Dresden") protocol achieved stiffening by the following process: corneal epithelial cell debridement, riboflavin application to the exposed corneal stroma to completely saturate it, followed by irradiation with ultraviolet (UV)-A light at 365 nm [2]. The UV energy is absorbed by stromal riboflavin, which results in a photochemical reaction that generates reduced riboflavin species and reactive oxygen species (ROS). These photoactivated molecules cause the formation of covalent bonds between the collagen fibers and the proteoglycans of the extracellular matrix [4, 5]. As the cross-linking

F. Hafezi (✉)
ELZA Institute, Dietikon/Zurich, Switzerland
e-mail: farhad@hafezi.ch

F. Hafezi · E. A. Torres-Netto
Laboratory of Ocular Cell Biology, Center for Applied Biotechnology
and Molecular Medicine, University of Zurich, Zurich, Switzerland

F. Hafezi · E. A. Torres-Netto
Faculty of Medicine, University of Geneva, Geneva, Switzerland

F. Hafezi
USC Roski Eye Institute, University of Southern California, Los Angeles, CA, USA

F. Hafezi
Department of Ophthalmology, University of Wenzhou, Wenzhou, China

E. A. Torres-Netto
Department of Ophthalmology, Paulista School of Medicine, Federal University
of Sao Paulo, Sao Paulo, Brazil

E. A. Torres-Netto
Department of Ophthalmology, University Hospital Zurich, University of Zurich,
Zurich, Switzerland

© The Author(s), under exclusive license to Springer Nature Switzerland AG 2022   159
A. Armia and C. Mazzotta (eds.), *Keratoconus*,
https://doi.org/10.1007/978-3-030-84506-3_9

procedure progresses, the riboflavin is 'consumed' by the light, and the longer the procedure (or the higher the intensity of light), the more riboflavin is consumed, and the deeper the effect of the reaction in the cornea. It is here where riboflavin serves another role: shielding the deeper corneal layers (in particular, the corneal endothelium) from UV-induced damage and apoptosis [4, 5].

The Dresden protocol specified that for CXL to be performed safely, corneas should have a minimum corneal thickness of 400 μm after epithelial debridement. In a 400 μm-thick cornea, the Dresden protocol cross-links the superficial ~330 μm of the stroma, leaving ~70 μm of unreacted riboflavin in the stroma, above the endothelial cell layer, as the safety margin (Fig. 1). This safety margin distance calculation was created based on riboflavin concentration estimates and the total amount of UV energy that would be delivered to the cornea, especially to the endothelial cell layer (which needs to be protected from receiving damaging amounts of UV irradiation). However, the consequence of this is that the 400 μm corneal thickness limitation excludes many corneas with corneal ectatic disease that would benefit from CXL, many of whom will eventually otherwise require keratoplasty.

Over the years, several modifications have been made to the Dresden protocol to overcome the 400 μm limit that involve artificially thickening the cornea (Fig. 1). Although feasible, these approaches are associated with drawbacks that may result in unpredictable outcomes, and consequently can reduce the subsequent efficacy of cross-linking [6–8].

Hafezi et al. developed the first approach for treating thin corneas in 2009 [6], which involved the preoperative swelling of the cornea with hypo-osmolaric riboflavin. Of the 20 eyes treated, keratectasia remained stable in all eyes after 6-months of follow-up, and no cases of endothelial cell loss were observed. However, the swelling effect using the same riboflavin soaking regime can be highly variable from one cornea to the next [9].

A later approach was Jacob et al.'s contact lens-assisted CXL (CA-CXL), which involves the use of an iso-osmolaric riboflavin-soaked contact lens, to artificially "thicken" the cornea [7]. While this form of treatment would conveniently allow the 400 μm corneal thickness limit to be reached before irradiation, this approach has the disadvantage that the diffusion of oxygen into the stroma is hindered by the contact lens [10]. Oxygen is an essential component of the cross-linking photochemical reaction, and this cross-linking method is associated with a ~30% reduction in cross-linking efficacy compared with Dresden protocol CXL, as measured by Brillouin microscopy thermal shrinkage tests and biomechanical stress–strain measurements [11, 12]. Repurposed small-incision lenticule extraction (SMILE) lenticules have also been used in a similar manner to the contact lens approach [13].

Mazzotta et al. [8] proposed "epithelial island cross-linking," where epithelial cells over the thinnest point of the cornea are not debrided. In this way, a thin area of the cornea would have the advantage of not losing 40–50 μm of additional thickness from epithelial removal. Furthermore, the riboflavin that accumulates in the epithelial cells attenuates the UV-A energy over these areas. Here, in addition to

Individualized UV fluence

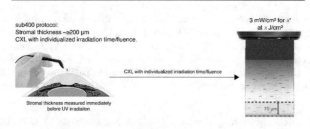

sub400 protocol:
Stromal thickness ~≥200 μm
CXL with individualized irradiation time/fluence.

CXL with individualized irradiation time/fluence

Stromal thickness measured immediately
before UV irradiation

3 mW/cm² for *x*′
at *x* J/cm²

70 μm

Artificially thicken the cornea

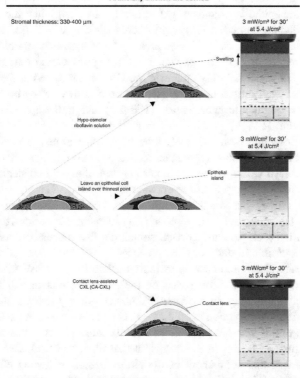

Stromal thickness: 330–400 μm

3 mW/cm² for 30′
at 5.4 J/cm²

Swelling

Hypo-osmolar
riboflavin solution

3 mW/cm² for 30′
at 5.4 J/cm²

Leave an epithelial cell
island over thinnest point

Epithelial
island

Contact lens-assisted
CXL (CA-CXL)

3 mW/cm² for 30′
at 5.4 J/cm²

Contact lens

Thickness-directed protocol choice

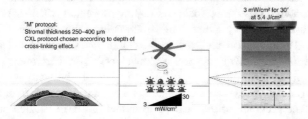

"M" protocol:
Stromal thickness 250–400 μm
CXL protocol chosen according to depth of
cross-linking effect.

3 mW/cm² for 30′
at 5.4 J/cm²

3   30
mW/cm²

◀**Fig. 1** Strategies to cross-link thin corneas: hypo-osmolaric riboflavin to swell the cornea prior to UV irradiation; leaving an island of epithelial cells over the thinnest part of the cornea, or the application of a riboflavin-soaked contact lens to artificially thicken the cornea (all of which can be used on corneas in corneal stroma as thin as ∼330 μm), or the sub400 protocol that uses a measurement of corneal thickness immediately before UV irradiation to determine the total UV fluence applied to the cornea, customized to each cornea by altering irradiation time accordingly (this can be used in corneas as thin as 200 μm, and still maintain a 70 μm non-cross-linked safety margin above the corneal endothelium)

the shielding effect that the epithelium would bring both from the point of view of oxygen, and also from the penetration of UV light, there have been concerns that the edges of the epithelial islands might refract UV-A energy into the intermediate stroma, introducing unpredictability in the cross-linking effect. As expected, this approach results in an unequal demarcation line between epithelialized and de-epithelialized areas [11]. It appears that the regions of the cornea where the epithelium is left intact not only attenuate the UV dose received in the stroma, but also restricts oxygen diffusion, which results in a shallower cross-linking effect in areas under the epithelium-intact region (150 μm) than in the epithelium-debrided regions (250 μm) [14–16].

These previous thin cornea cross-linking approaches aimed to increase stromal thickness, but logically, other approaches to constrain the depth of the cross-linking reaction could also work. In theory, increasing the riboflavin concentration in the anterior stroma should help limit the cross-linking effect to that region, and ensure that less UV energy penetrates through to the posterior stroma or the corneal endothelium. However, such an approach would require a customized riboflavin concentration for each patients' cornea, something that makes matters more complex and is unfeasible in daily clinical practice.

A logical alternative approach is to individualize the total UV irradiation (fluence) delivered to each patient, based on their corneal thickness. This approach requires simply shortening the irradiation time accordingly and has the advantage that a single riboflavin solution is all that is necessary. However, as sensible as this approach appears, it was not possible in 2009 because so little was known about riboflavin diffusion kinetics in the cornea at that time, and back then, the role of oxygen as an essential component of the biomechanical stiffening effect of CXL was not yet known [17, 18]. Recently, an approach called the "sub400" protocol has been developed that uses an algorithm that accounts for UV intensity, oxygen and stromal riboflavin levels during the cross-linking procedure [17, 18]. The algorithm predicts both the extent of biomechanical stiffening achieved after CXL and the duration of UV irradiation required to cross-link the stroma to the same safety threshold/ distance from the corneal epithelial cells. Furthermore, the algorithm takes into account Fick's law of diffusion estimates of riboflavin and oxygen diffusion, and UV energy exposure calculations using the Lambert–Beer law of light absorption. The accuracy of the theoretical model has been verified previously in pre-clinical experiments, where the predicted CXL concentration did strongly correlate ($R^2 = 0.95$) with the biomechanical stiffening in porcine, murine, and rabbit corneas [10].

The results of a clinical validation of the sub400 algorithm have recently been published [19], in which 39 patients with progressive keratoconus and stromal thicknesses ranging from 214 to 398 μm were treated epithelial debridement, followed by 20 minutes of stromal saturation with a 0.1% hypotonic riboflavin solution. UV irradiation was then performed at an intensity of 3 mW/cm^2 with the duration (and therefore the total fluence) being adapted to the intraoperative stromal thickness of each eye being treated. The individualized CXL with sub400 protocol successfully prevented keratoconus progression in these ultra thin keratoconic corneas in 90% of cases after 1 year of follow-up. Besides that, and in line with recent experimental evidence that suggests the current threshold of endothelial damage might have been overestimated for decades [20], no cornea showed clinical signs of endothelial decompensation. There was a significant correlation between demarcation line depth and irradiation time but no significant correlation between the depth of the demarcation line and change in Kmax.

Finally, an alternative approach proposed by Mazzotta et al. is the "M" protocol [21], which instead of developing an algorithm and clinically validating it, instead cross-references the depth of cross-linking achieved by previously published CXL protocols that use different technical settings (including protocols that use different intensities to the standard 3 mW/cm^2 settings defined in the Dresden protocol, pulsed and continuous light, and even iontophoresis) with the thickness of the thin cornea needing cross-linked, and suggests an appropriate cross-linking protocol for the cornea. This protocol matches in vivo scanning laser confocal microscopy and OCT morphological data from various studies, with the mathematical assessment of the cross-link concentration threshold according to the measured demarcation line, using the Dresden protocol as the benchmark. It demonstrates that the maximum interaction between UV-A, riboflavin, oxygen, and collagen-proteoglycans complex would be in the first 200 μm, where 70% of riboflavin-UV-A interactions occur, while the remaining 30% of the CXL photo-oxidative reaction would be dissipated in the deep stroma between 200 and 300 μm. This approach requires physicians to have access to a range of cross-linking technologies (as opposed to a simple 3 mW/cm^2 intensity lamp that is all that is required with the sub400 protocol) to be able to treat all thin corneas of a thickness between 250 and 400 μm.

In summary, new promising protocols have brought fresh perspectives for the treatment of thin corneas. Instead of artificially modifying corneal thickness, approaches such as individualized CXL using the sub400 protocol instead control the depth of cross-linking to a safe distance from the endothelium, by modifying UV illumination time based on patients' corneal thickness. Moving forward, this application can potentially be used in other corneal ectasias such as keratoglobus (Hafezi et al., in preparation), thereby expanding the number of patients who could benefit from the treatment and further reducing the number of people who experience further vision loss, or who ultimately require corneal transplantation.

References

1. Raiskup F, Theuring A, Pillunat LE, Spoerl E. Corneal collagen crosslinking with riboflavin and ultraviolet-A light in progressive keratoconus: ten-year results. J Cataract Refract Surg. 2015;41(1):41–6.
2. Randleman JB, Khandelwal SS, Hafezi F. Corneal cross-linking. Surv Ophthalmol. 2015;60 (6):509–23.
3. Wollensak G, Spoerl E, Seiler T. Riboflavin/ultraviolet-a-induced collagen crosslinking for the treatment of keratoconus. Am J Ophthalmol. 2003;135(5):620–7.
4. Spoerl E, Huhle M, Seiler T. Induction of cross-links in corneal tissue. Exp Eye Res. 1998;66 (1):97–103.
5. Zhang Y, Conrad AH, Conrad GW. Effects of ultraviolet-A and riboflavin on the interaction of collagen and proteoglycans during corneal cross-linking. J Biol Chem. 2011;286 (15):13011–22.
6. Hafezi F, Mrochen M, Iseli HP, Seiler T. Collagen crosslinking with ultraviolet-A and hypoosmolar riboflavin solution in thin corneas. J Cataract Refract Surg. 2009;35(4):621–4.
7. Jacob S, Kumar DA, Agarwal A, Basu S, Sinha P, Agarwal A. Contact lens-assisted collagen cross-linking (CACXL): a new technique for cross-linking thin corneas. J Refract Surg. 2014;30(6):366–72.
8. Mazzotta C, Ramovecchi V. Customized epithelial debridement for thin ectatic corneas undergoing corneal cross-linking: epithelial island cross-linking technique. Clin Ophthalmol. 2014;8:1337–43.
9. Wollensak G, Sporl E. Biomechanical efficacy of corneal cross-linking using hypoosmolar riboflavin solution. Eur J Ophthalmol. 2019;29(5):474–81.
10. Kling S, Hafezi F. An algorithm to predict the biomechanical stiffening effect in corneal cross-linking. J Refract Surg. 2017;33(2):128–36.
11. Wollensak G, Sporl E, Herbst H. Biomechanical efficacy of contact lens-assisted collagen cross-linking in porcine eyes. Acta Ophthalmol. 2019;97(1):e84–90.
12. Zhang H, Roozbahani M, Piccinini AL, et al. Depth-dependent reduction of biomechanical efficacy of contact lens-assisted corneal cross-linking analyzed by brillouin microscopy. J Refract Surg. 2019;35(11):721–8.
13. Sachdev MS, Gupta D, Sachdev G, Sachdev R. Tailored stromal expansion with a refractive lenticule for crosslinking the ultrathin cornea. J Cataract Refract Surg. 2015;41(5):918–23.
14. Deshmukh R, Hafezi F, Kymionis GD, et al. Current concepts in crosslinking thin corneas. Indian J Ophthalmol. 2019;67(1):8–15.
15. Kaya V, Utine CA, Yilmaz OF. Efficacy of corneal collagen cross-linking using a custom epithelial debridement technique in thin corneas: a confocal microscopy study. J Refract Surg. 2011;27(6):444–50.
16. Torres-Netto EA, Kling S, Hafezi N, Vinciguerra P, Randleman JB, Hafezi F. Oxygen diffusion may limit the biomechanical effectiveness of iontophoresis-assisted transepithelial corneal cross-linking. J Refract Surg. 2018;34(11):768–74.
17. Kling S, Richoz O, Hammer A, et al. Increased biomechanical efficacy of corneal cross-linking in thin corneas due to higher oxygen availability. J Refract Surg. 2015;31 (12):840–6.
18. Richoz O, Hammer A, Tabibian D, Gatzioufas Z, Hafezi F. The biomechanical effect of corneal collagen cross-linking (CXL) with riboflavin and UV-A is oxygen dependent. Transl Vis Sci Technol. 2013;2(7):6.
19. Hafezi F, Kling S, Gilardoni F, et al. Individualized corneal cross-linking with riboflavin and UV-A in ultrathin corneas: the sub400 protocol. Am J Ophthalmol. 2021;224:133–42.

20. Seiler TG, Batista A, Frueh BE, Koenig K. Riboflavin concentrations at the endothelium during corneal cross-linking in humans. Invest Ophthalmol Vis Sci. 2019;60(6):2140–5.
21. Mazzotta C, Riomani A, Burroni A. Pachymetry-based accelerated cross-linking: the "M Nomogram" for standardized treatment of all-thickness progressive ectatic corneas. Int K Kerat Ect Corn Dis. 2019;7(2):137–44.

Corneal Allogenic Intrastromal Ring Segments C.A.I.R.S

Vaishnavi Ravishankar and Soosan Jacob

1 Introduction

Corneal ectatic diseases such as keratoconus, pellucid marginal degeneration and post LASIK ectasia may impair both uncorrected and best corrected visual acuity in patients, irrespective of progression or not. Structural and morphologic distortion of any degree usually has a negative impact on quality of vision. Treatment of the same aims not only at arresting progression but also at enhancing functional visual quality. Corneal transplant (penetrating or lamellar) can be successful in advanced disease, however limitations include postoperative astigmatism, side effects from chronic topical steroid use, corneal graft rejection, and recurrence of keratoconus in the donor cornea. Intrastromal corneal ring segments (ICRS) are a form of treatment for mild to moderate grades of corneal ectatic disorders, especially in patients who have poor functional visual acuity with glasses or are contact lens intolerant. A clear central visual axis is a prerequisite for this procedure.

CAIRS, or corneal allogenic intrastromal ring segments, first introduced by one of the authors (SJ), is a relatively newer modality of therapy involving mid-peripheral intrastromal transplantation of donor cornea stromal segments in patients with keratoconus. It is an allogenic alternative to synthetic intra corneal ring segments providing numerous advantages over the same [1–18].

V. Ravishankar · S. Jacob (✉)
Dr. Agarwal's Refractive and Cornea Foundation (DARCF), Chennai, India
e-mail: dr_soosanj@hotmail.com

V. Ravishankar · S. Jacob
Dr. Agarwal's Group of Eye Hospitals, Chennai, India

A. Armia and C. Mazzotta (eds.), *Keratoconus*,
https://doi.org/10.1007/978-3-030-84506-3_10

2 Classification of ICRS

Intracorneal ring segments (ICRS) act as spacer elements between the bundles of corneal lamellae, producing a shortening of the central arc length as well as a regularization of topography. In normal eyes with a regular corneal thickness, there exists a uniform stress distribution. In nonuniform corneal thickness, such as in patients with corneal ectatic disease, there is a concentration of stress at the thinnest region. Once the segments are inserted, the curvature is decreased centrally, stress is redistributed and the biomechanical cycle of keratoconus is arrested or slowed.

Intracorneal ring segments (ICRS) may be classified into:

1. **Synthetic ICRS**
2. **CAIRS**

Synthetic ICRS are made of polymethylmethacrylate (PMMA) and are introduced at a 75–80% depth in the corneal stroma, to induce a change in geometry and refractive power. Theoretically, the thicker the segment and the closer the site of implantation to the centre of the cornea, the higher will be the flattening effect achieved.

CAIRS threads semi-circular segments of allogenic tissue into intracorneal channels cut either manually or by a femtosecond laser in the patient's mid-peripheral stroma to reinforce and reshape the corneal surface.

3 History

The technique was first conceived by the author, SJ in 2015 as an ideal procedure that would combine the morphological and biomechanical benefits of ICRS and negate the adverse effects such as stromal melt and necrosis, extrusion, exposure etc. associated with them by virtue of being synthetic.

The initial attempts involved manual stromal dissection of tissue, and these tissue segments were inserted into circular channels made at mid-stromal depth. Initially, the incision was made over the flat axis and a CAIRS segments was inserted to either side of the incision, straddling the incision. This was done in order to make insertion of segments easier but later, the technique evolved and underwent various modifications for ease of surgery. The incision was soon made on the steeper axis and an Intacs segment or a specially designed pigtail instrument was used to pull the segment completely into the channel on either side of the incision. By March 2017, it became apparent that broader channels helped easy insertion while continuing to give good effect. Hence, the Intacs pull-through technique was abandoned and instead, broader mid-depth channels were created that allowed the segments to be easily pushed in using a curved Y rod and drawn in from the opposite incision using a curved reverse Sinskey hook.

The CAIRS procedure is now increasingly being adopted all over the world due to a relatively simple learning curve, ease of surgery and effectiveness as well as the safety of the procedure. Manual dissection of tunnels has been used for creation of channels when femtosecond laser is not available.

Instruments:

The author SJ has also designed instruments for the CAIRS procedure (Fig. 1). The Jacob CAIRS Trephine (Madhu Surgicals), the CAIRS marker, the various CAIRS inserters (curved Y-rod, curved reverse Sinskey, Pigtail pull-through), the CAIRS smoothener and others are inventions and designs that are aimed at improving ease, accuracy and speed (Epsilon Eye Care).

Technique

The technique for CAIRS preparation and CAIRS procedure is described below (Figs. 2, 3, 4 and 5).

CAIRS PREPARATION:

CAIRS begins with creating the ring of donor stromal tissue. As explained in our initial published study,[1] CAIRS refers to ring segments created from allogenic

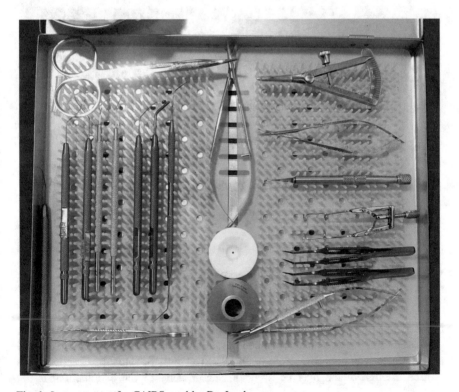

Fig. 1 Instrument set for CAIRS used by Dr. Jacob

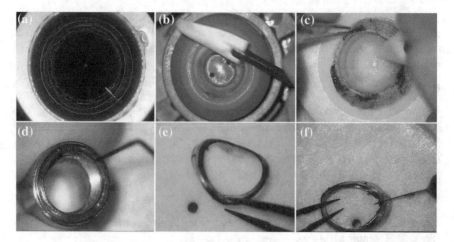

Fig. 2 **a** Femtosecond dissected channels are created in the keratoconic patient's eye; **b**- A donor cornea is debrided of epithelium; **c** Endothelium is also removed from the donor cornea; **d** The double bladed Jacob CAIRS trephine™ (Madhu Surgicals) is seen; **e** The CAIRS ring is seen punched out; **f** The ring is cut to the desired stromal length

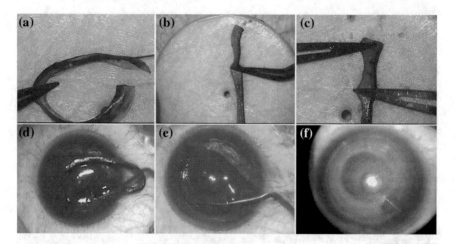

Fig. 3 **a** The ring is straightened out; **b, c** The CAIRS segment is flattened with a non toothed forceps; **d, e** It is inserted into the femtosecond channel. Being progressive keratoconus, this was followed by cross-linking; **f** The CAIRS segment is seen lying intra-stromally on the first post-operative day

tissue. This could be of any origin—donor corneal or scleral tissue, preserved or processed tissue or even bioengineered tissue. Commonly, screened and processed donor cornea with negative serology for HIV, Hepatitis B, Hepatitis C and syphilis is used, though others may be used too. The quality of the endothelium is not

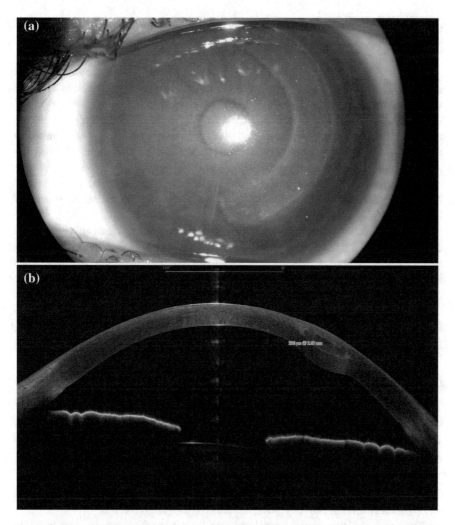

Fig. 4 Post-operative slit lamp appearance and anterior segment OCT of a single segment CAIRS

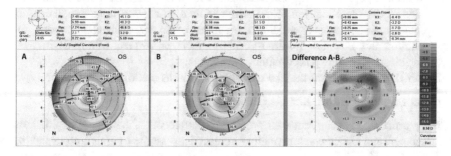

Fig. 5 Difference map pre and post CAIRS showing flattening and regularization of the topography and centralization of the cone together with improvement in the indices

important as it is not transplanted and therefore, older donor tissue can be used. The tissue should however be non-edematous with clear stroma.

CAIRS may be prepared and supplied by eye banks or created by the surgeon. When donor cornea is used, it is removed from the storage solution and mounted on an artificial anterior chamber. The epithelium is completely debrided and the center is marked and laid upside down on a Teflon block. The endothelium is stripped and the double-bladed Jacob Trephine is used to punch a ring of stromal tissue. This ring is cut in half to yield two segments of stromal tissue which may be trimmed to an appropriate size or it may be used uncut as a single long segment. The breadth and the thickness of these segments can be customized according to severity, type of cone, location of cone, refractive error, pattern of astigmatism and other factors. The trephine comes in different sizes, allowing for thicker or thinner segments of tissue.

When coupled with corneal collagen cross linking, as in cases of progressive corneal ectasia, the segments may be inserted after soaking in a solution of ribo-flavin for half an hour, following which they are ready for insertion. Alternately, as shown by Parker et al., the CAIRS can be stretched out and allowed to air dry. The dehydration shrinks and stiffens the tissue temporarily making it easier to insert into the intrastromal channels. Following insertion into the channel, the dehydrated CAIRS segments rehydrate immediately on theirv own. Parker et al. have also stained the segments with 0.06% Trypan blue to enhance visibility during implantation.

Cairs Insertion:

The procedure is done under topical anesthesia. Femtosecond laser-dissected channels or manually dissected channels are prepared in the keratoconic patient's eye. Depending on the patient's requirements, either single segment or double segments may be inserted.

CAIRS are inserted into the channels in one of the following ways:

1. A gentle push-in/pull-through technique may be used, with the aid of a curved Y-rod and reverse Sinskey hook, or curved 23- gauge forceps.
2. The Jacob CAIRS pig-tail instrument may be used to draw the segment out. It is introduced into the channel and the segment is tied or anchored to the tip of the instrument at the leading end once it reaches the opposite incision or the other side of the same incision. The inserter is then withdrawn from the other side, thereby simultaneously guiding the segment into the channel in a near circumferential manner. An almost 360° segment or segment of any desired arc length may be thus placed within the channels.
3. An INTACS segment may be use to draw it in as described previously.

Cairs combined with CXL/ CACXL:

If the procedure is being done for progressive keratoconus, the patient's epithelium is scraped and either conventional or contact lens–assisted corneal cross-linking

(CACXL) is performed depending on the minimum corneal thickness. This may be performed either simultaneously or sequentially.

Advantages Over Synthetic ICRS

Serious complications associated with synthetic ICRS have included:

- Segment migration
- Overriding of segments
- Stromal thinning leading to melt and necrosis
- Exposure or extrusion of segments
- Corneal neovascularisation
- Infectious keratitis.

In contrast, CAIRS segments do not hinder the passage of oxygen and nutrients unlike synthetic segments. The recipient cornea is more tolerant towards CAIRS as these are made of allogenic tissue such as donor stroma, which is easily integrated into host tissue.

CAIRS may not only be implanted in mild cases but also in patients with more advanced disease. Synthetic ICRS require a minimum requisite stromal thickness, generally 400 microns of tissue, above the synthetic segment in order to prevent stromal necrosis and melt. CAIRS, being allogenic and also less rigid, may be implanted into thinner corneas.

In addition, CAIRS also allow more customizability in terms of arc length, thickness, optic zone and depth of implantation and thereby allows better results while decreasing the need for maintaining a large inventory of synthetic ICRS. CAIRS recipients also experience less glare in comparison to patients with synthetic segments due to absence of any reflections.

Advantages Over Deep Anterior Lamellar Keratoplasty (DALK):

CAIRS has numerous advantages over DALK. It is a reversible procedure and does not take away the ability to perform a future DALK. CAIRS is less invasive and an easier surgery with good outcomes. The easy learning curve makes it amenable to be performed by general ophthalmologists too, unlike DALK which requires specialized and advanced corneal training. It thus makes treatment easily available to a larger pool of keratoconus patients even in areas where access to specialized corneal care may not be available.

In addition, it spares the visual axis unlike DALK and avoids suture induced regular and irregular astigmatism. It also avoids a large and deep incision on the cornea as well as suture and surface related problems. Since the corneal nerve plexus is breached circumferentially and at many levels in a DALK, there is a higher risk for surface related issues like dry eye, neurotrophic keratitis and persistent epithelial defect, which is not the case in CAIRS. CAIRS also has a lower risk of rejection due to a very low volume of stromal transfer compared to DALK. Lack of epithelial or endothelial transfer, rapid keratocyte repopulation from host stroma into the small amount of CAIRS tissue, negligible antigenicity, distant placement of the CAIRS from the limbus and limbal blood vessels and lack of sutures and therefore suture induced vascularization are other factors that decrease the risk of rejection. Absence of visual axis interface issues such as those that may arise in DALK is another advantage. In the remote possibility of haze or rejection of the CAIRS, there is still no effect on visual acuity as they are not placed in the visual axis.

CAIRS may also be economically more viable due to easy availability of donor cornea in many countries. Even in countries where donor cornea is expensive or difficult to procure, the use of one cornea can be maximized by using the central disc of tissue for a penetrating keratoplasty or DALK or by cutting the CAIRS segment after harvesting a DMEK or PDEK graft. CAIRS harvested from one cornea may be used for more than one patient. Eye banks can also maximize the use of corneas as CAIRS does not require endothelial viability. A manual technique of implantation can be used when femtosecond laser is not available to create the intra-stromal channel within the keratoconic patient's eye. CAIRS may be done in conjunction with the newer thin cornea cross-linking protocols such as CACXL or the sub 400 protocol.

Disadvantages

Unless effective cross-linking is also possible, extremely thin corneas may continue to progress and a DALK may eventually be necessary. Keratoconic corneas with central scarring do not benefit in terms of visual improvement with CAIRS.

4   Conclusion

Since it's conception, the technique of CAIRS has proven to be an uncomplicated and safe solution for treating keratoconus. Patients have shown to improve in uncorrected and best corrected visual acuity, with a reduction in the steepest keratometric value and irregular astigmatism with successful arrest of disease progression in conjunction with cross-linking techniques.

References

1. Corneal Allogenic Intrastromal Ring Segments (CAIRS) Combined With Corneal Cross-linking for Keratoconus: Soosan Jacob, MS, FRCS, DNB; Shaila R. Patel, DNB; Amar Agarwal, MS, FRCS, FRCO; Arvind Ramalingam, Boptom; A.I. Saijimol, BSc; John Michael Raj, MSc. J Refract Surg. 2018;34(5):296–303.
2. Jacob S. Corneal Allogenic Intrastromal Ring Segments (CAIRS), Sept 14th, 2018. AAO One Network Multimedia: https://www.aao.org/clinical-video/corneal-allogenic-intrastromal-ring-segments-cairs. Accessed 18 Apr 2020.

3. Jacob S. Allogenic Ring Segments for Keratoconus. 2017;AAO One Network Multimedia. https://www.aao.org/1-minute-video/allogenic-ring-segments-keratoconus. Accessed 9 May 2021.
4. Pandit TR, Jacob S. Corneal allogenic intrastromal ring segments for corneal ectatic disorders. 2017;AAO One Network Multimedia. https://www.aao.org/interview/allogenic-intrastromal-ring-segments-corneal-ectas. Accessed 9 May 2021.
5. Soosan Jacob, MD. Corneal allogenic intrastromal ring segments (CAIRS). 2019;ASCRS EyeWorld Magazine. https://www.youtube.com/watch?v=RWxUakc5Wz4&t=2s&ab_channel=EyeWorldMagazine. Accessed 9 May 2021.
6. Jacob S. CAIRS A new technique for Keratoconus and corneal ecstasias. 2017. https://www.youtube.com/watch?v=qF-9ycSQPq8. Accessed: 27 Apr 2021.
7. Jacob S. CAIRS (Corneal Allogeneic Intrastromal Ring Segments) for keratoconus, ectasias & irregular corneas. 2019. https://www.youtube.com/watch?v=SkxLwgP8cXA. Accessed 27 Apr 2021.
8. Larkin H. CAIRS for keratoconus. 2019. https://www.eurotimes.org/cairs-for-keratoconus/. Accessed 27 Apr 2021.
9. Jacob S. CAIRS for Keratoconus and PEARL for Presbyopia. Cataract and Refractive Surgery Today. 2019. https://crstoday.com/articles/2019-june/cairs-for-keratoconus-and-pearl-for-presbyopia/. Accessed 9 May 2021.
10. Dapena I, Parker JS, Melles GRJ. Potential benefits of modified corneal tissue grafts for keratoconus: bowman layer 'inlay' and 'onlay' transplantation, and allogenic tissue ring segments. Curr Opin Ophthalmol. 2020;31(4):276–83.
11. Srivatsa S, Jacob S, Agarwal A. Contact lens assisted corneal cross linking in thin ectatic corneas—a review. Indian J Ophthalmol. 2020;68(12):2773–8.
12. Parker JS, Dockery PW, Parker JS. Flattening the curve: a manual method for corneal allogenic intrastromal ring segment (CAIRS) implantation. J Cataract Refract Surg. 2020.
13. Parker JS, Dockery PW, Parker JS. Trypan blue-assisted corneal allogenic intrastromal ring segment implantation. J Cataract Refract Surg. 2021;47(1):127.
14. Torres Netto EA, Al-Otaibi WM, Hafezi NL, Kling S, Al-Farhan HM, Randleman JB, Hafezi F. Prevalence of keratoconus in paediatric patients in Riyadh, Saudi Arabia. Br J Ophthalmol. 2018;102(10):1436–41.
15. Kanellopoulos AJ, Pe LH, Perry HD, et al. Modified intracorneal ring segment implantations (INTACS) for the management of moderate to advanced keratoconus: efficacy and complications. Cornea. 2006;25:29–33.
16. Coskunseven E, Kymionis GD, Tsiklis NS, et al. Complications of intrastromal corneal ring segment implantation using a femtosecond laser for channel creation: a survey of 850 eyes with keratoconus. Acta Ophthalmol. 2011;89:54–7.
17. Jarade E, Dirani A, Fadlallah A, Antonios R, Cherfan G. New technique of intracorneal ring segments suturing after migration. J Refract Surg. 2013;29:855–7.
18. Alió JL, Shabayek MH, Belda JI, Correas P, Feijoo ED. Analysis of results related to good and bad outcomes of Intacs implantation for keratoconus correction. J Cataract Refract Surg. 2006;32:756–61.

All Surface Laser Ablation and Crosslinking

Miguel Rechichi, Marco Ferrise, and Samuel Arba Mosquera

The effectiveness of Corneal Collagen Cross-linking (CXL) to stop the keratoconus (KC) progression has been confirmed in several long-term studies [1–3].

Subsequently to CXL, many patients with unsatisfactory quality of vision have have benefited not only from the slowdown or arrest of the disease, but also from an improvement of refraction, visual acuity, topographic, and aberrometric outcomes, often caused by a flattening of the cone apex; however, these results were most of the times subject to an ample degree of unpredictability and variability [4].

A modern challenge in the management of keratoconus is to improve the refraction in these patients with significant ectasia and high degree of high-order ocular aberrations (HOAs) joining the CXL techniques with an excimer laser transepithelial (Trans prk) minimal stromal photoablation (Crosslinking Plus). These patients frequently have sub-par Best Spectacle Corrected Visual Acuity (BSCVA) because spectacles are unable to correct high irregular astigmatism, especially in peripheral keratoconus location, and a comfortable contact lens fitting sometimes is hard to reach, or not possible at all, and could cause corneal scarring and infections [5].

BSCVA and quality of vision could be improved by reshaping the corneal surface, regularizing as much as possible the corneal geometry in the central 4 mm zone, aiming to reduce vertical asymmetry and higher-order aberrations [6, 7].

The treatment of corneas with keratoconus using excimer laser machine was historically considered not appropriate because of further corneal thinning and possible weakening of corneal microstructure followed by iatrogenic ectasia worsening, but recent improvements in laser technology such as the development of Topography-guided (TG-PRK) and Wavefront-guided Photo-refractive keratec-

---

M. Rechichi
Centro Polispecialistico Mediterraneo, Sellia Marina, Catanzaro, Italy

M. Ferrise (✉)
Studio Oculistico Ferrise, Lamezia terme, Italy

S. A. Mosquera
SCHWIND Eye-Tech-Solutions, Kleinostheim, Germany

© The Author(s), under exclusive license to Springer Nature Switzerland AG 2022   177
A. Armia and C. Mazzotta (eds.), *Keratoconus*,
https://doi.org/10.1007/978-3-030-84506-3_11

tomy (WFG-PRK) procedures, together with a tracking system that compensates movements of the eyes on the X–Y–Z planes, as well as cyclorotation, have led to new options for dealing with ectatic corneas, introducing the concept of *customized treatments* [8–10].

The target of customized ablation is to improve the quality of visual acuity reducing not only the lower but also the higher-order aberration and irregular corneal astigmatism.

A sensible approach to the use of the excimer laser is based on the level of uncorrected distance visual acuity (UCVA) and Best Spectacle Corrected Visual Acuity (BSCVA), see Fig. 1.

If UCVA and/or BSCVA is satisfactory, only CXL is typically applied and the excimer laser is not employed. When the visual quality, UCVA and BSCVA have been reduced due to corneal irregularity then the use of the excimer laser may be indicated. The excimer laser is used to regularise the cornea and then, once this has been achieved, the cornea is stabilized with CXL.

Several adjuvant treatments may combine with CXL ("CXL-Plus") to offer a far wider reach of options. Topo-Guided PRK (TG-PRK), Trans-epithelial PTK (TE-PTK), intrastromal corneal rings (ISCR) implantation, and Toric Intraocular Lenses implantation are many of the refractive options that may be combined with CXL; this chapter will be focused on the use of All Surface Laser Ablation (ASLA) and Corneal CXL.

1 All Surface Laser Ablation

Photorefractive keratectomy (PRK) was introduced more than 30 years ago as a corneal refractive surgical technique using the excimer laser [11, 12].

There is a recognition that surface ablation has several potential advantages with regard to preserving corneal biomechanical integrity and avoiding intraoperative and late flap-related complications, leading to a resurgence in surface ablation techniques. The main limitations of PRK remain—postoperative pain, delayed epithelial healing, and postoperative stromal haze.

One of the main areas of interest has been the technique of epithelial removal.

The removal of corneal epithelium with the use of simple mechanical debridement, of alcohol, and the preservation of the epithelium as a flap (LASEKand Epi-LASIK) have all been assessed [13].

An alternative is transepithelial PRK, where epithelial removal is carried out with laser ablation, followed by a stromal laser refractive ablation [14].

This technique has several advantages, including no instrument contact with the eye and reduced time of surgery.

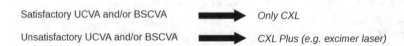

Fig. 1 Paradigm in the choice of treatment of corneal ectasia

Transepithelial PRK was born as a two-step procedure—an initial PTK pre-treatment for epithelial removal, followed by PRK [15].

In the latest iteration of the TransPRK technique, also referred as All-Surface Laser Ablation (ASLA), the epithelium is not ablated using an even or broad beam PTK profile. Instead a custom epithelial profile has been generated from population studies, since the epithelium does not have a uniform thickness [16].

The ablation profile generated from this population model thus targets 55 μm centrally, and 65 μm peripherally (users can individualize epithelial thickness values for center and periphery with a reference diameter), also considering the different ablation rate between epithelium and stroma. The ablation is not carried out as two distinct steps, but rather as a single continuous profile, to reduce operating time and the risk of dehydration between steps.

The refractive part of the treatment starts at the epithelium, whether or not partly reaching the stroma through the epithelium and Bowman membrane; the refractive-neutral part of the treatment etches the refractive contour down to the stroma; followed by the process of reepithelization.

With this approach, there is no need to recenter the treatment or repopulate the patient data. Continuous cyclotorsion control shaves time off the procedure, and stromal dehydration can be avoided.

This technique exploits the smoothing effect of the epithelium, since it is recognized that epithelial thickening occurs in areas of stromal irregularity as a compensation mechanism. This advantage is lost when the epithelium is removed before stromal ablation, exposing the underlying irregularity.

The diameter of the epithelial removal is calculated to match the total optical zone with the same centration reference, ensuring fast epithelial healing. Additionally, the healthy epithelial edge helps to speed recovery and visual rehabilitation.

There are several inherent advantages of TransPRK over PRK that make the former a desirable procedure to use and to improve, besides the catchy "no-touch, all-laser" marketing slogan.

TransPRK is patient friendly, because there is no risk of alcohol spillage and no extra manipulation, such as in mechanical debridement, thus reducing patients' stress during the procedure.

TransPRK also provides faster epithelial recovery due to a smaller, healthier, and neater epithelial edge, which translates to a shorter period of patient discomfort. Moreover, as opposed to alcohol and mechanical debridement, laser epithelial removal ensures that no area of Bowman membrane denuded of its epithelium is left untreated by the laser, as the epithelial removal zone is calculated to match the stromal ablation zone. This is an important protective factor against epithelial erosions postoperatively.

Another important advantage of a defined epithelial thickness ablation in TransPRK is seen in treating irregular corneas (eg, postkeratoplasty eyes, retreatment eyes, and keratoconic eyes in conjunction with CXL). In that last category of eyes, epithelial irregularities are usually much lower in magnitude than the underlying stromal irregularities.

However, in topography-guided or corneal wavefront-guided treatments, the treatment data are based on the epithelial topography and are lost when the epithelium is peeled, exposing a much more chaotic and unmeasured stromal surface.

TransPRK ensures that customized stromal ablation treats the topography measured, as the epithelial corneal surface imprint is translated to the stromal level by the defined-depth aspheric PTK ablation, see Fig. 2.

In irregular corneas, laser treatment using TransPRK may leave a smoother stromal surface for the epithelium to remodel over, compared with PRK with alcohol-assisted or mechanical epithelial debridement. The latter techniques remove the epithelium, exposing the more irregular stroma, whereas in TransPRK, the defined-depth aspheric PTK mode will copy the less irregular epithelial topography to the stromal surface, with better chances for the epithelium to remodel again and camouflage the stromal irregularities.

Because the cornea is measured preoperatively with the epithelium intact, it is logical to treat what is measured by the imaging devices. In conventional PRK, the epithelium is debrided, exposing a more irregular stroma. In TransPRK, the excimer pulses treat the epithelial topography exactly as measured by the preoperative topographer or aberrometer, so that the phototherapeutic keratectomy mode translates the treated shape faithfully to the stroma. The result is a perfect match between measured and treated aberrations. Correcting the treatment-induced spherical aberration and preexisting coma of any patient's cornea has the benefit of improving visual quality.

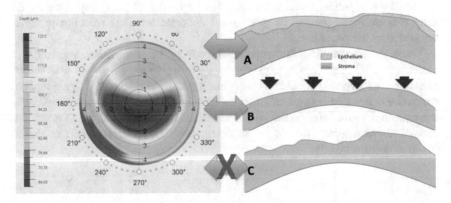

Fig. 2 a Masking effect of epithelium; **b** Smoother surface after Laser epithelial removal; **c** Uneven stromal surface after alcohol-assisted epithelial removal

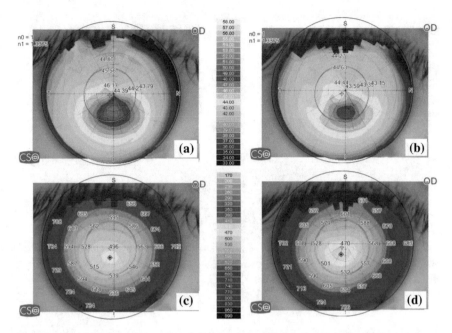

Fig. 3 Comparison between baseline (**a**, **c**) and at 1 year (**b**, **d**) after STARE-X anterior sagittal maps. In this patient the corrected distance visual acuity improved from 0.39 LogMAR to 0.1 LogMAR

2 Customized Treatments: The STARE-X Protocol for Corneal Regularization

In literature several approaches have been described combining different corneal collagen crosslinking and refractive surgery protocols performed at the same time (same-day) or in two surgical steps [17, 18].

The potential benefit of a combined ASLA plus CXL procedure is to directly reshape (regularize) the ectatic cornea and reinforce the reshaped cornea with cross-linking procedure that will further flatten the cornea in the following months.

To achieve this goal, an adjustable personalized protocol called "STARE-X" (Selective Trans-epithelial Ablation for Regularization of Ectasia and simultaneous cross-linking) was devised.

The protocol consisted of a combination of trans-epithelial topo-guided ablation treatment with Amaris laser platform (Schwind™ Eye Tech-Solution) and accelerated cxl performed with Avedro's (Waltham, Ma) KXL I™ cross-linker.

The Stare-X treatment may be proposed to patients with the following characteristics: age ≥ 21 years, grade I-II keratoconus (Amsler-Krumeich classification), progressive keratoconus (defined as an increase of at least 1 D in K-max over the 12-months preceding the treatment), the requirement of visual quality improvement, Rigid Gas Permeable (RGP) contact lens intolerance or altered fitting, corrected

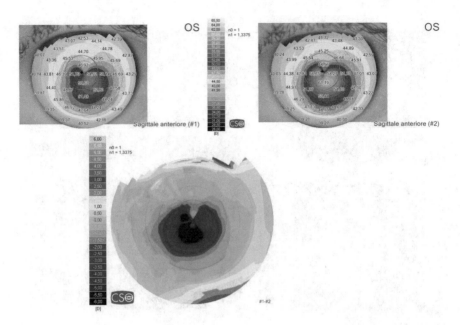

Fig. 4 Comparison between baseline (top right) and at 1 year (top left) after STARE-X anterior sagittal maps in advanced keratoconus. This patient, who was already scheduled for corneal transplant, after treatment reached 0.18 Logmar with an improved contact lens fitting

distance visual acuity (CDVA) $\leq 20/40$ or ≤ 0.6 decimal Snellen Lines, K-max ≤ 55 D, Optical Thinnest Point pachymetry ≥ 400 μm.

Factors that don't allow the use of this protocol are ocular Infections, history of interstitial keratitis, herpes simplex keratitis or other autoimmune diseases, presence of corneal scars, and any previous corneal procedure.

Step 1: Excimer laser corneal regularization

The first step of the Stare-X procedure is the Excimer laser corneal regularization.

The procedure consists of single-step corneal topography-guided trans-epithelial PRK with a starting planned optical zone (OZ) of 7 mm plus 0.6 mm transition zone (TZ) for central cone and 6.5 mm OZ plus 0.5 mm TZ for peripheral cone.

All treatments were planned by topographic data derived from the Optimized Refractive Keratectomy-Custom Ablation Manager software (ORK-CAM 5.1, SCHWIND eye-tech-solutions GmbH, Kleinostheim, Germany), considering the manifest refraction of the patient, corneal pachymetry, aberrometric and topographic parameters.

The eye tracker was checked intraoperatively before starting the treatment, considering the iris images taken in a supine position, to compensate for the cyclorotation that happens when a patient assumes a supine position, and comparing these preoperative images with repetitive images acquired throughout the treatment to determine the dynamic cyclotorsion (DC).

To provide an ablation precisely aligned with the preoperative plan, the dynamic cyclotorsion control (DCC) compensates the cyclorotation of the eye with the rotation of the ablation profile.

The principal parameters of the STARE-X protocol for the corneal regularization of keratoconus are the sequent: Epithelium removal of 55 μm in the center and 65 μm in the periphery of the selected ablation zone; stromal ablation depth limited at 50 μm, and optimized by excimer laser software for saving tissue; maximum correction of coma aberration, eventually limiting spherical and cylinder correction to not exceed the stromal ablation depth limit; ablation offset up to 1 mm from corneal vertex in the direction of the cone apex as measured manually on topography.

An important aspect of the of the individualization of the treatment are the possibility to reduce the optical zone in order to spare as much corneal tissue as possible. The stromal regulation plan to not exceed the ablation limit depth and to preserve a RST > 350 μm.

Furthermore, the treatment is not centered on the corneal apex; in fact the ablation was set 1 mm from the corneal vertex in direction of the cone apex, to center the ablation more on the cone apex respect to corneal vertex, and reducing stromal ablation over the cone apex. This allows a more focused subsequent CXL treatment on the area of ectasia, with improved regularization of the corneal simmetry after the flattening effect of the CXL takes place; this is even more useful in more peripheral cones.

It is this symmetric offset ablation strategy that enables Stare X protocol to define the ablation centered around the cone (beyond the actual corneal vertex and closer to the ectatic corneal apex, or to the thinnest corneal location). These settings allow the surgeon to center the ablation more on the cone with respect to the corneal vertex, reducing stromal ablation over the cone apex and further reducing coma aberrations. Using the cone/apex instead of vertex/pupil as ablation centre increases symmetry of the ablation profile.

Keratoconus ablations typically show a local ablation corresponding to the location of the cone, complemented by a superior wing opposite to the location of the cone. The ablation at the cone shall be reduced as shallow as possible. To do that classical strategies involve the reduction of the optical zone diameter down to 5.5 mm or so. By reducing optical zone size, both the ablation depth at the cone and at the wing generally reduces, however at the same time the size of the corneal regularized area is also severely reduced.

The corneal vertex in keratoconus and other ectatic diseases is naturally shifted towards the location of the ectatic cone, so that using a symmetric offset approach towards the corneal vertex reduces the ablation at the wing (by clipping its extension) and extends the ablation in the direction on the cone.

The rationale of using symmetric offset around the ectatic cone location is to try avoiding/reducing the superior wing (and potentially expecting a second wing to the outer side of the cone). So that the coma part of the cone (partly) converts into spherical aberration, and the coma part of the superior wing (partly) converts into astigmatism. By doing this, asymmetric aberrations (mainly coma and trefoil) are converted (due to the offset settings the ablation center towards the ectatic cone) into more regular aberrations (radially symmetric spherical aberration, and astigmatism).

Step 2: customized energy pulsed accelerated collagen crosslinking.

After excimer treatment, eyes underwent an epithelium-off pulsed light accelerated corneal collagen crosslinking (pl-ACXL) by using the KXL I UV-A source (Avedro Inc., Waltham, MS, USA).

The target residual stromal thickness (RST), planned before laser excimer corneal ablation, is considered to choose the UVA irradiation power and dose for CXL treatment.

We considered pulsed UVA irradiation (16 minutes, 15 mW/cm², pulsed 2:1 second, 5.4 J dose energy) if the RST is > 400 µm and pulsed UVA irradiation (8 minutes, 30 mW/cm², 7.2 J dose energy) if the RST < 400 µm.

The beam is carefully centered on the cone apex evaluated at the anterior tangential map for all the treatments.

A dextran-free riboflavin 0.1% with hydroxyl, propyl, methyl, and cellulose (VibeX Rapid, Avedro Inc., Waltham, MS, USA) was used, with 10 minutes of corneal soaking. Treated eyes were dressed by a soft contact lens bandage for 3 days and medicated.

3 All Surface Laser Ablation with Cross-Linking (ASLA-XTRA) for the Treatment of Myopia

The PTK and PRK treatments have also both been studied before in combination with corneal cross-linking (CXL) procedures in order to improve stability and refraction while reducing the HOAs cases of ectasia, in pathological eyes such as those with keratoconus [19–21].

It's been reported in literature [22, 23] that, after the CXL treatment, once the epithelial defect has fully healed, there is transformation and then apoptosis of the myofibroblasts, followed by subsequent repopulation by new keratocytes, and reabsorption of the myofibroblast derived abnormal collagen depositions and cell debris; this process seems to lead to an enhancement of corneal clarity.

Aslanides et al. proposed that this cellular process induced by CXL may have a beneficial effect on reducing subepithelial haze following ASLA transepithelial PRK in non pathological corneas, e.g. myopic eyes [24].

In their study, after the ASLA treatment was performed, an accelerated CXL treatment was performed using the Avedro KXL system (Avedro Inc., Waltham, MA). The riboflavin solution used was Vibex Rapid (Avedro Inc., Waltham, MA), the formulation of which is: 0.1% riboflavin, Saline, HPMC. The soaking time before the UV irradiation was 90s and the energy used 2.7 J/cm² (30 mW for 90 s).

The authors of the study reported in favor of the use of CXL in place of MMC in refractive laser ablation, finding similar reduction of fibroblast activity and haze formation as compared to Mytomycin C. Furthermore, the accelerated CXL can contribute to the postoperative biomechanical stability of the cornea and, as a result, a refraction that could potentially be more stable in the long term. Finally, the combination of riboflavin and UV radiation provides a sterilizing effect on the corneal surface that may reduce the possibility of postoperative infections.

In conclusion, the STARE-X protocol demonstrated effective results in halting keratoconus progression and improving corneal regularity with a safe and effective profile. STARE-X improved both visual acuity and corneal aberration in the middle term period 25. The effects were more evident in peripheral cone.

The next level of Stare X protocol will be the integration of epithelial map in the ablation profile. This will allow a more predictable ablation considering variation of epithelial thickness in keratoconic eyes.

References

1. Meiri Z, Keren S, Rosenblatt A, Sarig T, Shenhav L, Varssano D. Efficacy of corneal collagen cross-linking for the treatment of keratoconus: a systematic review and meta-analysis. Cornea. 2016;35(3):417–28. https://doi.org/10.1097/ICO.0000000000000723. PMID: 26751990.
2. Mazzotta C, Traversi C, Baiocchi S, Bagaglia S, Caporossi O, Villano A, Caporossi A. Corneal collagen crosslinking with riboflavin and ultraviolet A light for pediatric keratoconus: ten-year results. Cornea. 2018;37(5):560–6.
3. Kobashi H, Rong SS. Corneal collagen cross-linking for keratoconus: systematic review. Biomed Res Int. 2017;2017:8145651. https://doi.org/10.1155/2017/8145651. Epub 2017 Jun 11. PMID: 28691035; PMCID: PMC5485290.
4. Mazzotta C, Caporossi T, Denaro R, Bovone C, Sparano C, Paradiso A, Baiocchi S, Caporossi A. Morphological and functional correlations in riboflavin UV A corneal collagen cross-linking for keratoconus. Acta Ophthalmol. 2012;90(3):259–65.
5. Moschos MM, Nitoda E, Georgoudis P, Balidis M, Karageorgiadis E, Kozeis N. Contact lenses for keratoconus- current practice. Open Ophthalmol J. 2017;11:241–51.
6. Nilagiri VK, Metlapally S, Schor CM, Bharadwaj SR. A computational analysis of retinal image quality in eyes with keratoconus. Sci Rep. 2020;10(1):1321.https://doi.org/10.1038/s41598-020-57993-w.PMID:31992755;PMCID:PMC6987247.
7. Delgado S, Velazco J, Delgado Pelayo RM, Ruiz-Quintero N. Correlation of higher order aberrations in the anterior corneal surface and degree of keratoconus measured with a Scheimpflug camera. Arch Soc Esp Oftalmol. 2016;91(7):316–9.
8. Dawson DG, Randleman JB, Grossniklaus HE, O'Brien TP, Dubovy SR, Schmack I, Stulting RD, Edelhauser HF. Corneal ectasia after excimer laser keratorefractive surgery: histopathology, ultrastructure, and pathophysiology. Ophthalmology. 2008;115(12):2181–91. e1.
9. Arba-Mosquera S, Merayo-Lloves J, Ortueta de D. Clinical effects of pure cyclotorsional errors during refractive surgery. Invest Ophthalmol Vis Sci. 2008;49:4828–36.
10. Bueeler M, Mrochen M. Simulation of eye-tracker latency, spot size, and ablation pulse depth on the correction of higher order wavefront aberrations with scanning spot laser systems. J Refractive Surg. 2005;21:28–36.
11. Marshall J, Trokel S, Rothery S, Krueger R. Photoablative reprofiling of the cornea using an excimer laser: photorefractive keratectomy Lasers. Ophthalmol. 1986;1:21–48.

12. Trokel SL, Srinivasan R, Braren B. Excimer laser surgery of the cornea. Am J Ophthalmol. 1983;96(6):710–5.
13. Ghoreishi M, Attarzadeh H. Alcohol-assisted versus mechanical epithelium removal in photorefractive keratectomy. J Ophthalmic Vis Res. 2010;5(4):223–7.
14. Lee HK, Lee KS, Kim JK. Epithelial healing and clinical outcomes in excimer laser photorefractive surgery following three epithelial removal techniques: mechanical, alcohol, and excimer laser. Am J Ophthalmol. 2005;139(1):56–63.
15. Camellin M, Arba MS. Simultaneous aspheric wavefront-guided transepithelial photorefractive keratectomy and phototherapeutic keratectomy to correct aberrations and refractive errors after corneal surgery. J Cataract Refract Surg. 2010;36(7):1173–80.
16. Reinstein DZ, Archer TJ, Gobbe M, Silverman RH, Coleman DJ. Epithelial thickness in the normal cornea: three-dimensional display with Artemis very high-frequency digital ultrasound. J Refract Surg. 2008;24(6):571–81.
17. Kymionis GD, Grentzelos MA, Kankariya VP, Pallikaris IG. Combined transepithelial phototherapeutic keratectomy and corneal collagen crosslinking for ectatic disorders: cretan protocol. J Cataract Refract Surg. 2013;39:1939.
18. Kymionis GD, Grentzelos MA, Portaliou DM, Kankariya VP, Randleman JB. Corneal collagen cross-linking (CXL) combined with refractive procedures for the treatment of corneal ectatic disorders: CXL plus. J Refract Surg. 2014;30(8):566–76.
19. Mukherjee AN, Selimis V, Aslanides I. Transepithelial photorefractive keratectomy with crosslinking for keratoconus. Open Ophthalmol J. 2013;7:63–8.
20. Stojanovic A, Zhang J, Chen X, Nitter TA, Chen S, Wang Q. Topographyguided transepithelial surface ablation followed by corneal collagen crosslinking performed in a single combined procedure for the treatment of keratoconus and pellucid marginal degeneration. J Refract Surg. 2010;26(2):145–52.
21. Kymionis GD, Diakonis VF, Kalyvianaki M, Portaliou D, Siganos C, Kozobolis VP, et al. One-year follow-up of corneal confocal microscopy after corneal cross-linking in patients with post laser in situ keratosmileusis ectasia and keratoconus. Am J Ophthalmol. 2009;147 (5):774–8, e1.
22. Mencucci R, Marini M, Paladini I, Sarchielli E, Sgambati E, Menchini U. Effects of riboflavin/UVA corneal cross-linking on keratocytes and collagen fibres in human cornea. Clin Exp Ophthalmol. 2010;38(1):49–56.
23. Hafezi F, Kanellopoulos J, Wiltfang R, Seiler T. Corneal collagen crosslinking with riboflavin and ultraviolet a to treat induced keratectasia after laser in situ keratomileusis. J Cataract Refract Surg. 2007;33(12):2035–40.
24. Aslanides IM, Padroni S, Arba Mosquera S, Ioannides A, Mukherjee A. Comparison of single-step reverse transepithelial all-surface laser ablation (ASLA) to alcohol-assisted photorefractive keratectomy. Clin Ophthalmol. 2012;6: 973–80. https://doi.org/10.2147/OPTH.S32374. Epub 2012 Jun 27. PMID: 22815640; PMCID: PMC3399388.
Rechichi M, Mazzotta C, Oliverio GW, Romano V, Borroni D, Ferrise M, Bagaglia S, Jacob S, Meduri A. Selective transepithelial ablation with simultaneousaccelerated corneal crosslinking for corneal regularization of keratoconus: STARE-X protocol. J Cataract Refract Surg. 2021 Nov 1;47(11):1403–1410. https://doi.org/10.1097/j.jcrs.0000000000000640. PMID: 33770171.

IOL'S For Visual Rehabilitation in Stable Keratocounus

Ashraf Armia, Soheil Adib-Moghaddam, and Imane Tarib

1 Criteria of a Stable Keratoconus

1.1 Duration of Stability Evaluation

Patient monitoring for disease progression depends on multiple factors, such as the initial presentation of the ectatic disease at the time of diagnosis, patient's age as well as contact lens wear. There is a difference between progression in subclinical disease and progression in moderate to advanced disease that is taken into account as well [1].

Keratoconus can appear at prepubertal age, in puberty and progresses into the 3rd and 4th decade. Therefore, unless the patient's age is beyond this age group, the frequency of visits for patient follow-up depends on the physician and is modified according to the disease progression.

There is no consensus on an exact period of time upon which one can say that the ectatic disease is stable, a regular monitoring is necessary within the age group at risk. However, worsening factors such as eye rubbing, sleeping on the side and exerting pressure or compression on the eyelids have been studied in literature and

To my wife Vivian, my daughter Carol and my Son Karim. To my great father and mentor Armia. And to all our dear co-authors.

A. Armia (✉)
Ashraf Armia Eye Clinic, Giza, Egypt

A. Armia
Watany Eye Hospital and Watany Research and Development Center, Cairo, Egypt

S. Adib-Moghaddam
Ophthalmology Research Center, Farabi Eye Hospital, Tehran University of Medical Sciences, Tehran, Iran

I. Tarib
Ophthalmologist At Mohammed V University, Rabat, Morocco

© The Author(s), under exclusive license to Springer Nature Switzerland AG 2022
A. Armia and C. Mazzotta (eds.), *Keratoconus*,
https://doi.org/10.1007/978-3-030-84506-3_12

187

identified as a cause of progression of keratoconus [2]. Some recent studies suggest that the cumulative result of habits such as unilateral or bilateral eye rubbing, sleeping on the side and RGP wearing can be the origin of the biomechanical stress on the cornea leading to the appearance of ectatic disease [3].

Contrarily, disease progression in literature was defined as change in progression criteria, confirmed by consecutive examinations over different periods varying from 9 to 12 months.

However, this is not always an easy task, and it is important to distinguish a forme fruste of keratoconus in order to decide the proper treatment arsenal. Thus, various publications are studying repeatability and reliability of these progression criteria.

1.2   Corneal Biomechanics

Topographic progression criteria

The color maps in corneal topography provide a fast and efficient tool to reassure or ring an alarm for the physician. The software reports and compares the measured values with the mean and standard deviation values of a normal population. The color highlights the differences from normality for a rapid overview. Every minimum increase in one or more of these values magnifies a possible keratoconus progression. However, it is important to remember that the whole assessment is based entirely on anterior corneal surface topography, even though topography provides much more indexes and information than that, with various sensitivity and specificity, that need to be meticulously analyzed before concluding that the ectatic disease is stable or progressive [4].

Elevation maps provide data from both the anterior and posterior corneal surfaces showing the distribution of the differences in elevation between a reference sphere and the corneal anterior and posterior surfaces. The peaks are warm-colored, whereas the depressions are cold-colored. There has been more emphasis on the importance of posterior corneal changes in recent years, which may occur prior to changes in the anterior surface, in which case they allow to detect early keratoconus progression.

The pachymetric map shows physiological variability in thickness distribution (>520–540μ), with concentric morphology around the thinnest point. Thickness increase from center to periphery is evaluated by the corneal thickness spatial profile (CTSP) diagram. The percentage of increase of thickness (PIT) diagram shows the averages of thickness values of the points on imaginary circles centered on the thickness point with increased diameters from 0.4 to 8.8 mm. Keratoconic eyes usually show thinner corneas with less corneal volume. Also, CTSP and PIT of keratoconic eyes are different. The pachymetry gradient curve shows a faster increase from the thinnest point (TP) toward the periphery, when compared to normal corneas. Such presentations can indicate disease progression but have to be considered along other indices.

The numerical index value quantifies in an objective manner several aspects of corneal curvature. The numerical index value quantifies in an objective manner several aspects of corneal curvature: *Differential sector index (DSI), Surface asymmetry index (SAI), Irregular astigmatism index (IAI), Opposite sector index (OSI), Center-surrounded index (CSI), Corneal eccentricity index (CEI),* Symmetry vertical index (SI), Surface regularity index (SRI).

Progression of keratoconus can be detected by observing an increase of one or more of these indices in successive examinations taken at different times. Often, modifications in these indexes are synchronous with modifications in refraction as well.

The addition of a Scheimpflug camera allowed to provide indexes calculated on the basis of a tridimensional model from as many as 250,000 elevation points. Thus, ensuring high precision. The eight Ambrosio's indices are eight very sensitive values designed to disclose the development of keratoconus. Every index investigates in a peculiar manner the corneal anterior surface: *Index surface variance (ISV), Index of vertical asymmetry (IVA), KC index (KI), Center keratoconus index (CKI), Index of height asymmetry (IHA), Index of height decentration (IHD), Radius min and Topographical keratoconus classification (TKC).*

Some authors defined progression of ectasia as an increase in manifest refraction spherical equivalent of 0.50 diopters (D) or greater, Kmax increase of 1.00 D or greater, and corneal topographic refractive astigmatism increase of 1.00 D or greater, confirmed by two consecutive examinations over 9–12 months.

Scheimpflug system analyzers such as Pentacam, Sirius and Galilei reported to be highly reproducible and repeatable [5] both in differentiating keratoconus from normal corneas, as well as monitoring disease progression [6].

Others concluded to better parameters to differentiate between variability and true progression at low increments known as the ABCD staging system that consists of 5 stages, including a stage 0 referring to absence of disease. The parameters of this system are ARC anterior radius curvature (A), PRC posterior radius curvature (B), thinnest Pachymetry (C), distance best corrected vision (D) and deviation from normality indices [7]. These parameters averages have shown great repeatability and reliability allowing to determine disease progression. Thus, showing that progression can be underestimated in lower stages of the disease and overestimated in advanced stages.

1.3 Epithelial Thickness

The new generation OCT provides a precise corneal epithelial thickness map of the 6 mm surrounding the central corneal area. Modifications in the corneal epithelial thickness map is being more and more recognized as an early feature of keratoconus progression. The normal epithelial thickness value is about 50–55 μm. When the disease progression occurs, epithelial thickness on the cone apex decreases over the keratoconic protrusion [8, 9].

The SD-OCT corneal epithelial mapping was found valuable for detecting local thickness changes in eyes with keratoconus. Monitoring the corneal epithelial changes across the inferior area in patients with keratoconus was shown to be worthy for assessing disease progression in the recent literature [10]. It could even be an early occurrence in ectatic disease, way before topographic and refractive modifications appear [10].

1.4 Corneal Hysteresis

Alteration in mechanical stability is thought to be the initiating event of the ectatic disease. Therefore, Ocular Response Analyzer ORA was developed to measure corneal biomechanical properties in vivo. It examines corneal behavior during bidirectional applanation through a noncontact tonometer and produces an estimate of corneal hysteresis and corneal resistance factor.

The measurement process provided is based on the production of air pulse, which concaves corneal surface for a few milliseconds. Then, the air pump switches off, so that the applied force diminishes slightly, letting the cornea recur to its normal shape. Cornea passes through the phase of applanation twofold during the time of the measurement. Deformation of the elastic corneal surface is proportional to the pressure applied by the air-puff. ORA records the pressure twice, at a time of first and second corneal applanation point. The average of two obtained pressure values is Goldmann-correlated intraocular pressure (IOPg), and their difference is exactly corneal hysteresis (CH) [11].

There are currently additional keratoconus-specific parameters: the keratoconus match index (KMI) and the keratoconus match probability (KMP). Corneal hysteresis could be useful in evaluating keratoconus in early stages, as it was found in literature to be statistically lower in keratoconus patients [12]. However, it has not reached the gold standard statute.

The Corvis ST is another device that monitors the response of the cornea to an air pressure pulse using an ultra-high speed (UHS) Scheimpflug camera and uses the captured image sequence to produce estimates of IOP and deformation response parameters [13]. Several articles have demonstrated that corneal deformation parameters differ between normal eyes and keratoconic eyes [14], especially considering defined parameters such as deformation amplitude (DA), highest concavity, and corneal applanation velocity [15]. Corvis can be used in the evaluation of possible keratoconus progression: A deterioration of corneal biomechanics may be revealed with a numerical increase of this set of parameters [16]. New parameters, such as inverse concave radius (the maximal value of the inverse radius of curvature during the concave phase of the deformation) and deformation amplitude ratio (the ratio between deformation amplitude at the apex and at 2 mm) may increase the sensitivity of this novel instrument [4].

1.4.1 Refraction

Different methods of refraction in keratoconus patients have been compared in literature, and concluded that a superior CDVA is achieved using the manifest refraction [18] which is considered the gold standard to prescribe spectacles [19].

The technique consists of using autorefraction as starting values, based on which the physician or optometrist starts trying different lenses and asks the patient which ones provide the best visual acuity. It is best when it neutralizes accommodation and takes binocular vision into account [20]. Manifest refraction tends to be more different than autorefraction values in keratoconic patients given the high irregularities in their corneas.

The refraction is considered to be stable if there was a change in refraction of six subjective refractions within ± 0.50 D of spherical equivalent [21].

1.4.2 Visual Acuity

Poor visual acuity is the first reason for consultation and an important factor in surgical decisions in keratoconus patients [22]. The progressive decline in BCVA differs from a patient to the other, but continuous deterioration is synonym of disease progression.

More severe disease in eyes with steeper keratometry values, presence of corneal scars or vogt's striae showcase a more rapid deterioration in BCVA as keratoconus progresses. However, eyes with initial poor BCVA in severe disease do not report a similar rate of deterioration despite having more severe presentation. An explanation to this is that eyes with initial good visual acuity are more sensitive to small disease progression, contrarily to eyes with baseline poor visual acuity.

Best corrected visual acuity in keratoconus patients changes very quickly and can vary from a day to the other. Additionally to the corneal irregularities, it also depends on pupil size, lighting conditions and ocular surface abnormalities such as meibomian gland dysfunction MGD, which tends to occur more frequently in keratoconus patients along with greater tear film instability compared to a healthy population [23]. Thus, a stable visual acuity is a good sign of disease stability [23].

2 ICL in Keratoconus Patients

2.1 The Choice of ICL

ICL, a plate-haptic single-piece lens, is made of collamer which is a flexible, hydrophilic material consists of HEMA hydrogel, water and porcine collagen. It can be folded, implanted in posterior chamber through a 2.8–3.2 mm corneal incision, with a high degree of biocompatibility, good permeability of gases and metabolites,

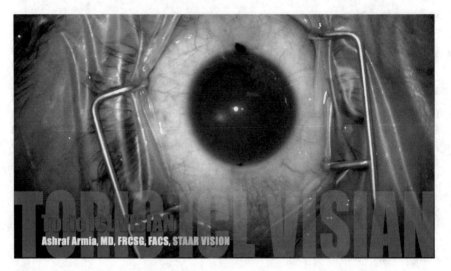

Fig. 1 Marking 0 and 180 degrees

absorption of ultraviolet. It is 6.0 mm wide and comes in five sizes (11.0, 11.5, 12.0, 12.5 and 13.0 mm). The lens has a central convex-concave optic zone with a diameter of 4.5–6.0 mm, and a power of −3.00 to −23.00 D [24]. The ICL design has been modified many times and the choice of using a toric ICL depends on the patients manifest refraction as well as the toricity provided by the STAAR surgical online formula.

The new design (Visian V4c) incorporates the KS-AquaPORT (STAAR Surgical), which is a hole of 360 mm in the center of the ICL optic, to optimize the flow of fluid within the eye. The CentraFLOW technology eliminates the need for a laser peripheral iridotomy or an intraoperative surgical iridectomy and might also reduce the incidence rate of cataracts or avoid the increase of IOP [25]. (Figs. 1, 2 and 3).

2.2 How to Refract

Although autorefraction remains a good place to start when assessing refractive error, it seems to be less accurate in keratoconus patients. The low repeatability of measurements in ectatic patients is a great indicator of this statement [26].

Studies have proven a great difference between autorefraction and manifest refraction, increasing as Kmax increases. Wavefront aberrometry is also being investigated as an exciting option to provide better refraction in keratoconus patients that present high order aberrations, given that this technique takes that latter

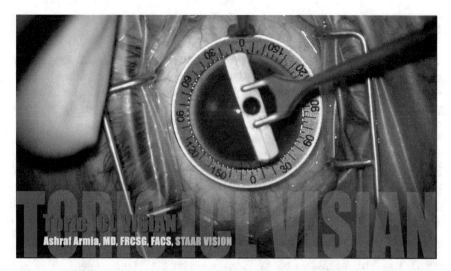

Fig. 2 Marking proper alignment

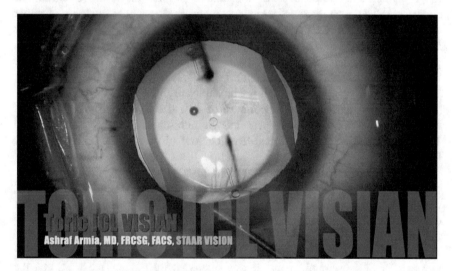

Fig. 3 Toric ICL in the proper position

into consideration, as well as tomography measurements. Currently, studies show a better achieved CDVA with subjective refraction rather than autorefraction [18], the latter varying from a measurement to another given the high irregularities in keratoconic eyes.

2.3   How to Measure ICL

The ICL power calculation is obtained from the manufacturer STAAR surgical, an online modified vertex formula is available for users. The variables in the formula are preoperative manifest spherical and cycloplegic refractive error, keratometric power, corneal thickness, horizontal visible iris diameter (HVID) or the white to white distance (WTW) and central anterior chamber depth (ACD).

WTW measurement is detailed in the following section, HVID can be obtained by the IOL Master, as for the keratometric power, corneal thickness and anterior chamber depth, they are measured using the pentacam. For the ACD, in cases of prominent corneal bulging, a subtraction of 0.2 mm is done from the reading.

Power and toricity are then measured by the company online calculator STAAR surgical.

2.3.1   Novel Technologies for More Accurate WTW Measurement

A very important factor in ICL implantation is size selection. Oversized or undersized ICLs can lead to various complications such as anterior chamber deformation, ICL rotation and decentration, final central vault deviations, cataract formation, mechanical trauma and pigment dispersion syndrome, refractive errors, glare and diplopia [27]. Authors compared the sulcus to sulcus (STS) and the white to white (WTW) methods for final optimized ICL length selection, they found that STS method provided higher vault predictability results.

Other studies analyzed the importance of ICL size selection over a period of time, and found a decentration measured via ultrasound biomicroscopy in up to 11% [28]. A similar study reported lens rotations of up to 18.5° in the first year [29].

These findings raised concerns regarding the stability of the toric ICL, which is crucial in yielding good refractive outcome. Thus, many studies analyzed different methods to measure either white to white, sulcus to sulcus or horizontal visible iris diameter in order to have optimal sizing of the ICL and therefore more stability of the implant.

A recent study showed the repeatability of WTW measurements using the Orbscan III [30]. In another one, it was suggested by Baumeister et al. that the horizontal WTW diameter is determined most accurately by the IOLMaster (Carl Zeiss Meditec). In this study, the mean rotation of the ICL was 0.9° [31]. In another study, it was reported that postoperative rotation after toric ICL implantation was less than 5° in 74% of eyes and less than 11° after 8 months [32].

Another study suggests that UBM valuation of STS distance results in more precise sizing of the ICL implant and consequently in more accurate refractive outcomes [33]. Effective lens position, reflected by postoperative lens vault may be a factor in postoperative refractive outcome. Residual refractive error was often the result of astigmatism in some patients.

The emerging anterior segment oct MS-39 uses SD-OCT and Placido-disk corneal topography to obtain measurements of the anterior segment of the eye. After autocalibration, the scanning process acquires 1 Placido top-view image and a series of 25 SD-OCT radial scans at a wavelength of 840 nm, with an axial resolution of 3.5 nm, a transverse resolution of 35 nm, and a maximum depth of 7.5 mm. Each scan is 16.0 mm long and includes 1024 A-scans. The ring edges are detected on the Placido image so that height, slope, and curvature data can be calculated using the arc-step method with conic curves. Profiles of the anterior cornea, posterior cornea, anterior lens, and iris are derived from the SD-OCT scans. Data for the anterior surface from the Placido image and SD-OCT scans are merged using a proprietary method. All other measurements for internal structures (posterior cornea, anterior lens, and iris) are derived solely from SD-OCT data. A repeatability study showed that the AS-OCT Placido topographer provided repeatable measurements supporting its use in clinical practice [34].

3 Cataract Surgery in Keratoconus Patients

3.1 IOL Selection

IOL selection depends on the manifest refraction, the subjective refraction and the findings of corneal topography. The refractive desires of the patient are also an important factor to make the right choice.

But as a general rule, in these patients, one should lean towards monofocal lenses, as multifocal IOLs cause contrast sensitivity loss that is higher in these patients than in normal patients, due to the corneal irregularities.

If the keratoconus is mild, the progression assessment shows stable disease, and the astigmatism is somewhat regular with the axis of manifest refraction being the same as that of corneal topography, a toric IOL can be implanted, and the power and the axis of the TIOL are determined according to the findings of topography as well as keratometry and refractive cylinder.

But if the patient presents with advanced disease, and the astigmatism is highly irregular and there are differences between the axes of manifest refraction and corneal topography, a monofocal IOL is chosen for implantation.

Other cases in which a monofocal is chosen in these patients are progressive or unstable disease, if they exhibit significant corneal distortion, if the patient intends to continue use of RGP postoperatively and if a PKP is anticipated.

In practice, the most widely used lenses for ectatic patients are the monofocal lenses. This is because we want to try not to induce more aberrations and, if we can, decrease them. Multifocal lenses are not recommended due to the high amount of higher order aberrations these corneas have; we would induce more aberrations and negatively affect the end result. Toric IOLs are becoming a popular option, but we have to know that for high astigmatisms in ectatic patients we will be debulking the astigmatism but not canceling it 100%. Toric IOLs are an option for carefully selected patients, and we should always have a detailed conversation in order to avoid unreasonable expectations and a good understanding of complications. We are going to offer a toric IOL only to patients that will not use toric contact lenses after the surgery.

3.2   IOL Power Calculation

Lens power calculation in KC patients is quite challenging, it requires more parameters to take into consideration given the irregularity of the cornea and the high astigmatism that accompanies it.

The location of the cone (central or paracentral) and the stability of the disease affect the calculation, and prior CXL or ICRS generally improve biometry measurements.

No formula is perfect, and often times comparing or averaging results of more than one equation is considered a good approach, using either standard or topography keratometry values.

In patients with previous implantation of ICRS, the k-reading are derived from the central optical zone.

KC patients usually present with longer axial length as well as deeper anterior chambers which also affect the effective lens position, and the use of capsular tension ring during surgery may decrease the risk of IOL rotation.

Target refraction depends on the surgeon's preference and the trend currently is towards slight myopia.

Regarding the IOL power calculation, the most challenging part is the accurate measurement of keratometric values (K values) due to the astigmatic power irregularity of the cornea itself between the cone apex and the peripheral cornea. This leads to considerable deviation in the IOL calculation and poor postoperative visual outcomes.

Three basic measurements are included in all the different formulas, the axial length, the corneal power and the estimated lens position. The steeper cornea and off-centered apex makes it difficult to obtain accurate keratometry readings. Ectatic eyes have higher axial lengths and deeper anterior chambers, making the effective lens position harder to estimate. As the apex is off-center it might not be in the visual axis, this means that the corneal Ks measured in the apex of the cornea might not be the k's we have to use for our calculations. We have to decide what optical zone we are going to use.

And always keep in mind that there is no specific rule to decide how large this zone should be; and that larger optical zones will overestimate Ks including the off-centered corneal apex in the calculation.

Ultrasound Biometry (UBM) is Inaccurate in ectatic patients. Optical biometry is preferred for axial length measurements due to the acquisition of it in the visual axis. Dr. Alio et al. enforced the importance of the accuracy of the AL in these patients showing a strong correlation between the pre-operative axial length and the post-operative spherical equivalent [35].

Optical biometry, such as the PCI IOL Master 700, yields results that will not be considered as absolute values. In fact, we might want to compare the K's with other devices (such as corneal tomography) and maybe use other K's for the calculations. IOL Master does not acquire all the measurements in one sweep; this is a disadvantage in ectatic eyes due to the big variations within small areas [36]. Contrarily, OLCR devices (Lenstar) LS900 has the advantage of taking all measurements in a single alignment and a single sweep, improving the accuracy of the individual measurements and increasing repeatability. Another advantage is that it incorporates the Barret toric calculator within its formulas. As in the IOL Master, the optical zone where the k values are calculated is good for a normal eye, but small for a patient with corneal ecta§sia. It also makes assumptions about the posterior curvature.

An important aspect to understand is that the total corneal power is given by the anterior and posterior cornea, meaning that measuring only the anterior cornea and assuming a fixed value for the posterior cornea will not be accurate enough.

Wide variety of devices are available to measure corneal power, but not all of them are reliable enough for these eyes. The automated and manual keratometry devices, the topography devices, IOLMaster and Lenstar will only measure the anterior corneal surface and make an assumption about the posterior curvature. It has been published that automated keratometry has bias overcorrecting or undercorrecting the corneal astigmatism in WTR (with the rule) astigmatism and ATR (against the rule) astigmatism respectively. Reaffirming the concept, the anterior and posterior corneal measurement is necessary for us to have accurate data.

1. Manual Keratometry:

Measures the central 3 mm of the cornea, measuring the radius of curvature of the anterior surface and making assumptions regarding the posterior surface.

In addition to the lack of data concerning the posterior cornea, the purkinje image will be distorted in ectatic eyes, making the calculations less reliable.

• Automated Keratometry:

Most devices measure the central 2.8–3.33 mm of the cornea. Due to the great variability in diopters within different areas in these corneas, measuring only one small area is not enough to have accurate results. Automated Keratometry has a better repeatability than the manual keratometry but we basically find the same problems as in manual keratometry [37].

• Corneal Topography:

It measures anterior corneal curvature and it will calculate elevation using Slope. It will make assumptions on the posterior corneal curvature assigning to it a fixed value. Ectatic corneas have multiple different elevations therefore calculating elevation from slope will not be accurate.

- Automated Keratometry:

Most devices measure the central 2.8–3.33 mm of the cornea. Due to the great variability in diopters within different areas in these corneas, measuring only one small area is not enough to have accurate results. Automated Keratometry has a better repeatability than the manual keratometry but we basically find the same problems as in manual keratometry.

- Corneal Tomography:

There is no doubt that up to now these devices are the gold standard to calculate K's in ectatic corneas. The main difference with the other devices is that it measures elevation in a direct manner, and it calculates curvature from it. The most commonly used devices are the Pentacam (Oculus GmbH, Wetzlar, Germany) Galilei (Ziemer Ophthalmic Systems AG) and Sirius Scheimpflug Analyzer (CSO, Costruzione Strumenti Oftalmici, Florence, Italy).; all these devices use the Scheimpflug technology to obtain their images. The Oculus Pentacam has one rotating camera, directly measuring elevation and calculating curvature. The Galilei has two rotating cameras and a built-in Placido disc, calculating corneal curvature by merging the Placido and the elevation data. With the tomography we are measuring the posterior corneal curvature and calculating the total corneal power without assumptions [38].

When using the Scheimpflug devices, we can overcome the problem of the off-centered corneal apex for K's calculation. You choose between a centration in the "Apex" or the "Pupil". This is useful because the apex might not be within the visual axis, and if we consider the high K's from it we will underestimate the power of the lens. These devices have the advantage of measuring elevation of the anterior and posterior corneal curvatures. Two maps generated from these devices of great value for us are: the True net power map and the Equivalent K-Readings (EKR).

- True Net Power Map

Will measure the refractive power of the anterior and posterior cornea assigning to each of them specific refractive indices. So Will put together many k readings in the area that we select, making it easier to select the k's we want to use for our IOL calculation.

- Equivalent K-Reading (EKR)

Will output the information in the way keratometers do (SimK), but including in the equation the anterior and posterior corneal power. EKR corrects keratometric values measured by the tomographer and adds the error that would be created using a single refraction index (1.3375) in a sagittal map. It allows us to evaluate the progression of power between the different areas and decide the K's we want to use in the area we desire between 1 and 7 mm.

Regarding formulas, due to the off-centered axis, optical measurement devices are preferred instead of ultrasound devices. The OLCR device in combination with the Barret toric calculator showed the best corneal astigmatism prediction error compared with a PCI device and other formulas. Dr D. Cooke showed in his publication comparing preinstalled formulas in PCI and OLCR devices that OLCR devices in combination with Olsen formula has the best results for long eyes [39]. Thebpatiphat et al. did a small study comparing three formulas, SRK, SRK-II and SRK-T and he concluded that the SRK-II formula might be the most accurate in mild Keratoconus [40].

Dr. S Bozorg and R Pineda in their review suggested that the Holladay 2 formula might be more accurate than other formulas when effective lens position is variable [41]. Dr Alio et al. did a retrospective study in which he operated with MICS and inserted toric IOL's in 17 eyes of 10 patients. He reported good results using the Hoffer Q formula in patients with average axial lengths and the SRK/T formula in longer eyes, with the last one having the best results [35]. Newer generation formulas like Barret Universal II, and the RBF calculator are promising but larger studies in ectatic corneas are needed.

- 4th generation formulas

Are theoretically considered an improvement over the previous formulas in order to calculate IOL power in all eyes but especially in abnormal ones. Holladay II, Haigis, Olsen, and Barrett are examples of this generation. An increased number of variables in these formulas could help to improve the ELP calculation. Holladay II formula created by Jack Holladay, adjusts the recommended IOL power more by including factors like AL, corneal power, white to white (WTW), ACD, lens thickness, age, and pre- operative refraction data. Although it remains theoretical, it has a strong base of 3500 patients in 35 study centers. It tends to be more precise in eyes with extreme findings, and it may also prove to be more accurate in variable ELP cases.

The Haigis formula requires the measured ACD value, and the Barrett formula needs lens thickness and WTW measurement. There are publications that suggest Holladay II formula to be more accurate than other formulas when ELP is variable. Newer generation formulas like Barrett Universal II and the radial basis function (RBF) calculator are promising, but larger studies in ectatic corneas are still needed.

So Mild Keratocouns SRK II formula may provide IOL power more accurately than other formulas, suggested in a retro- spective study by Thebpatiphat et al. SRK/T formula gives more accurate results in myopic eyes in comparison to SRK II; this concept is important because KCN and myopia are often linked together.

And Other stages Keratocouns SRK II formula showed the most reliable outcomes in all stages of KCN in their study, although the reliability was less in severe stages of KCN. Indeed, none of the formulas offer good predictability in advanced KCN. In these cases, a target postoperative refraction of 1.00 D could be considered (Fig. 4).

Modern database "IOLCon" promoting reliable IOL Calculation:

The first optical biometer was launched in 1999: Prof. Adolf F. Fercher's visionary ideas and patent laid the basis for the development of optical coherence tomography

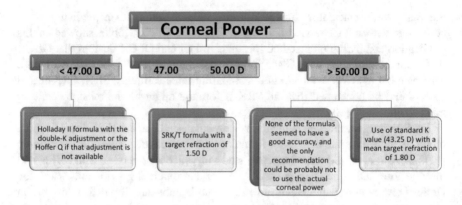

Fig. 4 Calculating intraocular lens power in eyes with keratoconus

used in ophthalmology in 1982. In 1999 the first optical biometer was launched by Zeiss and optical biometry revolutionized cataract surgery fundamentally together with Prof. Haigis ULIB database of intraocular lens constants. Prof. Achim Langenbucher developed Haigis' idea of an internet database for intraocular lens constants to meet modern standards and requirements by establishing a modern platform covering all IOL data and constants needed for appropriate IOL calculation. By establishing a state-of-the-art database for IOL constants that is internationally available, "IOLCon" provides essential data for a successful cataract surgery.

In combination with optical biometry, a database providing optimized constants for cataract surgery was needed. Haigis´ ULIB (User Group for Laser Interference Biometry) was the first database of its time to set a milestone in providing optimized constants for cataract surgery. From today's perspective, it no longer meets requirements as ULIB focused essentially on the Zeiss' biometer. Moreover, it did not offer an open interface—the direct download of data was only possible for the Zeiss IOL Master. In addition, there hasn't been an update of ULIB since 2016.

Therefore, Prof. Langenbucher started the development of IOLCon in 2015: He wanted to establish a database open to all lens and biometer manufacturers, its self-explanatory functionality providing users all relevant lens data at a glance by using XML as a public and documented data transfer format. Since its official commissioning in mid-2017, this international web-based platform IOLCon fulfills all of these requirements as well as the broad requirements of a modern biometry database: IOLCon is set up as a platform independent of specific devices, IOL manufacturers or surgeons. The data achieved in IOLCon is generated by two user groups: IOL manufacturers and ophthalmic surgeons. Download of technical data and constants as well as upload of information on biometry, the implanted IOL including its post-OP refraction needed for optimizing the constants is facilitated by an open data interface using the non-commercial XML download format with interface documentation.

IOLCon's data is used to provide both—global (all data of the respective IOL) and individual (e.g. for one surgeon) optimizations. Once registered for IOLCon, the ophthalmic surgeon can customize optimization, e.g. optimize his own data separately, optimizing for a particular biometer or patient's ethnicity. The method applied by IOLCon is characterized by "Intelligent IOL Constant Optimization" using e.g. statistical methods taking into account the measurement accuracies of the measuring instruments (e.g. biometers). Reliable traceability of the data is ensured by obligatory registration of all users. For the optical device industry, it is possible to upload own data as well as to transfer information provided by ULIB.

IOLCon, which is free of charge for ophthalmo-surgeons, is an essential tool for ophthalmology: It provides an up-to-date overview of available IOLs with all relevant technical, geometrical/optical and material characteristics. The search options of the database can easily be used in a variety of ways: data can be filtered regarding IOL- and biometer manufacturers, IOL materials, geometries, available powers and nominal or optimized constants, the data can be downloaded or printed in a convenient layout.

By launching IOLCon in 2017, a modern data base is worldwide available today which is open to all lens and biometer manufacturers. By its self-explanatory functionality, it provides its users with all relevant lens parameters. IOLCon fulfills the requirements of a modern biometry database and established itself as an indispensable tool for cataract surgeons. Since its official launch, IOLCon has grown steadily (for more information: https://iolcon.org/help.php). Biometer manufacturers already implemented the open XML interface to integrate IOLCon into their devices. Thus, by implementing this interface, a biometry database has been made available, which will also meet the future demands of ongoing developing ophthalmo-surgery. IOLCon offers much more than only a simple static table—it´s a global interactive up-to-date, modern internet platform that provides ophthalmo-surgeons with a documentation of all lens characteristics which are updated constantly. Today, IOLCon is regarded as gold standard data base for IOL parameters and constants, it´s a globally available internet-based platform which meets all requirements of state-of-the-art cataract surgery, it can be accessed at https://iolcon.org. [42, 17, 43, 44, 45, 46, 47, 48].

iTrace in Keratoconus:

The iTrace system utilizes placido disk plus ray tracing aberrometry to analyze complex eyes and display the information in easy to use and explain displays. For Keratoconus, some examples show how this useful diagnostic system can complement crosslinked corneas.

The following patient has been crosslinked and a Toric IOL has been implanted. The Chang Analysis shows the eye in component parts with High Order Aberrations displayed and separated into the Cornea, the Internal and the sum of these two which is the Total eye.

The surgeon can use the Toric Check display to see that location of the toric, versus the steep corneal axis plus the lens cylinder relative to the corneal astigmatism. In this example the surgeon has nailed the axis.

Using the patient's optics as measured, the surgeon can use visual simulation in the iTrace to see if a pinhole will help the vision. Pinhole treatments like small aperture contact lenses or the IC8 may be a valuable treatment option, but before offering the patient this plan, the surgeon can see if it will be successful.

The corneal optics of the patient with their scotopic pupil size of are quite poor, but with the pupil reduced to 2 or 2.5 mm, the vision below is much improved (Figs. 5, 6, 7, 8 and 9).

3.3 Incision

Early KC can be managed in a similar manner to normal cataract surgery. Severe KC with steep meridians and possible corneal scars can be troublesome. When the main incision is performed in a cornea with abnormal structural properties as in keratoconic eyes, post-operative K values and corneal shape can change in an unpredictable manner. Cataract main incision sites should be planned during preoperative examination according to the peripheral corneal thickness rather than the astigmatism axis. In the case of infero-temporal cone, the main incision should be placed superiorly or supero-temporal. Vice versa, in rare cases of rare superior steep cone the main incision should be placed temporally.

In the presence of corneal scarring which is common in advanced KC, the main incision should be placed 90 degrees apart from the scar location. In cases of inferior scarring, a superior approach is not advised as this will lead the phaco-probe to point inferiorly (underneath the scar) rendering all maneuvers more challenging due to the reduced intraocular visibility.

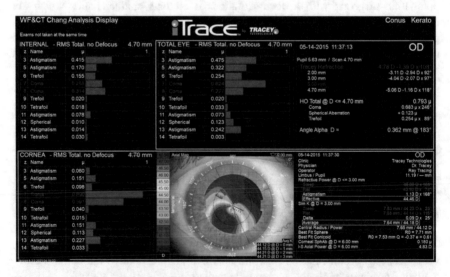

Fig. 5 The iTrace "Chang Analysis Display" screen showing a total High Order Aberrations value of 0.793μ (top right), coming mostly from the "coma" at the cornea, shown in the two long blue bars (bottom left), which is also displayed graphically in the axial map at the bottom

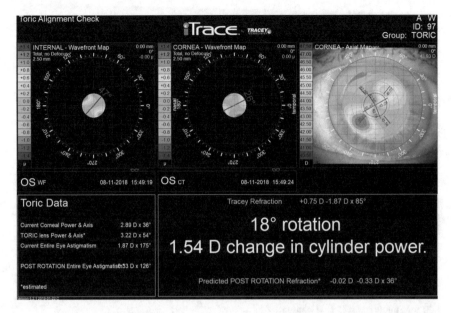

Fig. 6 The iTrace "Toric Alignment Check" screen showing the internal astigmatism flat axis of 47° (i.e. the orientation of the Toric IOL), and the corneal astigmatism step axis of 26°. Hence, the surgeon should rotate the Toric IOL 18° clockwise to get a decrease of the total eye's astigmatism from −1.87D to −0.33D

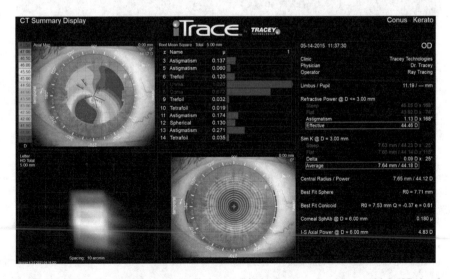

Fig. 7 The iTrace "Corneal Topography Summary Display" screen showing very high HOA's of the cornea (mainly coma—long blue bars) at 5.00 mm diameter, and also displaying a simulation on how the patient "sees" through a 5.00 mm pupil (blurred E at bottom left)

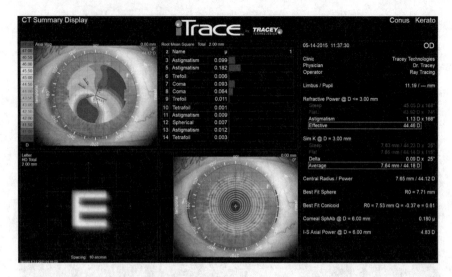

Fig. 8 The iTrace "Corneal Topography Summary Display" screen showing low HOA's of the cornea at 2.00 mm diameter, and also displaying a simulation on how the patient "sees" through a 2.00 mm pupil (sharper E at bottom left)

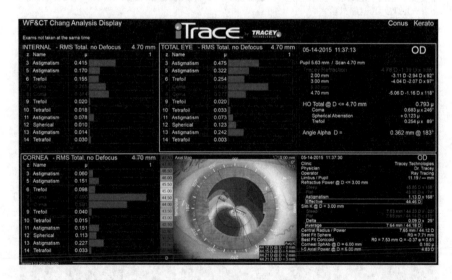

Fig. 9 The iTrace "WaveTouch Lens Order Display" screen showing precisely where the contact lens correction should be located, based on the ability of the iTrace to scan through an acquisition lens. This location, along with the exact aberration profile of the patient, is sent to a lathe program to create a customized scleral lens for this patient

Keratoconic corneas are thinner and floppier and therefore clear corneal wounds are more prone to leak after surgery. Thus, a well-constructed 2 steps sclero-corneal is advisable to reduce the risk of post-operative wound leak and to induce less change in corneal shape. So, the use of a corneal suture to secure the wound can be advisable.

An alternative to this can be cataract surgery through scleral tunnel incision, which will not only avoid possible worsening of the corneal geometry but also minimize contact with the corneal endothelium.

3.4   Particularities of Phacoemulsification

Surgical procedure: It is not a routine phacoemulsification and often requires extra steps to obtain optimal results, such as the use of generous amount of OVD to protect the endothelium, and sometimes the use of RGP contact lens intraoperatively to decrease image distortion during surgery and allow better visualization for the surgeon, in order to avoid possible complications, that can be due to bad visualization in certain cases.

In practice, preoperative cornea marking at the 0° and 180° positions was done, at slit lamp in vertical position with the patient sitting upright and looking forward.

In the presence of diffuse scars, the surgeon should expect a worse view under the surgical microscope compared with the slit lamp examination. This is due to the different light sources employed: a sharp oblique light at the ophthalmic slit lamp versus a central diffuse light under the surgical microscope. The latter will cause a light scattering together with shadows and reflections that will make the surgical steps more difficult.

To improve intraocular visibility and reduce image distortion due to the corneal irregularity it can be useful to spread a dispersive ophthalmic viscoelastic device such as the hydroxypropyl methylcellulose (HPMC) gel onto the cornea. This will improve the epithelial hydration rendering the corneal surface more regular and provide a mild magnification of the intraocular view. After making the corneal incisions, even in cases of good red reflex the use of capsular staining dye is recommended to enhance capsular visualization during continuous curvilinear capsulorhexis. During the surgery, it is also important to attempt to minimize the intraocular pressure by modifying the phacoemulsification machine parameters to reduce stress on the cornea (Fig. 10).

3.5   Post Operative Considerations

Given the high astigmatism induced by keratoconus, it can worsen after cataract surgery, most patients will require CL postoperatively, and a fitting consultation

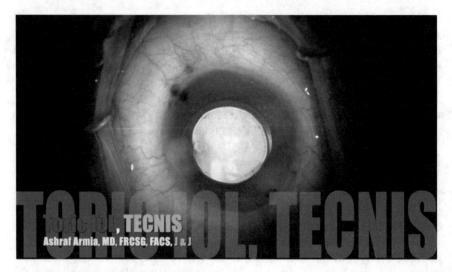

Fig. 10 Toric IOL, proper alignment

will have to take place in the days following the surgery to offer the patient the best VA possible.

3.6 Innovations in IOLs Technology

Small-aperture intraocular lens in keratoconus:

The small-aperture IOL implantation with severe corneal irregularities resulting in an increase of subjective and objective visual outcomes. As expected, the small aperture reduced visual distortion caused by corneal irregularities, leading to a better visual perception [49]. That a pinhole IOL can result in superior visual results is already known since the introduction of the add-on XtraFocus lens (Morcher) [50, 51].

Furthermore, XtraFocus is an IOL specifically designed for cases with corneal irregularities, whereas the IC-8 IOL was designed to function as an enhanced depth-of-focus IOL. However, in contrast to the add-on lens that has no optical power, the IC-8 IOL is placed directly in the capsular bag and can be used during standard cataract surgery. Similar to Grabner et al. [52] we could observe an increase in UDVA, UIVA, and UNVA. It is known that the small-aperture IOL shows superior results in UNVA and UIVA as compared to the monofocal IOL in healthy eyes. We could also observe an extended depth of focus with the IOL in our cohort with corneal irregularities. The defocus curve shows a clear plateau post-operatively as compared to the preoperative peak in visual acuity.

However, in contrast to other multifocal IOLs in which the complex optic can lead to an increase in optical phenomena such as glare and halo [53, 54], especially in patients with corneal irregularities, the pinhole system improves the visual quality with reducing occurrence of these phenomena. Nevertheless, in eyes with severe corneal irregularities, the pinhole IOL is not implanted primarily to achieve an extended depth of focus but to increase overall visual acuity. This increase in CDVA was most likely due to the IOL structure and not due to removal of existing opacities in the natural lens, as in most eyes cataract was, if present, at a very early stage. The IOL has therefore a high safety index and can be helpful in eyes with corneal irregularities. Another proof of this is the high patient satisfaction rate with the small-aperture IOL. Patients reported to perform better in daily tasks and a clear increase in their reading capabilities for distant and near signs. A challenge was IOL power calculation in these severely altered eyes. An extremely high variance could be observed in average keratometry ranging from 37 to 55 D with an astigmatism of up to 8 D within the central 3.0 mm corneal zone and is comparable to previous studies with advanced keratoconus or after keratoplasty [55, 56].

Knowing this, IOL power calculation was not possible with one of the used formulas because the resulted IOL would have been out of range. They targeted rather for a myopic outcome because this would be less harmful for a patient in the case of a residual refractive error. Overall, a sub- stantial amount of eyes had a myopic outcome with an average spherical equivalent of !1.22 D after 3 months. The most accurate results with the smallest mean absolute error was achieved with the Haigis formula [57]. The current range of the IOL power (15.5–27.5 D) is however a limitation. Several patients could not be included because they would have been out of range for the IOL power.

As compared to Hooshmand et al. [58], the PCO rate was higher in our cohort (12 vs. 7%). However, our cohort was substantially smaller, and no conclusion can be drawn on this basis. Both cases in which PCO was observed were treated with YAG- capsulotomy without further complications. Under red-free light examina- tion, it is possible to focus on the central part of the posterior capsule with the laser, even if the clear optics of the IOL is occupied by an inlay. In conclusion, the small-aperture IOL is a useful option in eyes with severe corneal irregularities. It has a high safety index, has a high patient satisfaction rate, and can lead to better visual quality. The main challenge remains the IOL power calculation and that further large population-based studies are required to choose the IOL power more accurately.

Custom intraocular lens design:

Custom IOLs are calculated and analyzed using personalized numerical ray tracing eye models. The models were built in the same way as those presented in a previous study [59], but had a modified corneal representation and virtual iris. Instead of the Zernike polynomial representation of the cornea, the mathematical description using a combination of Zernike polynomials and basis-splines was used. To cal- culate the IOL, the virtual iris was replaced by weighting each ray at the IOL's anterior surface. The weights were $\equiv 1.0$ in the inner 3 mm of the IOL and decreased linearly with the radius to zero at the IOL's edge (diameter: 6 mm). They were applied in addition to the weights at the corneal plane simulating the Stiles-Crawford effect.

Using two types of IOL: the aberration-neutral nIOL, and the fully aberration correcting cIOL. The nIOL was the Aspira-aA (HumanOptics AG, Erlangen, Germany), whose design data was provided by the manufacturer. The IOL power which produced the smallest wRMS was chosen in the same way as described previously [59]. The Cartesian x, y coordinates of the object point $z = -6$ m in front of the corneal apex were adjusted so that it produced the minimum wRMS at the position of the virtual fovea. The back surface of the IOL was kept and the front surface customized to calculate the cIOL.

During customization, the IOL's anterior surface was modified to nullify the optical path length differences in an iterative manner, similarly as described previously [59] for customization of the IOL's posterior surface. First, the ideal wavefront inside the IOL was calculated using backward numerical ray tracing from the virtual fovea through the IOL's posterior surface. The wavefront can easily be propagated inside the IOL, because the rays travel perpendicular to the wavefront. Using forward numerical ray tracing starting from the object point, the intersec- tion of each ray with the propagated wavefronts were computed and the corresponding propagation lengths were iteratively adjusted to minimize the optical path length differences. The coordinates of the IOL's ideal anterior surface were given by the intersection of the rays with the wavefronts propagated by the respective propa- gation lengths through the IOL. The cIOL's minimum thickness was imposed to be 5 to 8 μm thicker than the edge thickness of the nIOL to ensure mechanical sta- bility. The coordinates of the anterior IOL surfaces were fitted with a smooth mathematical surface description (comination of Zernike polynomial terms with $j \leq 22$ [60] and fourth order basis splines with $dx = dy = 0.375$ mm knot dis- tance) to enable numerical ray tracing. The precision of the fit was in the sub μm scale and sufficient to achieve root-mean-square wave-front errors of <0.0027 μm for all eyes.

The wRMS and the wavefront-error were used to verify successful optimization. Backward numerical ray tracing from the virtual fovea through IOL and cornea was used to calculate the wavefront in front of the eye, and the best-fitting sphere was subtracted from the wavefront to calculate the wavefront-errors. To analyze the dependency of wRMS on the iris diameter, the wRMSs were calculated without weighting the rays at the IOLs' surfaces. The iris diameter was simulated as cen- tered aperture stop placed at the anterior chamber depth.

An aberration-neutral IOL (nIOL) was chosen based on the wRMS for each eye. The anterior IOL surface was subsequently customized to correct the aberrations. The centered IOL with customized aberration-correcting front surface (cIOL) sucessfully reduced the wavefront-errors and the wRMS for normal cataractous eyes and even more for keratoconic eyes compared to the wavefront-errors and wRMS with the centered nIOL. This resulted in reduced dependency of the wRMS on the diameter of the virtual iris. The improvement was particularly high in the keratoconus group. Typically, the differences between the IOL surface elevation of nIOL and cIOL were larger for keratoconic eyes than normal eyes. The standard devia- tion (SD) of the difference between the anterior IOL surface elevation of nIOL and cIOL was 8.4 μm for NP and 29.3 μm for KP.

Whether eyes with keratoconic corneal tomography pattern could benefit more from aberration correction with custom intraocular lenses (IOLs) than normal cataractous eyes despite the effect of misalignment on the correction of aberrations. Custom IOLs (cIOLs) were calculated for twelve normal and twelve keratoconic eyes using personalized numerical ray tracing models. The Stiles- Crawford weighted root-mean-square spot-size (wRMS) at the virtual fovea was evaluated for cIOLs and aberration-neutral IOLs (nIOLs) in a simulated clinical study with 500 virtual IOL implantations per eye and per IOL. IOL misalignment (decentration, tilt, rotation) and pupillary ectopia (4.5 mm iris aperture) were varied upon each virtual implantation. IOL misalignment resulted in larger wRMS variations in the kera- toconus group than in the normal group. Custom freeform IOL-optics-design may become a promising option for the correction of advanced aberrations in eyes with non-progressive keratoconic corneal tomography pattern [61].

References

1. Moramarco A, Mastrofilippo V, Romano M, Iannetta D, Braglia L, Fontana L. Efficacy and safety of accelerated corneal cross-linking for progressive keratoconus: a 5-Year follow-up study. J Refract Surg. 2020;36:724–30. https://doi.org/10.3928/1081597X-20200819-01.
2. Carlson AN. Expanding our understanding of eye rubbing and keratoconus. Cornea. 2010;29 (2):245.
3. Gordon-Shaag A, Millodot M, Shneor E, Liu Y. The genetic and environmental factors for keratoconus. Biomed Res Int . 2015:795–738.
4. Vinciguerra P, Piscopo R, Camesasca F, Vinciguerra R. Progression in keratoconus. Int J Keratoconus and Ectatic Corneal Dis. 2016;5(1):21–31.
5. Shetty R, et al. Repeatability and agreement of three Scheimpflug-based imaging systems for measuring anterior segment parameters in keratoconus. Invest Ophthalmol Vis Sci. 2014;55 (8):5263–8.
6. Shetty R et al. Keratoconus screening indices and their diagnostic ability to distinguish normal from ectatic corneas. American Journal of Ophthalmology 2017. 181. https://doi.org/10.1016/j.ajo.2017.06.031.
7. Neuhann S, Schuh A, Krause D, et al. Comparison of variables measured with a Scheimpflug device for evaluation of progression and detection of keratoconus. Sci Rep. 2020;10:19308.
8. Kanellopoulos AJ, Aslanides IM, Asimellis G. Correlation between epithelial thickness in normal corneas, untreated ectatic corneas, and ectatic corneas previously treated with CXL; is overall epithelial thickness a very early ectasia prognostic factor? Clin Ophthalmol. 2012;6:789–800.
9. Li Y, Tan O, Brass R, Weiss JL, Huang D. Corneal epithelial thickness mapping by Fourier-domain optical coherence tomography XE "optical coherence tomography" in normal and keratoconic eye. Ophthalmology. 2012;119(12):2425–33.
10. Serrao S, et al. Role of corneal epithelial thickness mapping in the evaluation of keratoconus. Contact Lens and Anterior Eye. 42(6):662–665.

11. Fontes B, Ambrósio R, Velarde G, Nosé W. Ocular response analyzer measurements in keratoconus with normal central corneal thickness compared with matched normal control eyes. J Refract Surg. 2011;27:209–15.

12. Pniakowska Z, Jurowski P. Detection of the early keratoconus based on corneal biomechanical properties in the refractive surgery candidates. 2016. 64(2):109–13.

13. Bak-Nielsen S, Pedersen IB, Ivarsen A, Hjortdal J. Dynamic Scheimpflug-based assessment of keratoconus and the effects of corneal cross-linking. J Refract Surg. 2014;30(6):408–14.

14. Lanza M, Cennamo M, Iaccarino S, Irregolare C, Rechichi M, Bifani M, Gironi Carnevale UA. Evaluation of corneal deformation analyzed with Scheimpflug based device in healthy eyes and diseased ones. Biomed Res Int 2014;2014:748671.

15. Terai N, Raiskup F, Haustein M, Pillunat LE, Spoerl E. Identification of biomechanical properties of the cornea: the ocular response analyzer. Curr Eye Res. 2012;37(7):553–62.

16. Roberts, CJ. Biomechanics in keratoconus. Barbara, A., Textbook on keratoconus: new insights. New Delhi: Jaypee Brothers Medical Publishers; 2012. p. 29.

17. Scholtz S, Cayless A, Langenbucher A, Calculating the Human Eye, Basics on Biometry, in: Liu C and Bardan AS (Eds): Cataract Surgery, Pearls and Techniques, 978–3–030–38233–9, 459250_1_En, (Chapter 7), Springer, 1/2021, S. 87 – 114.

18. Soeters N, Muijzer MB, Molenaar J, Godefrooij DA, Wisse RPL. Autorefraction versus manifest refraction in patients with keratoconus. J Refract Surg. 2018;34(1):30–4.

19. Elliott DB. What is the appropriate gold standard test for refractive error? Ophthalmic Physiol Opt. 2017;37:115–7.

20. Momeni-Moghaddam H, Goss DA. Comparison of four different binocular balancing techniques. Clin Exp Optom. 2014;97:422–5.

21. Doroodgar F, Niazi F, Sanginabadi A, et al. Comparative analysis of the visual performance after implantation of the toric implantable collamer lens in stable keratoconus: a 4-year follow-up after sequential procedure (CXL+TICL implantation) BMJ Open Ophthalmology 2017;2:e000090.

22. Davis LJ, Schechtman KB, Wilson BS, Rosenstiel CE, Riley CH, Libassi DP, Gundel RE, Rosenberg L, Gordon MO, Zadnik K. The Collaborative Longitudinal Evaluation of Keratoconus (CLEK) study group; longitudinal changes in visual acuity in keratoconus. Invest Ophthalmol Vis Sci. 2006;47(2):489–500. https://doi.org/10.1167/iovs.05-0381.

23. Carracedo G, Recchioni A, Alejandre-Alba N, et al. Signs and symptoms of dry eye in keratoconus patients: a pilot study. Curr Eye Res. 2015;40(11):1088–94.

24. Srinivasan S. Phakic intraocularlenses: lessons learned. J Cataract Refract Surg. 2019;45:1529–30.

25. Li K, Wang Z, Zhang D, Wang S, Song X, Li Y, Wang MX. Visual outcomes and corneal biomechanics after V4c implantable collamer lens implantation in subclinical keratoconus. J Cataract Refract Surg. 2020;46(10):1339–45.

26. Davis LJ, Schechtman KB, Begley CG, Shin JA, Zadnik K; The CLEK Study Group. Repeatability of refraction and corrected visual acuity in keratoconus. Optom Vis Sci. 1998;75:887–896.

27. Boxer Wachler BS, Vicente LL. Optimizing the vault of collagen copolymer phakic intraocular lenses in eyes with keratoconus and myopia: comparison of 2 methods. J Cataract Refract Surg. 2010;36(10):1741–4.

28. Garcia-Feijoo J, et al. Ultrasound examination of posterior chamber phakic intraocular lens position. Ophthalmology. 2003;110:163–72.

29. Koivula A, Taube M, Zetterstro'm C. Phakic refractive lens: two-year results. J Refract Surg. 2008;24:507–15.

30. Sharma M, Jain N, Koshy AS, Arora V, Lalgudi VG. Repeatability of Orbscan III for anterior segment parameters in normal eyes 2020, Volume: 68, Issue Number: 12, Page: 2903–5.

31. Baumeister M, Terzi E, Ekici Y, Kohnen T. Comparison of manual and automated methods to determine horizontal corneal diameter. J Cataract Refract Surg. 2004;30:374–80.

32. Park SC, Kwun YK, Chung E-S, Ahn K, Chung T-Y. Postoperative astigmatism and axis stability after implantation of the STAAR Toric Implantable Col- lamer Lens. J Refract Surg. 2009;25:403–9.
33. Panda P, Ostrovsky A, Brodie S, Speaker M. Impact of Ultrasound Biomicroscopy (UBM) versus White-to-White (WTW) measurement on sizing of Visian Implantable Collamer Lens (ICL) and Residual Postoperative Refraction. Invest Ophthalmol Vis Sci. 2013;54(15):850.
34. Savini G, Schiano-Lomoriello D, Hoffer KJ. Repeatability of automatic measurements by a new anterior segment optical coherence tomographer combined with Placido topography and agreement with 2 Scheimpflug cameras. J Cataract Refract Surg. 2018;44(4):471–8. https://doi.org/10.1016/j.jcrs.2018.02.015 Epub 2018 Apr 25.
35. Alio JL, Garcia PP, Guliyeve FA, et al. MICS with toric intraocular lens in keratoconus: outcomes and predictability analysis of postoperative refraction. Br J Ophthalmol. 2014;98 (3):365–70.
36. Akman A, Asena L, Güngör SG. Evaluation and comparison of the new swept source OCT-based IOLMaster 700 with the IOLMaster 500. Br J Ophthalmol. 2016;100(9):1201–5. https://doi.org/10.1136/bjophthalmol-2015-307779.
37. Zhang L, Sy ME, Mai H, Yu F, Hamilton DR. Effect of posterior corneal astigmatism on refractive outcomes after toric intraocular lens implantation. J Cataract Refract Surg 2015; 41:84–9. Q 2015 ASCRS and ESCRS.
38. Lee H, Kim T-I, Kim EK. Corneal astigmatism analysis for toric intraocular lens implantation: precise measurement for perfect correction. Curr Opin Ophthalmol. 2015;26:34–8.
39. Cooke DL, Cooke TL, Prediction accuracy of preinstalled formulas on 2 optical biometers. J Cataract Refract Surg 2016; 42:358–62. Q 2016 ASCRS and ESCRS.
40. Thebpatiphat N, Hammersmith KM, Rapuano CJ, et al. Cataract surgery in keratoconus. Eye Contact Lens. 2007;33:244–6.
41. Bozorog S, Pineda R. Cataract and keratoconus: Minimizing complications in intraocular lens calculations. Sem Ophthalmol. 2014;29(5–6):376–9.
42. Larkin, IOLCon database awaits input, International internet database updates and optimises IOL constants, EuroTimes, March 2021, p. 19. https://www.eurotimes.org/iol-con-database-awaits-input/.
43. McCommon, IOLCon: Data Collaboration is the Future, CAKE Magazine, September 4, 2020. https://cakemagazine.org/iolcon-data-collaboration-is-the-future/.
44. Charters L, An international encyclopedic database for IOL specifications, The IOLCon platform optimizes intraocular lens constants, Ophthalmology Times Europe, April 2019, https://www.ophthalmologytimes.com/iols/international-encyclopedic-database-iol-specifications.
45. Scholtz S, Internet database "IOLCon", Biometry today, its challenges and the benefits, EUROPEAN OPHTHAMOLOGY NEWS (ESCRS), 9/2019, p. 2.
46. IOL constants database ready for use, EyeOnOptics, https://www.eyeonoptics.co.nz/articles/archive/iol-constants-database-ready-for-use/.
47. Scholtz SK (2019) Editorial. J Eye Stud Treat. 2019;(1): 31–2. https://ospopac.com/journal/eye-study-treatment/present-issue/Editorial-Journal-of-Eye-Study-and-Treatment
48. Scholtz S, Langenbucher A, (Un)avoidable errors in biometry, Eye Stud Treat. 2020;(1):73–75. https://ospopac.com/journal/eye-study-treatment/special-issue/UnAvoidable-Errors-in-Biometry.
49. Trindade BLC, Trindade FC, Trindade CLC, Santhiago MR. Phacoemulsi- fication with intraocular pinhole implantation associated with Descemet membrane endothelial keratoplasty to treat failed full-thickness graft with dense cataract. J Cataract Refract Surg. 2018;44:1280–3.
50. Trindade CC, Trindade BC, Trindade FC, Werner L, Osher R, Santhiago MR. New pinhole sulcus implant for the correction of irregular corneal astigmatism. J Cataract Refract Surg. 2017;43:1297–306.
51. Tsaousis KT, Werner L, Trindade CLC, Guan J, Li J, Reiter N. Assessment of a novel pinhole supplementary implant for sulcus fixation in pseudophakic cadaver eyes. Eye (Lond). 2018;32:637–45.

52. Grabner G, Ang RE, Vilupuru S. The small-aperture IC-8 intraocular lens: a new concept for added depth of focus in cataract patients. Am J Ophthalmol. 2015;160:1176-1184.e1.
53. Bellucci R. Multifocal intraocular lenses. Curr Opin Ophthalmol. 2005;16:33–7.
54. Shajari M, Steinwender G, Herrmann K, Kubiak KB, Pavlovic I, Plawetzki E, Schmack I, Kohnen T. Evaluation of keratoconus progression. Br J Oph- thalmol. 2019;103:551–7.
55. Shajari M, Friderich S, PourSadeghian M, Schmack I, Kohnen T. Character- istics of corneal astigmatism of anterior and posterior surface in a normal control group and patients with keratoconus. Cornea. 2017;36:457–62.
56. Hooshmand J, Allen P, Huynh T, Chan C, Singh R, Moshegov C, Agarwal S, Thornell E, Vote BJ. Small aperture IC-8 intraocular lens in cataract patients: achieving extended depth of focus through small aperture optics. Eye (Lond). 2019;33:1096–103.
57. Schröder S, Schrecker J, Daas L, Eppig T, Langenbucher A. Impact of intraocular lens displacement on the fixation axis. J Opt Soc Am A. 2018;35:561–6.
58. Zhu Z, Janunts E, Eppig T, Sauer T, Langenbucher A. Tomography-based customized IOL calculation model. Curr Eye Res. 2010;36:579–89.
59. Noll RJ. Zernike polynomials and atmospheric turbulence. J Opt Soc Am. 1976;66:207–11.
60. Schröder S, Eppig T, Liu W, Schrecker J, Langenbucher A. Keratoconic eyes with stable corneal tomography could benefit more from custom intraocular lens design than normal eyes. Sci Rep. 2019;9(1):3479.

Femtosecond-Laser Assisted Deep Anterior Lamellar Keratoplasty (F-DALK)

Gerald Schmidinger, Theo G. Seiler, and Ruth Donner

Due to the progressive nature of many corneal dystrophies and diseases, the indication for surgical intervention is often inevitable. With an incidence of 1/7.500 in northern European countries and a prevalence of up to 265 in 100.000 people, keratoconus is one of the major indications for corneal transplantation [1, 2]. About 10–20% of all patients diagnosed with keratoconus will eventually require keratoplasty [3, 4]. Of all corneal transplants performed today, approximately 20% are due to keratoconus [5, 6]. In the past, surgical intervention by means of transplantation entailed the replacement of all corneal layers. While the full-thickness transplantation of donor corneal tissue is always an option, partial-thickness transplantation techniques claim significant advantages over full-thickness transplantation. Most significantly, the rate of graft failure, secondary glaucoma, complicated cataracts, and continuous endothelial cell loss fall in favor of lamellar transplantation [7]. Prerequisite for partial-thickness transplantation is that the host cornea's endothelium is healthy. Some of the most common indications for anterior partial-thickness transplantation are keratoconus, pellucid marginal degeneration, post-LASIK ectasia, lattice, macular and granular stromal dystrophies, as well as stromal scars [8]. The AAO (American Academy of Ophthalmology) recognizes the deep anterior lamellar keratoplasty (DALK) technique as an alternative over penetrating keratoplasty with similar outcomes in terms of BSCVA and refractive error.

G. Schmidinger (✉) · R. Donner
Department of Ophthalmology, Medical University of Vienna, Spitalgasse 23, 1090 Vienna, Austria
e-mail: gerald.schmidinger@meduniwien.ac.at

R. Donner
e-mail: ruth.donner@meduniwien.ac.at

T. G. Seiler
Klinik Für Augenheilkunde, Universitätsklinikum Düsseldorf, Moorenstraße 5, 40225 Düsseldorf, Germany
e-mail: theo@seiler.tv

© The Author(s), under exclusive license to Springer Nature Switzerland AG 2022   213
A. Armia and C. Mazzotta (eds.), *Keratoconus*,
https://doi.org/10.1007/978-3-030-84506-3_13

Endothelial cell counts are higher at any postoperative point after DALK compared to PK (penetrating keratoplasty) [9]. Similar conclusions were drawn by the authors of a Cochrane review published in 2014 [10].

DALK Techniques:

Various forms of lamellar keratoplasty were trialed in the early development of lamellar keratoplasty. Anterior lamellar keratoplasty was soon associated with fewer intraoperative complications due to the maintenance of the globe's integrity, and a lower rate of graft rejection was observed. The complete removal of stromal tissue affected by severe cases of corneal dystrophies and degenerations led to the development of deep anterior lamellar keratoplasty. By the year 1984, Archila described the method of air injection into the stroma to facilitate preparation of a deep lamellar stromal resection plane [11]. Later, several renowned corneal surgeons described their methods to facilitate a safe and deep lamellar resection of the corneal stroma [12–15]. Anwar and Teichmann introduced the big-bubble technique in 2002, after Anwar had previously observed that the air injections during lamellar keratoplasty occasionally resulted in partial separations of the stroma from descemet's membrane (DM) [16]. While anterior lamellar keratoplasty might still be used in some cases, the big-bubble technique eventually gained dominance over other methods and is currently the most frequently used method.

With increasing use and popularity, the big bubble technique was refined and developed further. Varying characteristics of air bubbles were classified and their differentiation gained relevance due to the anatomic significance accompanied by each type of bubble [17]. Ideally, the plane of cleavage is created between the stroma and Dua's layer (DL), a structure that was discovered as a result of the big-bubble DALK technique (Type-1 Bubble). Alternatively, the air bubble may form between DL and DM (Type-2 Bubble); mixed bubbles are also possible [18]. Type-1 bubbles are desired in DALK due to their ability to produce a clean separation of the stroma as well as the high bursting resistance of DL, which reduces the risk of perforation [19]. This type of bubble can be identified by its tendency to spread from the center to the periphery in a well-circumscribed manner, usually spreading no larger than 8.5 mm in diameter. Type-2 bubbles are often large and spread from the periphery into the center. These are prone to bursting due to the DM's fragility [18]. To avoid DM perforation, the surgeon attempts to avoid producing a Type-2 bubble and favors the Type-1 bubble.

Achieving a big bubble is not guaranteed and is strongly dependent on the underlying corneal pathology and surgeon experience [20]. In the case of micro-perforation of the descemet membrane (DM), completing the surgery without complication is possible [21]. Larger perforations of the DM require the conversion from DALK to penetrating keratoplasty, as do cases with a persistent anterior chamber after DALK with micro-perforation [22].

Penetration into the anterior chamber with subsequent DALK failure can be caused by a variety of complications. DALK surgery might fail due to the unintentional penetration into the anterior chamber with a manual trephine. Failure of the big-bubble maneuver can also be caused by unintentional perforation with the big-bubble needle or canula, the spreading of injected air into the trabecular meshwork and into the anterior chamber, air returning through the canula's pathway, when the air bursts through the roof of the canula's stromal channel, or when the DM spontaneously ruptures and air escapes into the anterior chamber. While some of these failure etiologies are somewhat predestined by the underlying pathology (scarring etc.), the failure rate can be reduced by optimizing surgical technique. In an effort to decrease the risk of DM perforation, Sarnicola introduced the use of a blunt cannula in place of a needle, as was otherwise part of the standard procedure. Use of the blunt-ended cannula was shown to be an effective measure in reducing the rate of inadvertent surgeon-induced DM perforations and became the next widely accepted technical development in DALK [21].

The Use of a Femtosecond-Laser in Keratoplasty:

Manual trephination of donor and recipient tissue is still common in PK. Its quality is strongly influenced by the surgeon's experience, among other factors. The direction of trephination (epithelium to descemet or vice versa), keratometry readings, intraocular pressure or whether an obturator is used or not, will have considerable effects on the sidecut geometry, tilt, centration and circularity of the cut [23, 24].

These pitfalls can be overcome by the use of a FS Laser for corneal trephination (Femtolaser keratoplasty). Already by the year 2008, a 510(k) approval was granted by the FDA for the Intralase (Johnson & Johnson) Keratoplasty Software module. Today, several FS laser devices with KP modules are available (Table 1). The high level of precision achieved by femtosecond laser-assisted trephination contributes to its main advantage: the opportunity to reproducibly perform innovative sidecut geometries. Several different sidecut geometries have been described, including zig-zag, top-hat, mushroom (IntraLase, Johnson&Johnson, Ziemer) and decagonal incisions (Victus, Bausch + Lomb). These new sidecut geometries were introduced with the intention to increase wound stability, reduce astigmatism and to optimize incisions according to the indications of the surgery (pathology-focused transplanting technique) [25, 26].

In summary, results of published studies are difficult to compare, as different sidecut-designs, different lasers and different transplant diameters were used. Current investigations show a moderate improvement of visual and refractive outcomes and comparable complication rates. However, the level of evidence of available data is modest.

Femtosecond-DALK (f-DALK) Surgery:

The use of a femtosecond laser for DALK surgeries can be advantageous in two respects: firstly, the precision of the femtosecond laser incisions can facilitate a deep stromal dissection and vertical side-cuts without the risk of unintentional perforation. Secondly, the use of advanced side-cut geometries can reduce postoperative astigmatism, as previously described in femtosecond-laser penetrating keratoplasty [27, 32].

Table 1 Summary of Femtosecond-Laser devices for keratoplasty

Femtosecond-laser	Company	Interface	Speed	OCT	Software
IntraLase	Johnson&Johnson	flat	−150 kHz	−	multiple sidecut geometries possible
Victus	Bausch + Lomb	curved	−80 kHz	−	multiple sidecut geometries possible
Z6, Z8	Ziemer	flat	>1 MHz	+	top-hat, mushroom, LKP, DALK
Visumax	Zeiss	curved	−500 kHz	−	LKP, PKP
FS200	Alcon	flat	200 kHz	−	top-hat, mushroom, zig-zag

Table 2 Clinical outcome after femtosecond-laser keratoplasty

Visual acuity (logMAR) after femtosecond or manual KP					
Study	Design	N =	Femto	Manual	Sign
Farid et al. [28]	retro	57	0,1	0,18	n.s
Bahar et al. [27]	pros	94	0,32	0,39	0,4
Chamberlain et al. [29]	retro	100	0,26	0,34	0,47
Levinger et al. [30]	retro	59	0,31	0,32	0,91
Daniel et al. [32]	retro	141	0,2	0,4	**0,015**

In 2009, Farid and Steinert presented the first case where a big-bubble DALK surgery was performed using the IntraLase (Johnson&Johnson) femtosecond laser with a zig-zag sidecut profile [33]. The authors reported that the precise realization of the planned sidecut and lamellar cut helped to place the big-bubble needle at the correct plane. The precision of the femtosecond laser was thought to reduce the risk of unintentional perforation during trephination or lamellar preparation. One year later, Buzzonnetti et al. described the IntraBubble method, which added a guiding tunnel for the big-bubble maneuver [34]. A blunt canula was introduced into the guiding tunnel, which was calculated to end 50 μm above the endothelium. Using this method, the authors achieved a successful big-bubble maneuver in 8 of the 11 cases. In one of 11 cases the femtosecond laser induced a micro-perforation.

Studies evaluating the clinical outcome of f-DALK as opposed to manual DALK (m-DALK) are difficult to compare, since the surgical approaches vary considerably. Some studies showed advantages in the refractive outcome with f-DALK procedures [35], which were most likely related to the different anterior transplant diameters and not the femtosecond-laser itself. Others did not find differences in terms of BCVA between f-DALK and m-DALK [36].

OCT Guided Femtosecond—DALK Surgery:

Liu et al. recently described a technique using a femtosecond-laser with an intra-operative OCT, which allows for the depth of the corneal incisions and the big-bubble tunnel to be adjusted in real-time. The combination of improved planning with immediate OCT imaging and the ability of the femtosecond laser (FEMTO LDV Z8, Ziemer Ophthalmic Systems AG, Switzerland) to perform incisions precisely improves the overall level of control over the process of anterior stromal dissection, minimizing the risk for perforation of the DM and allowing for a more confident big bubble formation. The study showed that big-bubble tunnels can be produced with high precision. DALK surgery was successfully performed in 14 out of 14 cases. In recent years, the authors have been using this approach for DALK procedure. In the following we are going to present a retrospective analysis of clinical data.

Clinical Results of OCT Guided Femtosecond—DALK Surgery:

In a retrospective evaluation, the authors compared the intraoperative and postoperative outcome of f-DALK using the FEMTO LDV Z8 (Ziemer Ophthalmic Systems AG, Switzerland) to conventional manual big-bubble technique (m-DALK) in eyes with descemetic-DALK procedures. Intraoperative and postoperative results with a follow-up of more than 12 months were evaluated. Eyes with f-DALK (Group 1) were compared to eyes treated with m-DALK (Group 2) procedure.

For f-DALK procedures a guiding tunnel was created as previously reported by Liu et al. [37] Once the cornea was applanated and aligned, the built-in OCT was used to performed several scans for surgical planning. The depth of the end of the big-bubble tunnel was set to 50–80 μm above the endothelium, measured from the thinnest corneal point shown on the intraoperative OCT scan (Fig. 1). To avoid bias due to different transplant diameters in the two groups, a straight vertical side-cut with a diameter between 8.0 and 8.5 mm was chosen for f-DALK procedures. After removal of the anterior lamella using spatula and forceps, injection of air through the intrastromal tunnel was performed by inserting and carefully advancing a big-bubble canula connected to an air-filled 5-mL syringe (Fig. 2). Subsequently, DALK surgery was completed as conventional big-bubble procedure: the stromal wall of the bubble was punctured and blunt scissors were used to resect the residual stroma. The donor corneal button was then placed onto the recipient bed and aligned with 4 interrupted 10–0 nylon sutures. Two torque-antitorque sutures were then placed, and the interrupted sutures were removed. The procedure used in the control group (m-DALK) was in accordance with the protocol from Anwar et al. with big bubble creation by means of a sharp canula. Recipient trephination was performed with a vacuum-trephine with a diameter between 8.0 mm and 8.5 mm (0.2 mm smaller than the donor trephination).

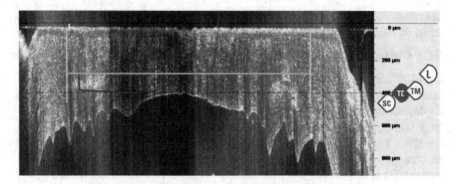

Fig. 1 OCT image with incision overlay during applanation using a femtosecond-laser to create a DALK incision. The green line demonstrates the planned side-cut depth, the orange line signifies the lamellar cut depth and the purple line displays the big-bubble tunnel. All endpoints can be adjusted in real-time using a touch-screen

In cases where a big-bubble Type-I was not achieved, a forced manual preparation of a descemetic-DALK (Dua-Layer or Descemet-membrane) was performed using the layer-by-layer method. Manual preparation was stopped when Dua-Layer or Descemet´s membrane was reached or a perforation occurred.

Results:

In this retrospective single center case series, a total of 96 patients underwent DALK surgery: 66 cases had a f-DALK and 30 cases had a m-DALK. The most frequent indication for DALK surgery was keratoconus, comprising 75% of cases. Most cases had advanced disease; significant stromal scarring was observed in 45% of keratoconus cases. The remaining cases had DALK surgery planned due to stromal scarring (17%) or stromal dystrophies (8%).

A successful Type I BB was achieved in a higher number of cases in the f-DALK group compared to the m-DALK group with 70% and 46%, respectively. Type II Bubbles were observed in 4,6% of the cases in the f-DALK group and in 10% of the cases in the m-DALK group. In the f-DALK group, conversion to PK was observed at a significantly lower rate compared to the manual group (19 and 46%). Perforation due to trephination was not observed in any case in the f-DALK group. The duration of the surgery did not differ between the two groups. The mean operative time was 68 ± 19 minutes in group 1 (f-DALK) and 65 ± 16 minutes in group 2 (m-DALK). A postoperative re-bubbling of the anterior chamber has been performed in one case in the f-DALK group (1,5%) and in one case in the m-DALK group (3,3%). Within the follow-up period, one case of stromal immune reaction was observed in the m-DALK group.

Mean keratometric readings after suture removal were slightly lower in the f-DALK group (49,5 dpt) compared to the m-DALK group (54,6 dpt), but this difference was not statistically significant. Seventy-two percent of the eyes in the f-DALK group had a BCVA of ≥ 20/40 compared to 60% in the m-DALK group.

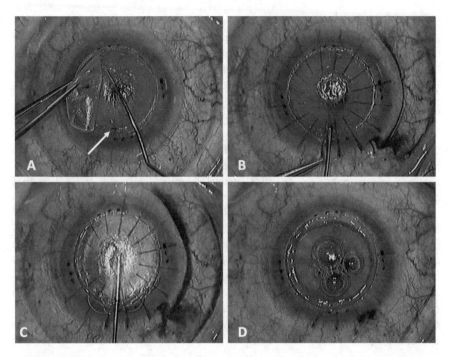

Fig. 2 Intraoperative steps after trephination using an OCT-guided femtosecond-laser. **a** Removing the superficial stroma. The white arrow marks the entrance point of the big-bubble tunnel. **b** Entering the big-bubble tunnel with a DALK canula (in this case a Sarnicola-canula was used). **c** Air bubbles in the anterior chamber are pushed to the periphery (red arrow), indicating that a Type-I bubble has been created. **d** Intraoperative situation after opening of the Type-I bubble and removal of the residual stroma

Discussion:

The results of this retrospective trial showed an increased success rate of big bubble maneuvers when using an OCT-guided femtosecond-laser trephination with a big-bubble guiding tunnel. The OCT-guided big-bubble tunnel close to the endothelium increased the number of successful big-bubble maneuvers from 46 to 70%. This increase led to a significant decrease of cases that had to be converted to penetrating keratoplasty. The surgeon in this trial had chosen an aggressive approach concerning the depth of preparation to guarantee optimal visual acuity results.[38] Cases with perforations of the Descemet's membrane were readily converted to penetrating keratoplasty. This explains the higher incidence of conversion to penetrating keratoplasty compared to some publications. On the other hand, very low numbers of re-bubblings were recorded in both groups. Primary graft failure or double anterior chamber was not observed in any of the cases. While improving the rate of successful big bubble dissections, long-term visual rehabilitation success, as measured by best corrected visual acuity after suture removal, did not differ between manual and femtosecond laser-assisted big bubble formation.

Postoperatively, keratometric values (Kmean, Kmax) did not differ significantly after manual versus femtosecond laser-assisted DALK. In these regards, DALK by either method is comparable and renders very good results. The key advantage found to using the femtosecond laser for DALK is the higher rate of successful intraoperative preparation and thus, fewer conversions to penetrating keratoplasty.

Summary and Outlook:

In and of itself, DALK is a demanding procedure and is only performed by comparably few surgeons. Femtosecond-laser assisted DALK potentially shortens the learning curve for surgeons, which benefits patients by reducing the invasiveness of the procedure, improving the odds against complications, and by maintaining patients' own, healthy endothelial tissue.

Despite its advantages, the femtosecond laser is a highly cost-intensive surgical aid that most likely cannot be afforded for widespread use and training. Also, its benefits are yet to be refined for optimal patient benefit. Despite these drawbacks, the benefits currently achieved with the femtosecond laser's use and the hopeful outlooks for its future improvement currently overpower its drawbacks. Further developments of femtosecond-laser devices with non-applanating patient interfaces [39] might combine the benefits of a high precision f-DALK trephination with the currently unmatched refractive outcome of a non-applanating excimer-laser trephination [40].

References

1. DA Godefrooij GA Wit de CS Uiterwaal SM Imhof RPL Wisse 2017 Age-specific incidence and prevalence of keratoconus: a nationwide registration study Am J Ophthalmol https://doi.org/10.1016/j.ajo.2016.12.015
2. H Hashemi 2020 The prevalence and risk factors for keratoconus: a systematic review and meta-analysis Cornea https://doi.org/10.1097/ICO.0000000000002150
3. M Romero-Jiménez J Santodomingo-Rubido JS Wolffsohn 2010 Keratoconus: a review Cont Lens Anterior Eye https://doi.org/10.1016/j.clae.2010.04.006
4. YS Rabinowitz 1998 Keratoconus Surv Ophthalmol https://doi.org/10.1016/S0039-6257(97)00119-7
5. Park CY, Lee JK, Gore PK, Lim CY, Chuck RS. Keratoplasty in the United States: a 10-year review from 2005 through 2014. Ophthalmology 2015. https://doi.org/10.1016/j.ophtha.2015.08.017.
6. Keenan TDL, Jones MNA, Rushton S, Carley FM. Trends in the indications for corneal graft surgery in the United Kingdom: 1999 through 2009. Arch Ophthalmol. 2012. https://doi.org/10.1001/archophthalmol.2011.2585.
7. Y Zhang S Wu Y Yao 2013 Long-term comparison of full-bed deep anterior lamellar keratoplasty and penetrating keratoplasty in treating keratoconus J Zhejiang Univ Sci B 14 5 438 450 https://doi.org/10.1631/jzus.B1200272
8. F Karimian S Feizi 2010 Deep anterior lamellar keratoplasty: indications, surgical techniques and complications Middle East Afr J Ophthalmol 17 1 28 37 https://doi.org/10.4103/0974-9233.61214

9. WJ Reinhart DC Musch DS Jacobs WB Lee SC Kaufman RM Shtein 2011 Deep anterior lamellar keratoplasty as an alternative to penetrating keratoplasty: a report by the American academy of ophthalmology Ophthalmology 118 1 209 218 https://doi.org/10.1016/j.ophtha.2010.11.002

10. Keane M, Coster D, Ziaei M, Williams K. Deep anterior lamellar keratoplasty versus penetrating keratoplasty for treating keratoconus. Cochrane Database Syst Rev. 2014;(7). https://doi.org/10.1002/14651858.CD009700.pub2.

11. EA Archila 1984 Deep lamellar keratoplasty dissection of host tissue with intrastromal air injection Cornea https://doi.org/10.1097/00003226-198706010-00012

12. J Sugita J Kondo 1997 Deep lamellar keratoplasty with complete removal of pathological stroma for vision improvement Br J Ophthalmol https://doi.org/10.1136/bjo.81.3.184

13. K Tsubota M Kaido Y Monden Y Satake H Bissen-Miyajima J Shimazaki 1998 A new surgical technique for deep lamellar keratoplasty with single running suture adjustment Am J Ophthalmol 126 1 1 8 https://doi.org/10.1016/s0002-9394(98)00067-1

14. GRJ Melles F Lander FJR Rietveld L Remeijer WH Beekhuis PS Binder 1999 A new surgical technique for deep stromal, anterior lamellar keratoplasty Br J Ophthalmol https://doi.org/10.1136/bjo.83.3.327

15. GRJ Melles L Remeijer AJM Geerards WH Beekhuis 2000 A quick surgical technique for deep, anterior lamellar keratoplasty using visco-dissection Cornea https://doi.org/10.1097/00003226-200007000-00004

16. M Anwar KD Teichmann 2002 Big-bubble technique to bare Descemet's membrane in anterior lamellar keratoplasty J Cataract Refract Surg https://doi.org/10.1016/S0886-3350(01)01181-6

17. Dua HS, Faraj LA, Said DG, Gray T, Lowe J. Human corneal anatomy rede fi ned a novel pre-descemet's layer (Dua's Layer). 2013;(Dl): 1778–85. https://doi.org/10.1016/j.ophtha.2013.01.018.

18. HS Dua T Katamish DG Said LA Faraj 2015 Differentiating type 1 from type 2 big bubbles in deep anterior lamellar keratoplasty Clin Ophthalmol 9 1155 1157 https://doi.org/10.2147/OPTH.S81089

19. Y Koçluk A Burcu EA Sukgen 2016 Demonstration of cornea Dua's layer at a deep anterior lamellar keratoplasty surgery Oman J Ophthalmol 9 3 179 181 https://doi.org/10.4103/0974-620X.192296

20. T Huang X Zhang Y Wang H Zhang A Huand N Gao 2012 Outcomes of deep anterior lamellar keratoplasty using the big-bubble technique in various corneal diseases Am J Ophthalmol 154 2 282 289.e1 https://doi.org/10.1016/j.ajo.2012.02.025

21. Sarnicola E, Sarnicola C, Sabatino F, Tosi GM, Perri P, Sarnicola V. Cannula DALK versus needle DALK for keratoconus. Cornea 2016;35(12). https://journals.lww.com/corneajrnl/Fulltext/2016/12000/Cannula_DALK_Versus_Needle_DALK_for_Keratoconus.3.aspx.

22. JC Reddy 2015 Clinical outcomes and risk factors for graft failure after deep anterior lamellar keratoplasty and penetrating keratoplasty for macular corneal dystrophy Cornea https://doi.org/10.1097/ICO.0000000000000327

23. Krumeich J, Binder PS, Knulle A. The theoretical effect of trephine tilt on postkeratoplasty astigmatism. CLAO J. 1988.

24. RJ Olson 1979 Variation in corneal graft size related to trephine technique Arch Ophthalmol https://doi.org/10.1001/archopht.1979.01020020065015

25. I Bahar I Kaiserman P McAllum D Rootman 2008 Femtosecond laser-assisted penetrating keratoplasty: stability evaluation of different wound configurations Cornea https://doi.org/10.1097/ICO.0b013e31815b7d50

26. P McAllum I Kaiserman I Bahar D Rootman 2008 Femtosecond laser top hat penetrating keratoplasty: wound burst pressures of incomplete cuts Arch Ophthalmol https://doi.org/10.1001/archopht.126.6.822

27. I Bahar 2009 Femtosecond laser versus manual dissection for top hat penetrating keratoplasty Br J Ophthalmol https://doi.org/10.1136/bjo.2008.148346

28. M Farid RF Steinert RN Gaster W Chamberlain A Lin 2009 Comparison of penetrating keratoplasty performed with a femtosecond laser zig-zag incision versus conventional blade trephination Ophthalmology 116 9 1638 1643 https://doi.org/10.1016/j.ophtha.2009.05.003

29. WD Chamberlain SW Rush WD Mathers M Cabezas FW Fraunfelder 2011 Comparison of femtosecond laser-assisted keratoplasty versus conventional penetrating keratoplasty Ophthalmology https://doi.org/10.1016/j.ophtha.2010.08.002

30. Levinger E, Trivizki O, Levinger S, Kremer I. Outcome of 'Mushroom' pattern femtosecond laser–assisted keratoplasty versus conventional penetrating keratoplasty in patients with keratoconus. Cornea 2014;33(5). https://journals.lww.com/corneajrnl/Fulltext/2014/05000/Outcome_of__Mushroom__Pattern_Femtosecond.9.aspx.

31. K Kamiya H Kobashi K Shimizu A Igarashi 2014 Clinical outcomes of penetrating keratoplasty performed with the VisuMax femtosecond laser system and comparison with conventional penetrating keratoplasty PLoS ONE https://doi.org/10.1371/journal.pone.0105464

32. MC Daniel D Böhringer P Maier P Eberwein F Birnbaum T Reinhard 2016 Comparison of long-term outcomes of femtosecond laser-assisted keratoplasty with conventional keratoplasty Cornea https://doi.org/10.1097/ICO.0000000000000739

33. M Farid RF Steinert 2009 Deep anterior lamellar keratoplasty performed with the femtosecond laser zigzag incision for the treatment of stromal corneal pathology and ectatic disease J Cataract Refract Surg https://doi.org/10.1016/j.jcrs.2009.01.012

34. L Buzzonetti A Laborante G Petrocelli 2010 Standardized big-bubble technique in deep anterior lamellar keratoplasty assisted by the femtosecond laser J Cataract Refract Surg 36 10 1631 1636 https://doi.org/10.1016/j.jcrs.2010.08.013

35. R Shehadeh-Mashor CC Chan I Bahar A Lichtinger SN Yeung DS Rootman 2014 Comparison between femtosecond laser mushroom configuration and manual trephine straight-edge configuration deep anterior lamellar keratoplasty Br J Ophthalmol https://doi.org/10.1136/bjophthalmol-2013-303737

36. Alio JL, Abdelghany AA, Barraquer R, Hammouda LM, Sabry AM. Femtosecond laser assisted deep anterior lamellar keratoplasty outcomes and healing patterns compared to manual technique. Biomed Res Int. 2015;2015:397891. https://doi.org/10.1155/2015/397891.

37. YC Liu 2019 Intraoperative optical coherence tomography-guided femtosecond laser-assisted deep anterior lamellar keratoplasty Cornea https://doi.org/10.1097/ICO.0000000000001851

38. Schiano-Lomoriello D, et al. Descemetic and predescemetic DALK in keratoconus patients: a clinical and confocal perspective study. Biomed Res Int. 2014;2014:123156. https://doi.org/10.1155/2014/123156.

39. S Siebelmann A Händel M Matthaei C Cursiefen B Bachmann 2020 Femtosecond laser-assisted (triple-)deep anterior lamellar keratoplasty with a novel liquid interface J. EuCornea https://doi.org/10.1016/j.xjec.2020.06.001

40. G Tóth N Szentmáry A Langenbucher E Akhmedova M El-Husseiny B Seitz 2019 Comparison of excimer laser versus femtosecond laser assisted trephination in penetrating keratoplasty: a retrospective study Adv Ther https://doi.org/10.1007/s12325-019-01120-3

SLAK: Stromal Lanticule Addition Keratoplasty

Leonardo Mastropasqua, Mario Nubile, and Manuela Lanzini

1 SLAK: Background and Rationale

The idea of reshaping corneal morphology basing on intrastromal lenticule implant starts from the introduction of Femtosecond Laser (FSL) in corneal surgery, in particular in refractive surgery. FSL is an ultrafast pulse laser that allows the dissection of tissues inducing a process of photodisruption and plasma cavitation formation [1].

Differently from the excimer laser photoablation, which vaporizes tissues, FSL performs stromal cuts by collagen lamellae separation; in this way the corneal stroma can be remodelled according to the desired shape. FSL was at first mainly used in LASIK surgery for flap creation; subsequently in refractive surgery the procedure of lenticule extraction (ReLEx; Carl Zeiss Meditec, Jena, Germany), was introduced in alternative to LASIK surgery to correct refractive errors [2]. This innovative approach in refractive surgery is based on stromal refractive lenticule removal performed with one single FSL laser. The refractive lenticule is created with pre-determined power within the anterior corneal stroma.

ReLEx surgery is now performed without a flap creation and the refractive lenticule is extracted through a small stromal incision. This technique, Small Incision Lenticule Extraction, rapidly spread in clinical practice and is known as SMILE [3].

To treat myopia the refractive lenticule presents a concavo-convex profile. The anterior surface is determined by the planar cap dissection while the posterior surface curvature correlated with the amount of refractive error to be corrected. The higher thickness of the lenticule is located the center and gradually reduces in the periphery [2, 3].

L. Mastropasqua · M. Nubile · M. Lanzini (✉)
Ophthalmic Clinic, G D'Annunzio University of Chieti-Pescara, Chieti, Italy
e-mail: m.lanzini@unich.it

223

Subsequently a specific nomogram of SMILE procedure has been introduced for the treatment of hyperopia, [4]. The hyperopic lenticule presents higher curvature in posterior surface compared to the anterior one. The lenticule thickness is maximum at the periphery and the thinnest point is located at the center of the lenticule [5].

It has been shown that extracted lenticule can be cryopreserved maintaining their structure and the possibility of reimplant refractive lenticule to correct refractive errors has been proposed [6].

The possibility of lenticule extraction and reimplantation was described with good results in animal models [7, 8].

In particular re-implantation of myopic lenticule, obtained with SMILE procedure, was proposed in humans as an additional procedure to treat hyperopia. In fact, the implantation of a myopic lenticule, with maximum thickness at the center, generates an increasing of central corneal curvature with consequent myopic shift of the patient's refraction [9, 10].

This scientific evidences originated the idea of remodelling corneal shaping by implanting in ectatic corneas stromal hyperopic refractive lenticule obtained by SMILE procedure.

In fact, implanting a negative meniscus hyperopic lenticule, with an inverted thickness profile that gradually becomes thicker from the center toward the periphery of the optical zone, can cause central corneal flattening and thickening in an ectatic cornea (Fig. 1).

The theoretical mechanism of action of SLAK (Stromal Lenticule Addiction Keratoplasty) is similar to the intra-corneal ring segments (ICRs);

In fact both techniques provide material addition and local profile elevation in the mid-periphery [11].

ICRs are polymethylmethacrylate elements implanted at 80% of stromal depth creating spacing between the collagen lamellae with consequent shortening of the central arc that is proportional to the ring thickness. Differently the implantation of hyperopic refractive lenticule is performed in anterior stroma and should cause less tension on the corneal lamellae [12].

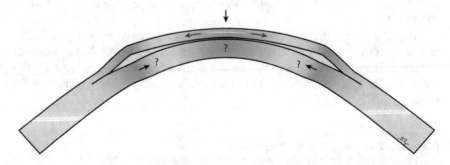

Fig. 1 Representative images of hyperopic, negative meniscus shaped refractive lentoid implanted in a stromal pocket. The obtained effect is a central corneal flattening and increasing thickness

At the light of these principles SLAK was proposed as a feasible and reproducible procedure for obtaining central corneal flattening while increasing the
stromal thickness in corneal ectasia.

2 Surgical Technique

2.1 Lenticule Preparation

Lenticules for implantation are obtained from human eye bank donor cornea suitable for transplantation. To avoid the effect of storage-induced stromal oedema on
FSL cut, it is useful to store tissue in dextran-enriched storage medium, so that
central corneal thickness (CCT) can be maintained lower than 600 μm.

The corneoscleral buttons were rinsed with balanced salt solution and mounted
on an artificial anterior chamber with standardized pressure. Corneal epithelium is
gently removed using a blunt spatula under a surgical microscope. Than a FLEx
procedure with a hyperopic profile is performed with a 500-kHz femtosecond laser
to sculpt the stromal lenticule into the donor cornea.

The femtosecond laser parameters are set as follows: repetition rate of 500 kHz
and spot separation between 2 and 2.5 μm for the lamellar cuts and 3 μm for the
side cuts. The spot energy is between 135 and 150 nJ.

In the donor cornea the flap thickness is set to 110 μm with a diameter of 8 mm.
Lenticule is planned for 8.00 D of hyperopic refractive correction with a 6-mm
optical zone.

This surgical planning provides a maximum lenticule thickness of 148 μm
located in periphery and the minimal lenticule thickness of 30 μm located in the
center. The overall transition zone in the periphery of the lenticules was 0.70 mm in
diameter.

After the femtosecond laser dissection procedure, the flap is lifted as in the
LASIK procedure. Then the underlying lenticule is separated and isolated using a
thin blunt stromal dissector. It is important to check under the surgical microscope
with high magnification that the isolated lenticule is intact, without ruptures or
tearing [13] (Fig. 2).

2.2 Lenticule Implantation Technique

A modified femtosecond laser flap-cut procedure is performed on the patient's
cornea to create an intrastromal pocket that will host the donor lenticule. The
surgical procedures is performed under topical anaesthesia. To obtain a single small
superior incision of 4 mm, the flap hinge length is set to 21.7 mm. The incision side
cut is angled at 100° from the surface layer. The stromal pocket diameter is set to

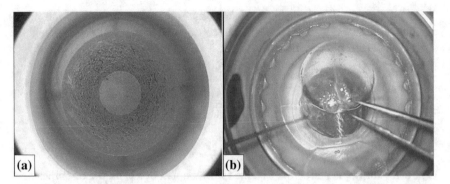

Fig. 2 Surgical procedure of lenticule preparation: the donor cornea is mounted on artificial anterior chamber. Lenticule is produced by a FLEx procedure (**a**) The flap is then lifted and lenticule dissected from residual stroma (**b**)

8.2 mm in order to make it 1.5 mm larger than the total diameter of the donor lenticule. The depth of the stromal pocket is set at 120 μm from the corneal surface.

Laser settings parameters included an energy cut index of 35 nJ and a spot separation of 5 μm.

The intrastromal pocket's cut is centred on the patient's cornea by the corneal fixation-based centration described by Reinstein et al. for SMILE surgery [14].

After FSL procedure is completed, the correct location and depth of the dissection cut is assessed with an AS-OCT scan prior to proceeding with lenticule implantation. The patient is now moved under a surgical microscope and the FSL incision is opened with a Seibel spatula. The pocket stromal layer is dissected using a SMILE dedicated spatula in order to open eventual residual tissue bridges. Correct lenticule orientation is obtained by distending the lenticule into a keratoplasty spoon-shaped glide.

Lenticule implantation is performed with dedicated designed forceps. This specific surgical instrument, with a cross-action opening, allows to drag the lenticule inside the pocket and, at the same time, stretch out the tissue while maintaining the grip in a single step. The edge of the lenticule is grabbed with the forceps and gently inserted into the pocket through the superior incision. The correct orientation of the lenticule, with the anterior surface located superiorly, is maintained. The lenticule's centration is carefully fixed onto the apex of the cone (Fig. 3).

A gentle centrifugal-oriented massage on the corneal surface is performed after insertion in order to avoid incomplete unfolding at the lenticule edges, striae, or micro-distortions of the tissue.

At the end of the procedure, the surgeon assesses the distension and centration of the lenticule under the surgical microscope, thus patient undergo AS-OCT, and topography in order to check the morphological result obtained. In case of incorrect centration with respect to the apex of the cone the lenticule is dragged to the target position by a blunt spatulas and spread out again. Once the right centration is

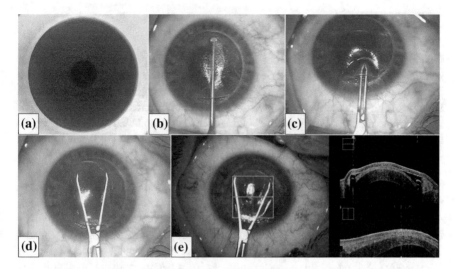

Fig. 3 The recipient cornea underwent FSL intrastromal pocket creation (**a**). The lamellar cut is dissected by a blunt spatula (**b**). The lenticule was positioned near the incision of recipient cornea and pushed inside the pocket (**c**). Proper distention of the lenticule was achieved by means of dedicated forceps (**d**). All the procedure may be performed with the aid of intraoperative OCT to check the correct morphological outcome (**e**)

obtained, the incision is dried with a sterile sponge to eliminate residual fluid from the interface and finally a bandage contact lens was applied. Total operation times range from 15 to 35 minutes.

Postoperatively the patients receive topical antibiotic and steorids for 8 weeks.

3   SLAK Results

3.1   Ex-vivo Morphological Results

Preliminary investigations were performed on human cadaver corneas not suitable for transplantation [13]. These experimental model showed that stromal negative meniscus lenticules can be successfully obtained by means of hyperopic-FLEx surgery and intrastromal pockets can be obtained by means of a modified flap-cut standardized procedure. The corneal topography showed a consistent central corneal flattening (7.3D), together with a peripheral increase of corneal curvature. An increased corneal thickness, congruent to the lenticule morphometry have been observed. The linear AS-OCT scans showed modifications both in anterior and posterior corneal surfaces.

3.2   Clinical Results in Humans

First clinical results of SLAK procedure were reported in patients affected by stable keratoconus at stage 3–4 [15]. The postoperative follow-up period considered was 6 months. No relevant intraoperative or postoperative complications were observed. Biomicrosopical examination showed a complete transparency of corneal stroma with regular anterior and posterior interface of the implanted lenticule (Fig. 4). During the first days after surgery it is possible to reveal few lenticular folds that disappear in the first postoperative week.

Uncorrected and Best Corrected Visual Acuity showed a significant improvement. These modifications were detectable during the first postoperative weeks and remained stable at 6 months.

The Q value, expression of corneal asphericity, decreased significantly indicating a more phisiological prolate corneal profile. Central corneal thickness increased significantly consistently with the local thickness of the implanted lenticule (Fig. 5).

Extended follow-up in a larger number of patients showed a stability of refractive postoperative results that remained stable up to 24 months after treatment.

Anterior segment OCT allows identification of anterior and posterior surface of the intrastromal lenticule implanted across the whole diameter in recipient cornea (Fig. 6). The OCT analysis shows that lenticule differential thickness was consistent with the expected values programmed for FSL cut [16].

The corneal epithelium, typically thinnest at the cone apex, signifcantly increases during the first 3 postoperative months after SLAK procedure [16]. Epithelial remodelling usually develops in an attempt to regularize corneal curvature [17].

It was reported that the fattening effect on the anterior corneal surface resulting from the lenticule implantation was associated with an epithelial remodelling that restored the central epithelial thickness values close to normality.

Fig. 4 Normal stromal transparency end interface regularity 12 months after SLAK

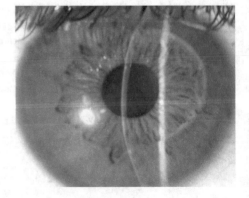

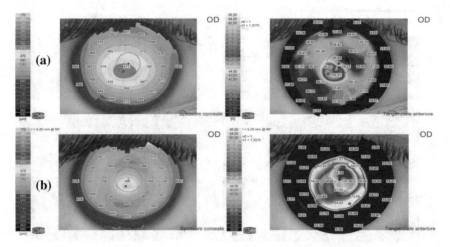

Fig. 5 Preoperative (**a**) and 12 months postoperative (**b**) corneal topography after SLAK procedure. Central corneal flattening is evident together with increased thickness

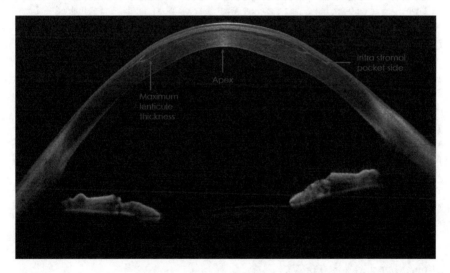

Fig. 6 OCT wide-field scan shows the morphometric outcome of SLAK procedure and allows to clearly evaluate the refractive lenticule implanted in the stromal pocket

3.3   In Vivo Confocal Microscopy Morphological Outcomes

Inflammatory response after SLAK was studied by means of In Vivo Confocal Microscopy (IVCM). No modifications of dendritic cell population, typically activated in rejection reaction, was observed after surgery; this finding correlates with clinical postoperative course, in fact no corneal rejection was reported in

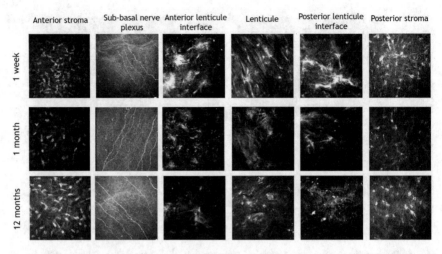

Fig. 7 IVCM representative images of different corneal layers at 1 week, 1 months and 12 months after surgery. Anterior and posterior stroma show normal keratocyte density and transparency of extracellular matrix. Mild reduction of sub-basal nerve fiber density was detected at 1 week after surgery but a fast recovery was detected at 1 months and remained stable at 12 months after SLAKAnterior and posterior lenticule interface show morphological regularity. Inside the lenticule a decreased cellularity is observable with normal transparency of the matrix

literature, indicating that the immunological stimulation after SLAK might be at least similar, if not lower, with respect to the DALK one [18].

IVCM studies revealed that Femtosecond lamellar cuts in SMILE surgery only partially affect sub-basal nerve density and nerve fibers [19] Similarly, after SLAK, a mild reduction of subepithelial nerve fiber density was reported immediately after surgery, but a recovery of normal nerve fiber density was documented during the first postoperative months.

Increased keratocyte reflectivity was observed after SLAK together with extracellular oedema that rapidly resolved in one month. Keratocyte density of recipient cornea remained stable.

Similarly to SMILE, a regular and hypo-reflective interface was documented after SLAK both at the anterior and posterior surface of the lenticule without stromal opacification (Fig. 7).

4   Future of SLAK

Scientific literature shows that SLAK is a safe procedure and implanted tissue is well tolerated by the recipient cornea; The procedure is effective in regularization of central corneal curvature, with consequent improving of visual performance in patients affected by corneal ectasia. Moreover this procedure could improve contact lens fitting, thus reducing the need of traditional corneal transplantation. Possible future evolution of this technique may lead to the creation of custom-made lentoids, to produce tailored refractive and structural effects in ectatic corneas. Moreover, SLAK procedure may be combined with collagen cross-linking obtaining in the same time a reshaping of corneal curvature and the stabilization of keratoconus progression.

The main advantages of SLAK surgery is the minimal invasiveness of the procedure and the possibility of reducing corneal curvature, adding stromal tissue with possible beneficial biomechanical effects.

References

1. Kymionis GD, Kankariya VP, Plaka AD, Reinstein DZ. Femtosecond laser technology in corneal refractive surgery: a review. J Refract Surg. 2012;28(12):912–20.
2. Sekundo W, Kunert K, Russmann C. First efficacy and safety study of femtosecond lenticule extraction for the correction of myopia: six-month results. J Cataract Refract Surg. 2008;34:1513–20.
3. Moshirfar M, McCaughey MV, Reinstein DZ, Shah R, Santiago-Caban L, Fenzl CR. Small-incision lenticule extraction. J Cataract Refract Surg. 2015;41(3):652–65.
4. Blum M, Kunert KS, Voßmerba¨umer U, Sekundo W. Femtosecond lenticule extraction (ReLEx) for correction of hyperopia—first results. Graefes Arch Clin Exp Ophthalmol. 2013;251(1):349–55.
5. Liu YC, Ang HP, Teo EP, Lwin NC, Yam GH, Mehta JS. Wound healing profiles of hyperopic-small incision lenticule extraction (SMILE). Sci Rep. 2016;6:29802.
6. Mohamed-Noriega K, Toh K-P, Poh R, Balehosur D, Riau A, Htoon HM. Cornea lenticule viability and structural integrity after refractive lenticule extraction (ReLEx) and cryopreservation. Mol Vis. 2011;17:3437–49.
7. Liu H, Zhu W, Jiang AC, Sprecher AJ, Zhou X. Femtosecond laser lenticule transplantation in rabbit cornea: experimental study. J Refract Surg. 2012;28(12):907–11.
8. Riau AK, Angunawela RI, Chaurasia SS, Lee WS, Tan DT, Mehta JS. Reversible femtosecond laser-assisted myopia correction: a non-human primate study of lenticule re-implantation after refractive lenticule extraction. PLoS One. 2013;8(6):e67058.
9. Sun L, Yao P, Li M, Shen Y, Zhao J, Zhou X. The safety and predictability of implanting autologous lenticule obtained by SMILE for hyperopia. J Refract Surg. 2015;31(6):374–9.
10. Ganesh S, Brar S, Rao PA. Cryopreservation of extracted corneal lenticules after small incision lenticule extraction for potential use in human subjects. Cornea. 2014;33(12):1355–62.
11. Vega-Estrada A, Alio JL. The use of intracorneal ring segments in keratoconus. Eye Vis (Lond). 2016;3:8.
12. Ganesh S, Brar S. Femtosecond intrastromal lenticular implantation combined with accelerated collagen cross-linking for the treatment of keratoconus—initial clinical result in 6 eyes. Cornea. 2015;34(10):1331–9.
13. Mastropasqua L, Nubile M. Corneal thickening and central flattening induced by femtosecond laser hyperopic-shaped intrastromal lenticule implantation. Int Ophthalmol. 2017;37:893–904.
14. Reinstein DZ, Gobbe M, Gobbe L, Archer TJ, Carp GI. Optical zone centration accuracy using corneal fixation-based SMILE compared to eye tracker-based femtosecond laser-assisted LASIK for myopia. J Refract Surg. 2015;31:586–92.

15. Mastropasqua L, Nubile M, Salgari N, Mastropasqua R. Femtosecond laser–assisted stromal lenticule addition keratoplasty for the treatment of advanced keratoconus: a preliminary study. J Refract Surg. 2018.
16. Nubile M, Salgari N, Mehta JS, Calienno R, Erroi E, Bondì J, Lanzini M, Liu YC, Mastropasqua L. Epithelial and stromal remodelling following femtosecond laser–assisted stromal lenticule addition keratoplasty (SLAK) for keratoconus. Sci Rep. 2021;11:2293.
17. Salomão MQ. Role of the corneal epithelium measurements in keratorefractive surgery. Curr Opin Ophthalmol. 2017;28:326–36.
18. Mastropasqua L, Salgari N, D'Ugo E, Lanzini M, Aliò del Barrio JL Aliò JL, Cochener B, Nubile M. In vivo confocal microscopy of stromal lenticule addition keratoplasty for advanced keratoconus. J Refract Surg. 2020;36(8):544–50.
19. Li M, Niu L, Qin B, et al. Confocal comparison of corneal reinnervation after small incision lenticule extraction (SMILE) and femtosecond laser in situ keratomileusis (FS-LASIK). PLoS One. 2013;8(12):e81435.

Donor-Recipient Crosslinking-Assisted Manual Deep Anterior Lamellar Keratoplasty: DRXL-DALK

Marco Zagari, Cosimo Mazzotta, Silvio Zagari, and Ashraf Armia

1 Introduction

Cornea transplant surgery for ectasia disorders has undergone significant changes in the last ten years, revolutionising the approach and prognosis of the disease.

During the late 1990s, Melles et al. [1] revolutionised the history of lamellar keratoplasty, proposing the major fundamentals of DALK (Deep Anterior Lamellar Keratoplasty) which were modified and proposed by Anwar et al. [2] in the so called "*Big Bubble*" DALK technique. In the next years, Tan et al. [3], Fogla et al. [4], Sarnicola et al. [5] made further changes to the technique, using suitable surgical instruments for the formation of the "*bubble*" and converting the "*air bubble*" procedure into an "*air-visco-bubble*" to make the technique even safer [5, 6].

The Big Bubble technique represents properly a "pneumatic delamination" of the corneal stroma and the Descemet's membrane (DM) plane, blowing air beneath the central corneal stroma, through a pre-cut channel to separate the layers [5], followed by the manual removal of the overhead stroma. The aim of DALK [1–3] is to achieve visual results similar to penetrating keratoplasty, reducing the risk of

M. Zagari · S. Zagari
Acicastello and Clinica Oculistica Vampolieri, Ophthalmology Unit, Poliambulatorio Centro Europeo, Catania, Italy

C. Mazzotta (✉)
Departmental Ophthalmology Unit, Alta Val D'Elsa Hospital, Campostaggia, Siena, Italy
e-mail: cgmazzotta@libero.it

C. Mazzotta
Siena Crosslinking Center, Siena, Italy

A. Armia
Ashraf Armia Eye Clinic, Giza, Egypt

A. Armia
Watany Eye Hospital and Watany Research and Development Center, Cairo, Egypt

© The Author(s), under exclusive license to Springer Nature Switzerland AG 2022   233
A. Armia and C. Mazzotta (eds.), *Keratoconus*,
https://doi.org/10.1007/978-3-030-84506-3_15

Table 1 Indications and purposes of DALK

Tectonic	Optical	Therapeutic	Cosmetic
Descemetocele	Ectasia (keratoconus, keratoglobus, etc.)	infections	Opacity
Pellucid marginal degeneration	Scarring	Dermoid cysts/ tumours	
Terrien's marginal Degeneration	Dystrophies	Perforations	
ulcers	Degenerations		
	Post-operative complications		

postoperative immune rejection and of early or later failure of the corneal graft. Moreover, being a "closed bulb eye surgery", this technique notably reduces the risk of complications such as supra-choroidal haemorrhage and the risk of glaucoma and endophthalmitis. One of the limit of the technique involves a long learning curve and standardization, although much progress has recently been made in this direction [3]. DALK [1–5] can be indicated in advanced ectasia not suitable of conservative management or not suitable of contact lens correction, opacities where the corneal endothelium is healthy and can be spared with significant biological benefits such as endothelial rejection, Table 1.

Advanced corneal ectasia increasing irregular corneal curvature, inducing extreme thinning with resulting reduction in visual acuity, Fig. 1, is one of the main indication for DALK surgery, where there is no need to replace the endothelium [3].

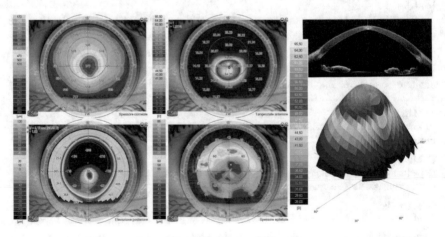

Fig. 1 Spectral domain corneal OCT shows anatomical and developmental characteristics of advanced Keratoconus suitable for DALK. The anterior and posterior elevation maps show prominent positive islands of elevation (>55 Dioptres). The thinnest point on the corneal thickness map is 348 μm. AS-OCT show apex degeneration

Table 2 Advantages of DALK

DALK advantages
Increased long-term graft survival
Reduction/annulment of late graft failure
Reduced complications correlated to prolonged use of steroids
Earlier removal of sutures
Saving on donor tissue (it is possible to use tissue with lower cellularity)
Reduced risk of rejection
Prevention of open globe eye surgery complications

Table 2 shows the major advantages of DALK compared to penetrating keratoplasty (PK) in treating advanced ectatic disorders [6, 7].

2 Our DRXL-DALK Technique

The original big bubble (BB) technique[2] included the trephination of approximately 300 μm and Descemet Membrane (DM) or pre-DM tissue layer separation through manual injection of air in the deep the stroma, creating a large air bubble forced to induce a "*pneumatic delamination*" separating the deeper stromal layers, followed by their careful manual excision using specific designed surgical spatula, forceps and scissors [5, 6]. This technique involves a steep learning curve and its final functional outcome will depend on many factors including the depth and regularity of the DM plane or pre-DM interface, homogeneous tensioning of the sutures and optimal healing of the cut, including stability of the donor-recipient joint. The surgical steps of our personal DALK in keratoconus are displayed in Table 3.

Table 3 Our personalized DRXL-DALK fundamental steps

DRXL-DALK steps
A. Circular donor recipient accelerated crosslinking (CDR-ACXL)
B. Keratoconus area identification, localization and marking
C. Manual trephination
D. Identification of the innermost stroma
E. Pneumatic Stromal Delamination (PSD) through air bubble generation
F. Bubble test
G. Debulking
H. Brave cut & stromal opening and excision
I. Donor-recipient sizing
J. Graft suture

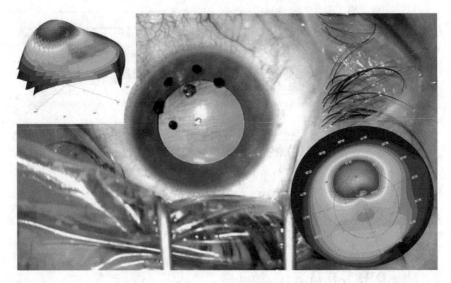

Fig. 2 Intraoperative view of manual localization of KC topography and identification of its topographic limits, highlighting the apex

A. Keratoconus Identification and Location

Keratoconus (KC), as represented in preoperative corneal tomography, must be localized compared to the geometric centre of the cornea thus identifying its confines, since its correct localization defines the diameter of the trephination that should take into account the pupillary dilation and the extreme edges of the KC compared to the geometric centre of the cornea, in order to eradicate the stromal component affected by disease (Fig. 2).

B. Trephination

After identifying the diameter of the transplant, the next step is trephination, which must take into account 80% of the thickness in the thinnest point (i.e. the apex of keratoconus).

To date, it is possible to carry out partial stroma trephination, using different types of trephines, with specific pre calibrated or manual pre-set.

C. Identification of the inner stroma

In order to achieve a good level of compromise between trephination depth and location of the border between the inner stroma and endothelium, we usually colour the stromal border within the trephination. A deep pre-cut is made with a crescent knife blade and a 27G [4] spatula in the deeper stroma (Fig. 3).

D. Pneumatic Stromal Delamination (PSD) and Bubble Types

The bubble is formed by injecting air causing an "*unstable air propagation*" between the stroma and DM, through a 27G needle cannula into a preformed

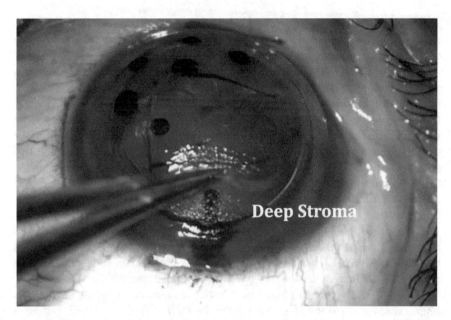

Fig. 3 The image shows the bluish colour inside the wound from trephination, showing the depth of the incision

channel with a specifically designed guide punch or needle. The tip of the needle is directed towards the corneal apex by approximately 4 mm; then the air-bubble injected with the hole of the cannula pointing downwards, causes what we properly prefer to name "*pneumatic stromal delamination*" (PSD) of the corneal layers, exploiting the lower deep lamellar cohesion of the pre-descemetic deep stroma (also

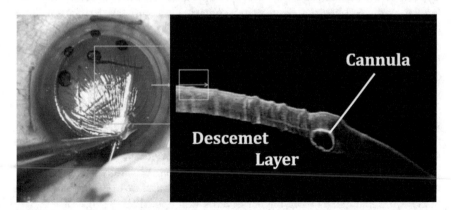

Fig. 4 Image AS-OCT Rescan—Zeiss intraoperative OCT. It is possible to directly visualize the position of the "*Fogla's cannula*" inside the stroma, near to the peripheral post 9mW/5.4Jcm^{2}ACXL demarcation line (DL) that offers a guide, just before air injecting

known as weak stroma) compared with the stiffer anterior-mid stroma, trapping the air above the DM or pre-DM layers. DM separation generally stops on the margin of the trephination, with emphysema of the above and surrounding stroma (Fig. 4).

After air-bubble injection, there is the possibility that 2 types of bubbles and a mixed type are formed, with different genesis, aspects and relative implications.

Generally, like most corneal surgeons, we prefer the advent of a *Type 1 Bubble* formation, between the pre-DM *"Dua's layer"* [7, 8] and the overlying deep stroma; the air forms a limited bubble, up to 8.5 mm in diameter, starting from the centre and gradually expanding outwards [19]. The type 1 bubble allows the surgeon to carry out a keratectomy using spatula and scissors, more securely, using the Dua's layer to protect the DM [7, 8]. In Mazzotta's opinion, this eventuality is comparable to the protection offered by the lens cortex after hydro-delineation during cataract surgery towards the posterior capsule rupture.

Differently from type 1, the *Type 2 Bubble* is a large and very thin bubble beginning at the peripheral cornea and expanding very quickly towards the centre. It is located between *Dua's layer* [7] and Descemet's membrane and there is a higher risk of DM perforation because no protection is offered towards the DM [9–13].

Different factors are related to type 1 bubble formation, including trephination depth, absence of scarring evaluated by AS-OCT examination and slit lamp observation) and stage I to III keratoconus [9–13]. In some cases, it is possible to create mixed-bubbles; in this case, according to some authors, it is recommended to open the type 1 bubble and leave the type 2 bubble intact [13, 14]. The mixed-bubble can be solved with greater safety by moistening the residual stroma for several minutes using trypan blue to highlight the residual stroma which takes on a bluish colour, while the DM will remain transparent [15, 16]. Moreover, by colouring the stroma we better remove any stromal residues from the type 1 bubble [1].

E. Bubble Test

The role of the bubble test [4–6] (*B-test*) is essential, since the air bubble injection through peripheral anterior chamber paracentesis highlights the detachment limits of the Descemet's membrane. This generally occurs up to the edge of trephination. Moreover, the *B-test* serves to identify the type of bubble formed. In our experience, before carrying out a bubble-test, it is advisable to decompress the anterior chamber due to the increased intraocular pressure caused by bubble genesis.

F. Debulking

Manual debulking of the stroma takes place using a crescent knife-blade to remove the majority of the stroma and prepare the residue stroma for the *"brave cut"*. This surgical time may even be bypassed in case the stroma is particularly thin. Intra-operative real time OCT may help the decision. Generally good functional outcome is achieved if pre-DM stroma thickness is inferior to 80 μm and particularly if the interface is more regular in the 4 mm optical zone (Fig. 6).

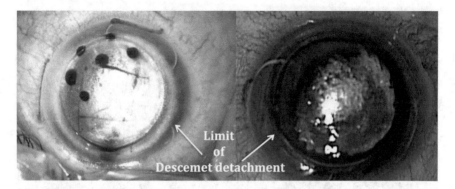

Fig. 5 Bubble test in two different types of bubble. The Left image shows a *Type 1 Bubble*, and the Right image, a *Type 2 Bubble*

G. Brave Cut, Stromal Opening and Excision

The big bubble confined between the stroma and the DM is perforated with a 30° blade, Fig. 5; to control the rapid air discharge from the chamber formed by DM-stroma, some viscoelastic is deposed over the stroma before making the cut, which slows the air and reduces the risk of accidental DM perforation. Sarnicola et al. [5] proposed converting the air bubble to an "*air visco-bubble*" by injecting viscoelastic through the aperture, which would make the bubble test positive rather than negative and allow the residual stroma to be more securely divided into quadrants before excision [5, 6] (Fig. 7).

Fig. 6 Debulking

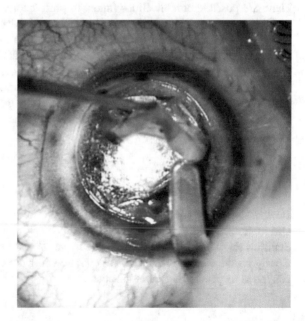

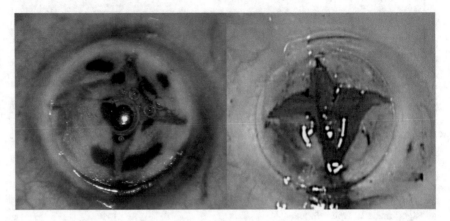

Fig. 7 Intraoperative image of opening in quadrants after *"Air-Visco Bubble"*

H. Donor-Recipient Sizing

In our experience, the preference, where possible, is to maintain the same size between donor and recipient, but according to refraction in cases of high myopia or higher peripheral prolapsed corneas, we prefer to slightly undersize the donor flap (<0.25 mm). Donor oversizing may not allow the correct alignment of the junction between Descemet's membrane and stroma, with the potential formation of a double chamber.

I. Graft Suture

There are possible complications linked to graft sutures [20–22].

Stitches are placed in the four cardinal points, at a depth of 90% of the thickness [17–19] to prevent the dehiscence of the wound. Sutures can be continued with 8–12 or more separate stitches, or with a single or double anti-torsional running sutures according to surgeon preference and practice. There are several suture techniques: separate sutures only, single running suture, double running suture, mixed suture, all of which in our opinion are valid methods [18]. The essential criteria for the sutures concerns the correct alignment between epithelium and stroma [17–19] (Fig. 8).

3 Repairing Descemet's Ruptures

DM ruptures are very frequent during the surgeon's corneal learning curve [20–22]. Statistics show that perforation is decidedly variable from 4 and 31% and it depends closely on the experience of the surgeon, however not all DM ruptures need to be converted to penetrating keratoplasty.

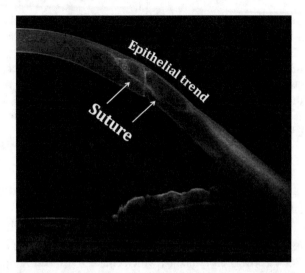

Fig. 8 Corneal Spectral Domain OCT documenting sutures in line with epithelial trend. The corneal suture is placed at a depth of 50% of stromal thickness, equidistant from the donor and recipient cornea

The timing of the identification of the micro/macro perforation is essential in recovering function and allowing for an excellent outcome. Management of DM ruptures is a highly debates topic, since some authors have shown how

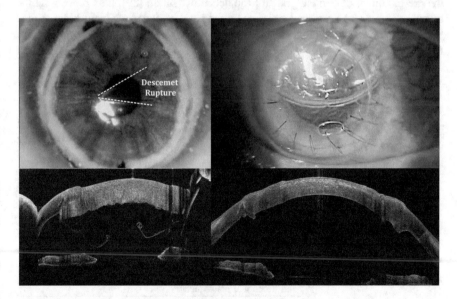

Fig. 9 Spectral domain corneal OCT and Anterior Segment picture show iatrogenic macro ruptures of the DM in the centre. The perforation has been repaired by injecting air into the eye anterior chamber; the second picture shows the total repair with no loss of tissue

intraoperative conversion to PK gives excellent results [20–22]. On the other hand, it is safer to manage DM ruptures with air bubble injection into the anterior chamber [20–22].

In our opinion, DM ruptures can be repaired in the majority of cases, by injecting air into the anterior chamber. Intraoperative ruptures may be micro or macro perforations, with possible loss of endothelial tissue; iatrogenic ruptures are generally linear without tissue loss, meaning it is sufficient to put air into the AC and to extend the endothelial flap, as in a DMEK operation [20] (Fig. 9).

4 Corneal Cross-Linking (CXL) as Adjuvant Treatment in DALK Surgery

Solid scientific evidence is paving the way for the multiple benefits of combining Riboflavin UV-A corneal crosslinking with corneal transplant surgery [23–26]. Some of the feasible and proved advantages of this combination are displayed in Table 4. Recently, Mazzotta et al. demonstrated that also accelerated crosslinking (A-CXL) at 9mW/5.4 J/cm^2 has the ability to stabilize ectasia progression trough a biomechanical and biochemical stiffening effect [28]. A secondary effect of CXL proved by in vivo confocal microscopy is cellular apoptosis and keratocytes repopulation with deposition of new higher resistant collagen fibres and increased resistance against collagenase activity. Some authors have suggested to use CXL in the pre-treatment of corneal graft for the decellularization [29], thus preventing the rejection [30, 31]. In our protocol we use the circular donor-recipient bidirectional 9 mW/5.4 J/cm^2 Accelerated CXL [27] and we named this approach proposed by Mazzotta "*Circular Donor-recipient Accelerated Crosslinking*" or CDR-ACXL and

Table 4 CDR-ACXL and DRXL-DALK advantages	CDR-ACXL and DRXL-DALK advantages
	Decellularization of the graft minimizing rejection
	Stiffening of the donor and the recipient corneas
	Facilitation of the recipient cornea trephination
	Demarcation line OCT guide for punch and cannula insertion in the deep stroma
	Facilitation of Type 2 Bubble formation
	Higher early and late "bidirectional" Stability of the Wound
	Early removal of the suture preventing wound dehiscence
	Prevention of spontaneous early and later wound dehiscence
	Reduction of post traumatic wound dehiscence morphologic and functional consequences
	Minor irregular progressive astigmatism and decay of Visual Acuity

the surgical technique Zagari-Mazzotta *"Donor-Recipient Crosslinking-assisted Deep Anterior Lamellar Keratoplasty"* or DRXL-DALK.

The innovation of our technique consists in applying for the first time a peripheral [25] or annular *"doughnuts-shaped"* Accelerated 9mW CXL [28] pre-operatively in both the donor [23] and the recipient corneas [25] with different timing. The rationale of this "donor-recipient" named by Zagari and Mazzotta the Donor-Recipient X-Linked Deep Anterior Lamellar Keratoplasty technique (DRXL-DALK). This original preoperative *"two-way"* whose acronym we gave is *"Circular Donor-Recipient Accelerated CXL"* (CDR-ACXL) prior to DALK surgery, enables us to reduce peripheral keratolysis [27, 29] and consequent thinning with wound displacement and secondary progressive irregular astigmatism after corneal transplant. This result is achieved moreover, stiffening of both recipient's and donor's peripheral ring [26] while sparing the transparency of donor central cornea and preserving the recipient's cornea from unnecessary scar alterations that could negatively affect the formation of the bubble in the area surrounding the localization of the keratoconus. Basically, in our experience this new approach is favourable to DALK early and late outcome. First of all, it stabilizes the progression of the peripheral ectatic process in the recipient cornea after the lamellar transplant, also inducing a crosslinking dependent biochemical and biomechanical reinforcement of the whole donor-recipient junction, thus definitively stabilizing the wound and preventing its late dehiscence and the relative progressive irregular astigmatism often occurring for the slowly continuous thinning of the peripheral recipient ectatic cornea. ACXL on the recipient cornea is performed one month before the DALK surgery session, while the peripheral donor cornea is cross-linked in the same day before DALK surgery.

The "peripheral *"doughnut shaped"* 9 mW/5.4 J/cm^2 ACXL [27] treatment is performed in the recipient cornea under topical anaesthesia (4% Oxibuprocaine chlorydrate 1.6 mg/0.4 mL drops), applied 10 min before the treatment. After applying a closed valves eyelid speculum, epithelium is removed circularly between 6 and 10 mmutes sparing the limbus, with a blunt metal spatula. A dextran-free plus hydroxyl-propyl methylcellulose (HPMC) disposable 0.1% riboflavin isotonic solution is instilled for one drop every minute for 10 minutes of corneal soaking, before starting continuous light UV-A irradiation. During UV-A-irradiation we use a specifically designed mask named Zagari-Mazzotta (ZM Marker) ® whose bleu 3D printed prototype is visible in the Fig. 12 (the prototype offers a central shield of 6 mm, allowing a "doughnuts shaped A-CXL" irradiation between 6 and 10 mm. Two drops of riboflavin solution are administered every 2.5 min for a total of 10 minutes of UV-A exposure at 9mW/cm^2 of UV-A power and at standard Fluence of 5.4 J/cm^2. At the end of the UV-A irradiation, the cornea is washed with balanced saline solution (BSS) and medicated with preservative-free netilmicin plus dexamethasone, cyclopentolate eyedrops and dressed with a therapeutic bandage soft contact lens for 4 days. After therapeutic contact lens removal, fluor-ometholone 0.2% eye-drops (tapered 3 times/day) and sodium hyaluronate 0.2% lacrimal substitutes are administered for 4–6 weeks until DALK surgery, Fig. 10.

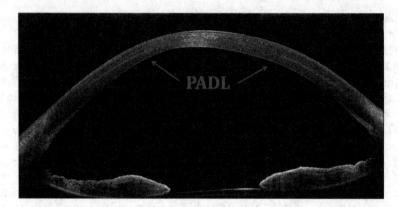

Fig. 10 Spectral Domain OCT scan after 15 days from the Circular-Donor-recipient Accelerated Crosslinking (CDR-ACXL) developed by Mazzotta and Zagari and performed on the recipient prior to DRXL-DALK. A *"Peripheral Annular Demarcation Lines"* (PADL) is clearly detectable and measurable

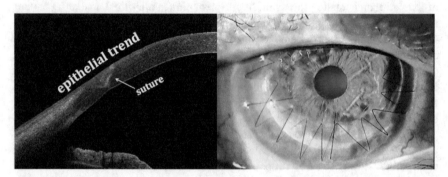

Fig. 11 Spectral Domain OCT scan and anterior segment image show the perfect donor-recipient junction alignment 15 days after the Zagari-Mazzotta DRXL-DALK Technique with clearly visible *Peripheral Annular Demarcation Lines* (PADL) of the donor, perfectly aligned with the recipient's stroma favoured by the preoperative CDR-ACXL

The 9 mW/5,4 J/cm^2 ACXL procedure is carried out on the donor cornea the day of surgery using the ZM marker®. After irradiation the epithelium is completely removed, the donor flap punched and sutured on the recipient (Fig. 11).

In addition to the early and later advantage of stabilizing the wound on both the donor and recipient side preventing spontaneous [30, 31] and maybe reducing the consequences of post-traumatic wound dehiscence [32] after keratoplasty, the CDR-ACXL technique performed prior to DALK in our experience has proven to be useful during the trephination phase, which in this case it occurs on a compacted tissue resulting more facilitated and precise.

Another advantage we found is the higher rate of Type 2 bubble formation in the DRXL-DALK. The CDR-ACXL induced tissue compaction seems to facilitate

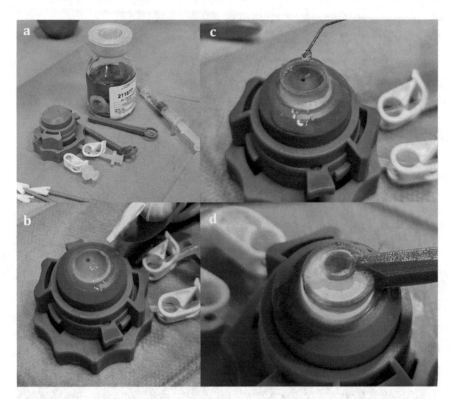

Fig. 12 DRXL-DALK surgery with pre DALK CDR-ACXL. **a** donor cornea; **b** donor cornea placed in the test chamber at manual epithelial removal. **c** placement of silicone ring, soaking the donor cornea with isotonic riboflavin solution for 10 minutes. **d** Zagari-Mazzotta ZM-Marker® 3D printed blue prototype with 6 mm central shield and limbus anular shield during the CDR-ACXL phase

the genesis of a type 2 bubble and the separation of layers, if we consider that the PADL can be a point of reference for bubble genesis. Another observation is that during the surgical removal of the peripheral tissue, the margins appear particularly smooth, transparent and show no irregularities. Moreover, the CDR-ACXL giving higher stability to the corneal wound, facilitates the passage and sealing of the sutures and reduces early and late postoperative edema around the suture. Considering the CXL-induced apoptosis lowering the levels of immunogenicity just from 15 days after the DALK, [28] the CDR-ACXL could be useful in reducing the probability of rejection [25, 26].

Another feature that must be considered is that the cross-linked hyper-reflective tissue and relative demarcation lines [28] has characteristics that can be easily visualized intraoperatively by anterior segment OCT. In our experience the PADL obtained after CDR-ACXL and visualized during the DALK allows a greater precision for the punch depth insertion and during forming the intra-corneal tunnel acting as guide for cannula insertion at the right depth.

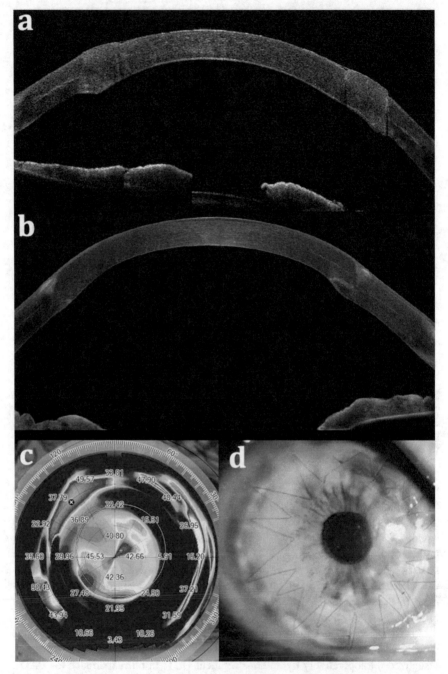

Fig. 13 a AS-OCT 24 h after Doughnut-shape CXL-DALK surgery: the red arrows show the evident DL of the recipient. **b** AS-OCT same patient, 50 days later: the red arrows show the presence of PADL in donor and recipient, with partial stroma alignment in proximity to the lines of demarcation. The corneal topography shows the flattened peripheral margin of the flaps with regular astigmatism

The corneal suture is also consistently more adherent after CDR-ACXL, improving and maintaining the alignment between the donor-recipient tissues conferring a wound higher stability. In the light of our experiences and preliminary data after the combination of CDR-ACXL and DALK in the so called DRXL-DALK technique, the use of preoperative donor-recipient peripheral crosslinking could contribute to the progressive standardization of corneal lamellar surgery for the benefit of surgeons and patients so the state of the art can still be improved (Fig. 13).

References

1. Melles GR, Remeijer L, Geerards AJ, Beekhuis WH. The future of lamellar keratoplasty. Curr Opin Ophthalmol. 1999;10(4):253–9. https://doi.org/10.1097/00055735-199908000-00006 PMID: 10621532.
2. Anwar M, Teichmann KD. Big-bubble technique to bare Descemet's membrane in anterior lamellar keratoplasty. J Cataract Refract Surg. 2002;28(3):398–403.
3. Tan DT, Anshu A. Anterior lamellar keratoplasty: 'Back to the Future'—a review. Clin Exp Ophthalmol. 2010;38(2):118–27.
4. Fogla R. Deep anterior lamellar keratoplasty in the management of keratoconus. Indian J Ophthalmol. 2013;61(8):465–8. https://doi.org/10.4103/0301-4738.116061.PMID:23925339; PMCID:PMC3775089.
5. Muftuoglu O, Toro P, Hogan RN, Bowman RW, Cavanagh HD, McCulley JP, Mootha VV, Sarnicola V. Sarnicola air-visco bubble technique in deep anterior lamellar keratoplasty. Cornea. 2013;32(4):527–32.
6. Sarnicola V, Toro P. Blunt cannula for descemetic deep anterior lamellar keratoplasty. Cornea. 2011;30(8):895–8. https://doi.org/10.1097/ICO.0b013e3181e848c3 PMID: 21464706.
7. Dua HS, Faraj LA, Said DG, Gray T, Lowe J. Human corneal anatomy redefined: a novel pre-Descemet's layer (Dua's layer). Ophthalmology. 2013;120(9):1778–85.
8. Dua HS, Katamish T, Said DG, Faraj LA. Differentiating type 1 from type 2 big bubbles in deep anterior lamellar keratoplasty. Clin Ophthalmol. 2015;26(9):1155–7.
9. Fogla R, Padmanabhan P. Results of deep lamellar keratoplasty using the big-bubble technique in patients with keratoconus. Am J Ophthalmol. 2006;141(2):254–9.
10. Borderie VM, Werthel AL, Touzeau O, Allouch C, Boutboul S, Laroche L. Comparison of techniques used for removing the recipient stroma in anterior lamellar keratoplasty. Arch Ophthalmol. 2008;126(1):31–7.
11. Borderie VM, Touhami S, Georgeon C, Sandali O. Predictive factors for successful type 1 big bubble during deep anterior lamellar keratoplasty. J Ophthalmol. 2018;13(2018):4685406. https://doi.org/10.1155/2018/4685406.
12. Michieletto P, Balestrazzi A, Balestrazzi A, Mazzotta C, Occhipinti I, Rossi T. Factors predicting unsuccessful big bubble deep lamellar anterior keratoplasty. Ophthalmologica. 2006;220(6):379–82.
13. Scorcia V, Giannaccare G, Lucisano A, Soda M, Scalzo GC, Myerscough J, Pellegrini M, Verdoliva F, Piccoli G, Bovone C, Busin M. Predictors of bubble formation and type obtained with pneumatic dissection during deep anterior lamellar keratoplasty in keratoconus. Am J Ophthalmol. 2020;212:127–33.
14. Jafarinasab MR, Feizi S, Javadi MA, Hashemloo A. Graft biomechanical properties after penetrating keratoplasty versus deep anterior lamellar keratoplasty. Curr Eye Res. 2011;36 (5):417–21.

15. Sharma N, Jhanji V, Titiyal JS, Amiel H, Vajpayee RB. Use of trypan blue dye during conversion of deep anterior lamellar keratoplasty to penetrating keratoplasty. J Cataract Refract Surg. 2008;34(8):1242–5.
16. Livny E, Bahar I, Hammel N, Nahum Y. Blue bubble' technique: an ab interno approach for Descemet separation in deep anterior lamellar keratoplasty using trypan blue stained viscoelastic device. Clin Exp Ophthalmol. 2018;46(3):275–9.
17. Eve FR, Troutman RC. Placement of sutures used in corneal incisions. Am J Ophthalmol. 1976;82(5):786–9.
18. Guimaräes RQ, Rowsey JJ, Guimaräes MF, Reis PP, Castro RD, Tirado BR. Suturing in lamellar surgery: the BRA-technique. Refract Corneal Surg. 1992;8(1):84–7.
19. Rowsey JJ. Prevention and correction of corneal transplant astigmatism. Trans New Orleans Acad Ophthalmol. 1987;35:35–51.
20. Kodavoor SK, Deb B, Ramamurthy D. Outcome of deep anterior lamellar keratoplasty patients with intraoperative Descemet's membrane perforation: a retrospective cross-sectional study. Indian J Ophthalmol. 2018;66(11):1574–9.
21. Ziaei M, Ormonde SE. Descemet's membrane macroperforation during interface irrigation in big bubble deep anterior lamellar keratoplasty. Oman J Ophthalmol. 2017;10(3):241–3.
22. Jhanji V, Sharma N, Vajpayee RB. Intraoperative perforation of Descemet's membrane during "big bubble" deep anterior lamellar keratoplasty. Int Ophthalmol. 2010;30(3):291–5.
23. Arafat S, Robert M, Shukla A, et al. UV crosslinking of donor corneas confers resistance to keratolysis. Cornea. 2014;33:955–9.
24. Huang T, Ye R, Ouyang C, Hou C, Hu Y, Wu Q. Use of donors predisposed by corneal collagen cross-linking in penetrating keratoplasty for treating patients with keratoconus. Am J Ophthalmol. 2017;184:115–20.
25. Ziaei M, Gokul A, Vellara H, Patel D, McGhee CN. Peripheral cornea crosslinking before deep anterior lamellar keratoplasty. Med Hypothesis Discov Innov Ophthalmol. 2020 Summer;9(2):127–34.
26. Lammer J, Laggner M, Pircher N, Fischinger I, Hofmann C, Schmidinger G. Endothelial safety and efficacy of ex vivo collagen cross-linking of human corneal transplants. Am J Ophthalmol. 2020;214:127–33.
27. Mazzotta C, Raiskup F, Hafezi F, Torres-Netto EA, Armia Balamoun A, Giannaccare G, Bagaglia SA. Long term results of accelerated 9 mW corneal crosslinking for early progressive keratoconus: The Siena eye-cross study 2. Eye Vis (Lond). 2021;8(1):16.
28. Mazzotta C, Hafezi F, Kymionis G, Caragiuli S, Jacob S, Traversi C, Barabino S, Randleman JB. In vivo confocal microscopy after corneal collagen crosslinking. Ocul Surf. 2015;13(4):298–314.
29. Spoerl E, Wollensak G, Seiler T. Increased resistance of crosslinked corneaagainst enzymatic digestion. Curr Eye Res. 2004;29:35–40.
30. Wang X, Liu T, Zhang S, Qi X, Li S, Shi W, Gao H. Outcomes of wound dehiscence after penetrating keratoplasty and lamellar keratoplasty. J Ophthalmol. 2018;8(2018):1435389. https://doi.org/10.1155/2018/1435389.
31. Mannan R, Jhanji V, Sharma N, Pruthi A, Vajpayee RB. Spontaneous wound dehiscence after early suture removal after deep anterior lamellar keratoplasty. Eye Contact Lens. 2011;37(2):109–11.
32. Lee WB, Mathys KC. Traumatic wound dehiscence after deep anterior lamellar keratoplasty. J Cataract Refract Surg. 2009;35(6):1129–31.

Index

© The Editor(s) (if applicable) and The Author(s), under exclusive license to
Springer Nature Switzerland AG 2022
A. Armia and C. Mazzotta (eds.), *Keratoconus*,
https://doi.org/10.1007/978-3-030-84506-3

Printed in the United States
by Baker & Taylor Publisher Services